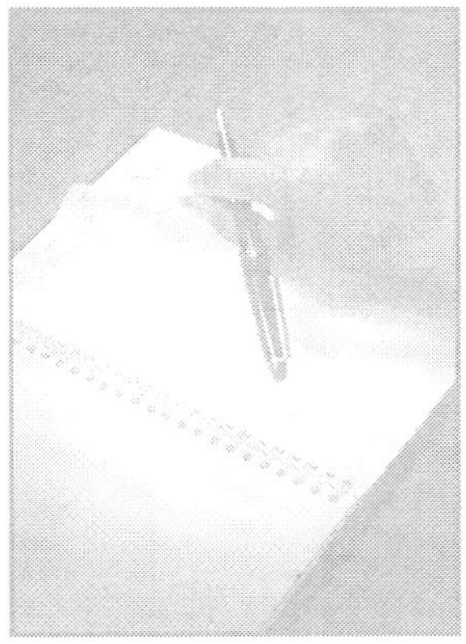

ACNM Exam Prep Workshop
Salt Lake City, UT 2006

Margaret A. McGill, CNM, MN
Randi Beth Singer, CNM, MSN, WHNP

Workshop co-presented with:
Lindsey O'Neill Hill, MSN, CNM
Angela Wilson-Liverman, MSN, CNM

AMERICAN COLLEGE *of* NURSE-MIDWIVES®
With women, for a lifetime®

ISBN 0-914324-14-4

To order additional copies of this book and other ACNM publications, access the ACNM Web site at www.ShopACNM.com.

American College of Nurse-Midwives
8403 Colesville Rd., Suite 1550
Silver Spring, MD 20910-6374

Printed in the United States

The original workbook authors wrote in 2005:

We would like to acknowledge the following

All midwives, since they were once students—faced with the task of learning enormous amounts of information, caring for women and families and successfully passing a certification examination. Many of them were responsible for the ground swell requesting an examination preparation course.

Deanne Williams and ACNM for their openness to hear the requests and desire to meet them.

All previous students, especially at the Parkland School of Nurse-Midwifery who, while learning, continue to teach the midwives who teach them.

And women and families who are the ultimate teachers of all……

Writers of the 2006 edition would like to add our gratitude to:

Mary Brucker and her colleagues who developed the first ACNM exam prep workshop and materials

Students, graduates, and faculty of the Vanderbilt University Nurse-Midwifery Program

ACNM Production: Caity Byrne, Production Editor
Nancy Dickerson

Exam Prep 2006 -- Table of Contents

Chapter I- Primary Care (continued)

Chapter II- Antepartum Care (continued)

Exam Prep 2006 -- Table of Contents

Exam Prep 2006 -- Table of Contents

Chapter VI- Family Planning/Gynecology (continued)

Exam Prep 2006 -- Table of Contents

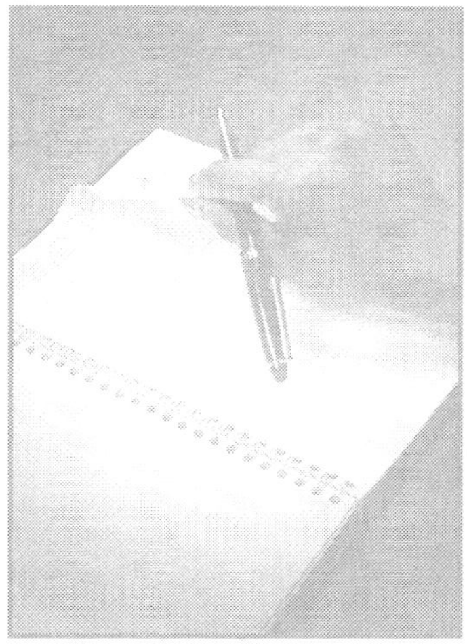

ACNM Exam Prep 2006
Introduction

The Certification Examination

Exam purpose and background

Formal certification examinations have been administered to graduate nurse-midwives/midwives for more than 30 years, initially by the American College of Nurse-Midwives Division of Certification. Testing format has gone from observation of clinical skills to short answer written exams to multiple-choice written exams to the present computer-based format. In 1991, ACNM contracted with the ACNM Certification Council, Inc. (ACC) to develop and conduct certification of graduates of ACNM Division of Accreditation (DOA) accredited institutions, and to maintain certificate renewal. The intent of certification and certification maintenance is to verify to the profession and the public that an individual is a safe beginning practitioner, and that the midwife maintains a safe level of knowledge. State licensure is the legal basis for practice; many states and institutions require certification by ACNM, ACC, or the certification body designated by ACNM for practice privileges. *In 2005, ACC changed its name to the American Midwifery Certification Board, Inc. (AMCB).*

AMCB has various rules and safeguards.

- **Be sure to read the Candidate's Booklet and understand the specifics.** For example, you will need 2 forms of identification in order to be admitted to the test. Note that the booklet specifies that its contents, including policies, procedures, and fees are *subject to change without notice*.
- If you are seeking CNM certification, **your nursing license must be current *at the time of the exam,* not when you apply.**
- Some states may have additional requirements, such as taking the first available examination following graduation. AMCB requires you to take the certification examination within 12 months of the date of completion of your program, and you must pass the exam within 24 months of graduation. For AMCB purposes, **"date of completion" is the date indicated by the program director. This is not necessarily the day of graduation, pinning, or other completion ceremonies.**

American Midwifery Certification Board, Inc.
849 International Drive, Suite 205
Linthicum, MD 21090
Phone **(410) 694-9424**
Fax **(410) 694-9425**
www.amcbmidwife.org

Relationship between ACNM and AMCB

AMCB is a separate corporate entity from ACNM. ACNM has designated AMCB as the certification body, and contracts with them to write and administer the national certification exam. At this time, it is the AMCB that awards nurse-midwifery/midwifery certification to eligible candidates.

Eligibility criteria to sit for the AMCB exam

For the Certified Nurse-Midwife (CNM) credential:

- Licensure as Registered Nurse in one of the 50 states, the District of Columbia, or US territories, with notarized proof of license active on date of examination (web verification is not acceptable proof).
- Satisfactory completion of a nurse-midwifery program (or in a Master's Program, satisfactory completion of all basic nurse-midwifery theoretical and clinical requirements of the nurse-midwifery component) accredited or preaccredited by the ACNM DOA.
- Verification by the director of the nurse-midwifery program attesting that the candidate has satisfactorily completed the nurse-midwifery component of the program and the date it was completed. The verification must be on the institution's official letterhead.

For the Certified Midwife (CM) credential:

- Satisfactory completion of a midwifery program accredited or preaccredited by the ACNM DOA.
- Verification by the director of the midwifery program that the candidate has satisfactorily completed the midwifery component of the program and the date it was completed. The verification must be on the institution's official letterhead.

Examination construction

The exams are composed of questions written by midwives in a variety of clinical practice and/or education settings around the country, with answers validated in current literature sources. Each question is written independently of the other questions and a minimum passing standard is set for the question.

Standard setting

A standard is determined for each question by a group of experts in midwifery (practice and education). This process determines the degree of difficulty of the question, and evaluates each alternative answer. Because of this process, the cut score or standard for a particular test varies from test to test. For example, you cannot say that to pass you must reach a score of any particular percentage because the individual questions on the test allow the cut score to be uniquely calculated for each examination. For more information about the grading process, see the article in the reference list at the end of this chapter: Fullerton JT, Parker KW, & Severino R. (1997). Development and outcomes of the multiple-choice format national certification examination in nurse-midwifery and midwifery. *Journal of Nurse-Midwifery, 42*(4), 349-54.

Content of certification exam

The content areas covered by the certification exam and the percentages of the total represented by each area are:

I. Primary Care	**5-10%**
II. Antepartum	**25-30%**
III. Intrapartum	**25-35%**
IV. Postpartum	**5-10%**
V. Neonatal	**5-10%**
VI. Family planning/gynecology	**15-20%**
VII. Professional issues	**Up to 5%**

The blueprint and specific questions are based on periodic midwifery job analyses, the most recent of which is described in the second article included in the reference list at the end of this chapter: Fullerton JT, Johnson P, & Oshio S. (2000). The 1999 AMCB task analysis of nurse-midwifery/midwifery practice phase I: the instrument development study. *Journal of Midwifery & Women's Health, 45*(2), 150-6.

The organization of the ACNM exam preparation workshop and the accompanying book are based on the test blueprint supplied by the AMCB.

Question format

The AMCB certification exam questions are in multiple choice format. Questions are presented in random order, not grouped according to content area, to simulate full-scope clinical practice in which the midwife encounters a variety of patient care issues throughout the day. There are three or four options from which you must choose the single best response. Included in the 175 questions are some that are being pretested for future use. These questions are not counted in the scoring, are not identifiable by the test taker, and are scattered throughout the exam.

- The AMCB exam is computer-based. Items (questions) are presented one at the time, and you can go back and forth to change answers if desired. You will be oriented to the testing environment and will have a short exercise (not midwifery questions) to become familiar with the program. There is a clock on the computer screen, and the computer terminates the exam when the time limit of 4 hours has lapsed.
- The questions test your knowledge and judgment of both normal and deviations in all core competence clinical areas. ***Approximately two-thirds of the content for each clinical area is devoted to normal phenomena and one-third to deviations from normal.***
- **At least two-thirds of the content for each clinical area is devoted to items testing clinical judgment, with the balance made up of items testing knowledge.**

Entire Test	Normal	Abnormal
Knowledge	23%	11%
Judgment	44%	22%

Number of questions and time to complete the exam

There are a total of 175 questions on the exam, including questions being pretested for future use. You will have 4 hours to complete all 175 questions and critique the exam.

Items to bring to the exam

- Arrive at the testing site at least 15 minutes before the scheduled time. **Bring 2 current official forms of identification with your name and signature. One ID must be government-issued with a recent photograph, such as a driver's license, passport, military ID, or city, county, or state-issued ID card.** Temporary ID cards, even with photo and signature, are not accepted. The second ID can be a valid credit card, social security card, student ID – anything with your current name printed and a legible signature. FIRST and LAST names must match on the identification cards and on the application.
- You may keep eyeglasses with a case and a watch with you.

What NOT to bring to the exam

- Personal digital assistants (PDAs, e.g., Palm Pilot), purses, briefcases, hats, papers, and writing implements should be left at home or in your car. Scratch paper and a pencil will be provided; the paper must be signed and returned after the exam.

Exam critique

- The AMCB welcomes feedback about questions. This is extremely advantageous to you. You do not have to depend upon a question having poor statistical behavior for them to take a second look at it. You may comment on individual items throughout the exam. There will be an online posttest questionnaire about your experience, not individual questions. Critique is voluntary. Any question that is substantively criticized will be reviewed by the AMCB after the test, in conjunction with the statistical analysis. AMCB has calculated that the 4-hour examination time limit is sufficient for the test to be completed and critiques recorded, so no additional time is provided for critique. USE THE CRITIQUE OPTION. You have nothing to lose. However, do not simply write, "answer is unclear." Instead, write something like, "stem refers to 'pregnancy diet' and it is not clear if this is the average diet for all women, or for certain women, e.g., those with cultural limitations or allergies, Thus, option a or b could be correct." In other words, give a short rationale why the question posed a problem for you.

Guessing

- There is no penalty for guessing on the exam. It is to your advantage to answer every question.

Further information about the AMCB examination

- Go to the AMCB web site for more details (www.amcbmidwife.org). The booklet available on the AMCB website, "Information for Candidates of the National Certification Examination in Nurse-Midwifery and Midwifery" describes the exam blueprint and has sample questions included. You should download a copy of the booklet soon and read it cover to cover. Be sure to review it before you register for the exam, as the contents and policies may change. If you have questions that are not answered by a careful review of the booklet or on the web site, call the AMCB at 410-694-9424 and ask for help.

Preparing for the Certification Exam

There are many excellent resources to help determine the best way to study based on your personal learning style, and many are available free on the web. A partial list is provided on page 15. There are also tried and true test-taking strategies. Of course, you didn't get this far without some study and test-taking skills! But, if you are feeling overwhelmed at the prospect of being tested on your entire body of midwifery knowledge, or if you suspect that your study skills would benefit from some structure, read on.

Proven study strategies

- **Develop a study schedule and stick to it.**
  - Budget the time you have available to prepare, remembering to maintain healthy habits such as a nutritious diet and regular exercise.
  - Establish daily and weekly study goals -- don't just plan to crawl in bed with your Varney every night and see how far you get.
  - Condition yourself to study in a specific setting that is conducive to concentration, with good lighting, comfortable seating, and few distractions.
  - Determine when during the day you are alert and study then.
  - Use a checklist or outline to make sure you cover all the content areas.
  - Studying for short periods is more effective than one marathon session.
- **Review your midwifery program materials, especially areas that challenged you.**
- **Use standard texts** (e.g., *Varney's Midwifery, Williams Obstetrics).*
- **Do not lose time by surfing the web for obscure information.**
- **Do not ignore areas you "think" you know well.**
- **Do not rely on any ONE source.** Answers to questions are validated in a variety of sources, and at least two current references are usually required.
- **As you study and review, make up questions. Remember the majority of the test content is on healthy women and in judgment format—so think application. For example**:

If studying	*Ask yourself*
Antepartum nutrition	If a pregnant woman is a vegan, how does that change my counseling?
Contraception	If a woman has a history of thrombophlebitis, what methods of contraception can she use?
Gynecology	When is partner treatment recommended for vaginitis?
Postpartum	How does breastfeeding affect postpartum weight loss?

- **Study as if you are practicing IRL (in real life), but remain aware that correct answers are based on current literature, not the policies in your particular practice.**

- **Be aware of differences between practices in your area/region and nationally**. The exam tests knowledge of national practices and standards, not regional or local.
- **If possible, review tests from your program**. Such reviews help you verify content knowledge, and also realize how you learn. For example if there is a test on which you did not do well, why? Was it because you glossed over the material or didn't study it (information gap), could not remember it (retention gap), incorrectly understood it (misinterpretation), did not connect the dots between pieces of content (synthesis gap), failed to understand the vocabulary (vocabulary gap), rushed to an answer (jumping to conclusions), misread, miskeyed, or failed to check the answers (carelessness)? If you changed an answer, did it help or hurt your score? Knowing what you did wrong can help you avoid similar mistakes on the certification examination.
- **Resist any temptation not to prepare for the exam** no matter how well you did in your basic program, and no matter how experienced you are.
- **Do not underline or highlight everything**. Highlighting or underlining everything you read becomes counterproductive. Same with taking notes as you read – don't write down everything. Read the section or chapter first and then outline it or return to highlight important concepts.
- **Take a self-test and analysis, and get suggestions for studying strategies based on your learning style at http://www.vark-learn.com/english/index.asp**. Do you know what type of learner you are – audial, visual, kinesthetic, or read/write? The visual learner enjoys flash cards; taking notes and outlining is for the read/write learner. Or try mapping.
- **Only develop mnemonics if they help you**. It probably takes as much energy to develop and memorize something silly like "Detectives extensively criticize police standards" as to know that the Bishop's Score consists of "Dilation, Effacement, Consistency, Position and Station". It might be more helpful to you to know that four of the five factors of the Bishop's Score describe the cervix, and the last one refers to the pelvis.
- **Use worksheets if they help you**. For example, consider developing a worksheet on all the CDC treatments for sexually transmitted diseases. Worksheets allow you quickly to see similarities and differences -- in this case, which treatments are different for a pregnant woman compared to a nonpregnant woman. (Thus, enabling you to learn one list of treatments with only one or two variations for pregnancy.)
- **If you are confused about a point, ask a CNM/CM** (e.g. faculty, colleague).

- **Get a study buddy.** Research has indicated that studying at least some of the time with another person enhances your performance. You may know some item cold (or so you think) until the study partner asks you about it in his or her words. Study partners help you look at material differently. And, if you can teach the material to someone, then you know that you know it.
- **Do not expect to be able to anticipate all the questions.**
- **Some information just has to be memorized, and that is hard work.**

Suggestions for the AMCB exam

- **Focus on normal health!** The majority (two-thirds) of the exam questions are focused on normal health issues like childbirth, contraception, etc. Only one-third will be on complications.
- **As you focus on the normal, make certain you can recognize deviations from normal, and beware that you do not normalize abnormal conditions.** It is unlikely that many answers will be “consultation” or “referral”, but you need to know when that may be the best response.
- **Think about the knowledge and judgment one needs to be a safe practitioner**. For example, contraindications to commonly used medications such as contraceptives or drugs that are not safe for pregnant or nursing women.

Test-Taking Strategies: On the Day of the Exam

- Get started early, so you have plenty of time to prepare yourself and get to the site without rushing.
- Eat a nourishing breakfast that includes protein and fruits. Go easy on the refined carbohydrates – 4 hours is a long time when your sugar high is gone!
- Wear comfortable clothes that you can sit in for 4 hours. Dress in layers, and bring a sweater or jacket in case the room is cool. Do not overdress in case the room is warm.
- Be sure you know the where the testing site is, and arrive early for the exam. Use any extra time to relax, think positively, focus your mind, and empty your bladder.
- There may be other people taking tests in the same room as you. Their exams may be shorter or longer than yours, and they may be using the keyboard or calculators. Request earplugs from the supervisor if you think you may be distracted.
- Do not spend the minutes before the test trying to do a last minute studying with friends. You are more likely to confuse yourself at that point.

How to handle anxiety

- Be well prepared!
- Acknowledge outside pressures, including the consequences of the exam. Remember, though, that this is a test of your knowledge, judgment, and ability to take a computer-based exam on midwifery material. Failure may be humiliating (and expensive), but it does not mean you're a bad person.
- Accept that you will experience some anxiety. Some is to your advantage. It energizes you.
- Approach the exam with confidence, using whatever strategies have been successful in the past: visualization, logic, talking to yourself, practice, journaling, etc.
- Don't cram.
- **Avoid speaking with anyone who expresses negativity about the exam or the experience.**
- Exercise regularly.
- Get a good night's sleep before the exam.
- Eat a healthy meal before the exam, avoiding sugar and any foods that may cause gastrointestinal distress.
- Use deep breathing—remember the old Lamaze and Dick-Read breathing.
- During the test—focus on each question. Do not attempt to calculate how you are doing.
- Realize that it is likely that you will block at some points. Expect that lapse of memory. It does not mean you are having a permanent memory loss, just information overload. Expect it-- go on to another question.

> Suggestion: The exam has 175 questions. Each question is worth one point. You might target completing them in 3 hours, and allow yourself the additional hour for review and feedback. Roughly, that is a question a minute. Plan so that you can check after one hour that you are on question 60, at the end of two you should be question 120, etc. There will be a clock on the computer, but you may use your own watch.

When the Exam Begins

- Read instructions carefully and follow them.
- Take full advantage of the practice exercise before you start.

Taking the test

- Stay focused.
- Take one question at a time, without worrying about the last one or the next one.
- Maintain a steady pace, budgeting your time.
- Change your position frequently.
- Read the question carefully and look for words such as "and", "or", "best", etc. that impact your choice.

- Read each question with the intention of answering it before you read the answer options. This increases your concentration and helps you read the question more clearly. You also are less likely to be fooled by a wrong answer.
- Read all the options before selecting your answer, even if you find an answer you think is correct.
- Check your response at the end of each question to ensure that you indicated the answer you intended.
- Note important information in the stem. This is particularly true with judgment questions. For example, an antepartum question about a woman who is 35 years old may immediately alert you to a genetics option.
- Be <u>especially</u> careful if a question has negative phrases (e.g., not, except); make sure you remember what really is being asked when you choose your response.
- Do not read into questions. Use common sense. Questions are not meant to trick you.
- Budget your time.
- If you find a difficult question, do not waste time agonizing over it. Take a best guess quickly and make a note to come back to it. Do this for several reasons:
    - Expect that you will miss some questions
    - Other questions can help trigger your memory
    - You do not want to waste time
- Do not look for a pattern in the answers. Even if you find 5 questions with "b" as your answer in a row, do not change them. Certification examinations do not have patterned answers. Distracters are arranged in numerical order, alphabetically, or by some other arbitrary method.
- Do not be alarmed if it takes the full 4 hours to complete the exam – you don't get extra points for finishing early!
- Critique questions as needed, but be aware of how much time you spend on this process.
- If you find yourself becoming tense or anxious during the test:
    - Relax and try to regain control; take deep, slow breaths and visualize yourself receiving positive results.
    - Do not allow yourself to think about the fear. Think about the task at hand, one question at the time.
    - Give yourself some positive reinforcement – you have successfully completed a rigorous midwifery program; your program director and faculty believe you are capable of further success; you're smart, you're good looking, and darn it, people like you!

What about practice/information that is on the cutting edge?

- Remember if "intervention (or information) X" is very new to you, perhaps it isn't even an option. Read the options and choose the best of them, even if you now think "intervention X" might be better than any of those listed.
- If "intervention (or information) X" is available, choose it. Although you may not have heard of it before, few options really are brand new. However, if it is listed, make certain you take advantage of AMCB's policy of encouraging a candidate to critique the questions. This is extremely advantageous. You do not have to depend upon a question having poor statistical behavior. You may be the only SNM/SM who has seen the new article. You need to alert AMCB, and this method of feedback allows you to give rationale for your response or suggest that the available answers are not currently correct. Your entry might read something like this: *per new issue of JMWH, intervention X is the best, but this is recent information and X is not listed.*

Controversial Issues

- Many SNMs/SMs are uncertain how to study controversial areas or subjects without clear rights and wrongs. For example, in the question of hormone replacement therapy (HRT) for menopause and ovarian cancer: one large randomized clinical trial suggests an association, but 15 case controls analyzed by CDC fail to show an association. Do not attempt to diminish a controversy by simply choosing one side, as in a debate. Odds are that the test will not include questions that force you to choose a side when controversy exists. If you feel that a question could be logically answered by either of two options, again, use the feedback mechanism with the critique option.

Bottom Line:
Answer questions based on your knowledge today. Do not try to second guess the test makers. Feel free to reflect any issues you have in feedback to AMCB.

What if (you are CERTAIN that) more than 1 option is correct?

If you find a question with two or more valid answers, choose the one you believe is better. Then be sure to provide feedback to AMCB, remembering to give rationale with your critique.

If you do not know the answer

- Do not spend excessive time on the question.
- Use the process of elimination when you do not know the answer immediately. Usually, you can eliminate two options relatively quickly, increasing your chance to a 50:50.

- **Beware of "negative" questions, and pay special attention**. Note the negative word (e.g. EXCEPT, all BUT, does NOT). You are being asked to eliminate true responses, not false ones. When looking for negative options, remember to look for extreme modifiers (e.g. always, never, all).
- If in doubt, critique the question when you have time. Certification exam questions generally are written very well, but you have nothing to lose if you have to guess.
- Guessing strategies:
  - **If there are two similar answers, it is likely that one of the two is the correct answer.**
  - **If applicable, the option that is longest and most descriptive is most likely the answer.**
  - **When numbers are each option—choose one of the middle range.**
  - **If the stem needs a plural option—you then can eliminate singular options or vice versa**. In general, the answer will be the choice that grammatically completes the sentence.
  - An option with an absolute qualifier—e.g. **always, never -- can <u>almost</u> always be omitted.**
  - **Sometimes you can get a clue from other questions.**
  - **All other things being equal, if one of the options is to refer the woman outside midwifery care, it may be incorrect** because the examination heavily tests on the action of the midwife, not physician or other provider.
  - If the question has a drug option with dosage, remember it is not meant to be tricky. **If in doubt, assume that the dosage is correct, and look primarily at whether or not the drug in question is appropriate.**

When you are finished with the exam

- Check that you have answered every question. It is amazing how many individuals skip a question and ultimately forget to complete it. Even if you simply choose "c", you have a 25% chance. By not answering it at all, you have a 0% chance.
- Have you done a critique? Sometimes a candidate is simply too tired to comment on a problem question. But remember, it is to <u>your</u> advantage to do so. Do not depend on other test takers. In addition to possibly helping yourself, you may help the exam committee, and ultimately, the profession of midwifery.
- Take a deep breath! Consider doing something special for yourself. You deserve it.

PLEASE DO NOT TALK ABOUT THE QUESTIONS WITH ANYONE, INCLUDING YOUR FACULTY. TEST SECURITY IS IMPORTANT TO OUR PROFESSION.

After the test

You will receive a provisional score immediately after taking the exam to document that you took it. Your official results will be mailed to the address on your application within 8 weeks, along with your certificate. If you did not pass, you will receive an analysis of your results, which will help you prepare to retake the exam no sooner than one month after the first exam.

- Program directors do not receive notification of whether an individual candidate passed or did not pass the examination. You are encouraged to share your success with your faculty – after all, they helped prepare you for the exam. They want to congratulate you if you passed, and they will be very supportive if you did not.

References

Fullerton, J.T., Johnson, P., & Oshio, S. (2000). The 1999 ACC task analysis of nurse-midwifery/midwifery practice phase I: the instrument development study. *Journal of Midwifery & Women's Health, 45*(2), 150-6.

Fullerton, J.T., Parker, K.W., Gross L.J. (2000). Examination adaptation: translating the national nurse-midwifery/midwifery certification examination. *Journal of Midwifery & Women's Health, 45*(4):330-6.

Fullerton, J.T., Parker, K.W., Severino R. (1997). Development and outcomes of the multiple-choice format national certification examination in nurse-midwifery and midwifery. *Journal of Nurse-Midwifery, 42*(4), 349-54.

Fullerton, J.T., Roberts, J.E., Valhoff, W.L. (1996). Recent developments in professional midwifery education and credentialing. *Journal of Nurse-Midwifery, 41*(4), 322-7.

Fullerton, J.T., Severino, R. (1995). Factors that predict performance on the national certification examination for nurse-midwives. *Journal of Nurse-Midwifery, 40*(1), 19-25.

Gloe, D. Study habits and test-taking tips. *Dermatology Nursing, 11*(6), 439-43, 447-9.

Mullen, C.A. (1996). Strategies for success: preparing for the certification examination. *Journal of Perianesthesia Nursing, 11*(5), 324-9

Rea, K. (1998). Preparing for the home health nurse certification examination. *Home Healthcare Nurse, 16*(5),331-7.

Sample Web Resources

http://www.vark-learn.com/english/index.asp

Guide to learning styles with self test, analysis, and suggestions for studying strategies based on your specific learning style: read/write, aural, kinesthetic, or visual.

http://www.harvardwestlake.com/students/studyskills/

Chapters 1, 3, 4, 5, and 6 are applicable. Not specific to midwifery, and surely you have some of the skills, but you may find some good ideas for organizing your study and approaching a test of this nature.

http://www.ucc.vt.edu/stdysk/stdyhlp.html

Time management, study skills, strategies for difficult questions.

http://www.studygs.net/

Index study system, review tools including mapping and flashcards, dealing with test anxiety.

NOTES

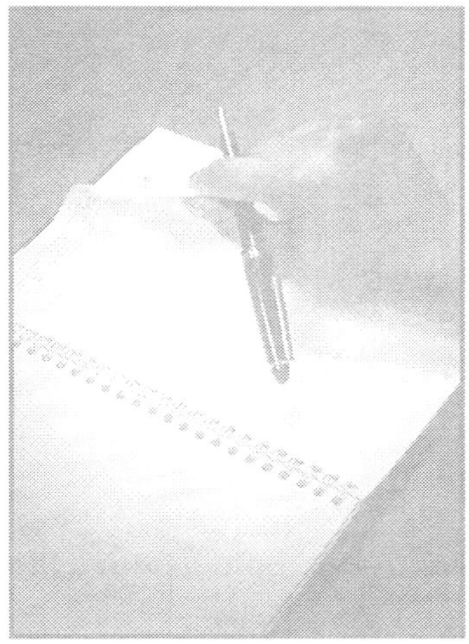

Chapter I

Primary Care

I. Primary Care (5%-10%)

A. **Physiology**

B. **Pathophysiology**

1. **Genetic**
2. **Infection**
3. **Immune conditions**
4. **Cancer**
5. **Substance abuse**
6. **Environmental exposures**
7. **Food-borne and nutritional disease**

C. **Pharmacology (includes alternative/complementary therapies)**

D. **Assessment of the well woman**

1. **History**
2. **Physical examination**
    a. Head, eyes, ears, nose, and throat
    b. Heart and lungs
    c. Breast
    d. Abdomen/costovertebral angle tenderness
    e. Pelvic exam (bimanual/speculum)
    f. Skin/extremities
    g. Neurologic
    h. Vital signs
3. **Cultural factors**

E. **Health promotion and disease prevention**

1. **Behavioral screening and counseling**
    a. Sexually transmitted infection
    b. Breast self-exam
    c. Substance abuse
    d. Domestic violence
    e. Exercise/nutrition
    f. Injury prevention
    g. Depression
2. **Laboratory tests and procedures**
    a. Pap smears, STD testing
    b. Mammograms
    c. Bone density screening
    d. Colon cancer screening

e. Lab tests, e.g. cholesterol, thyroid function

3. Assessments indicated by status of the woman

4. Immunizations

F. Deviations from normal: Assessment, management and indications for consultation, co-management or referral

1. Cardiovascular

a. Hypertension
b. Mitral valve prolapse
c. Hyperlipidemia
d. Anemias

2. Dermatologic

a. Carcinomas
b. Acne vulgaris
c. Rosacea
d. Dermatoses
e. Skin infections
f. Infestations

3. Endocrine

a. Obesity
b. Thyroid disease
c. Diabetes
d. Metabolic syndrome

4. Head, eye, ear, nose, and throat

a. Viral upper respiratory infections
b. Throat infections
c. Allergic rhinitis
d. Vasomotor rhinitis

5. Gastrointestinal

a. Hepatitis
b. Gastroesophageal reflux disease
c. Peptic ulcer disease
d. Constipation
e. Diarrhea
f. Irritable bowel syndrome
g. Hemorrhoids
h. Vomiting

i. Gallbladder disease

6. **Musculoskeletal**
    a. Osteoarthritis
    b. Low back pain
    c. Carpal tunnel syndrome
    d. Osteoporosis
7. **Neurologic**
    a. Headaches
    b. Seizures
8. **Respiratory**
    a. Bronchitis
    b. Pneumonia
    c. Tuberculosis
    d. Asthma
9. **Urinary**
    a. Infection

I. Primary Care

Primary care includes health promotion, disease prevention, health maintenance, counseling, patient education, diagnosis, and treatment of acute and chronic conditions in a variety of health care settings (e.g., office, inpatient).

In 1992, ACNM issued a position statement describing the role of the CNM in primary care. Federal agencies, such as the National Health Service Corps and the Office of Rural Health, recognize certified nurse-midwives (CNMs) as primary care providers, and state Medicaid agencies have the option of utilizing CNMs as primary care case managers. The statement was revised in 1997.

Components of midwifery care outlined in the *Core Competencies* include the primary health care of women, specifying management of common health problems, health promotion and disease prevention. (http://www.midwife.org/display.cfm?id=484).

A. Physiology

1. Respiratory System

a. Composed of lungs, trachea, bronchi

b. Functions

1) Keep body supplied with oxygen and eliminate excess carbon dioxide by moving air in and out
2) Gas exchange occurs across the alveolar-pulmonary capillary membranes
3) Chemoreceptors in the medulla oblongata and the carotid body respond to changes in hydrogen ion concentration (pH) in the blood and spinal fluid
4) Excess levels of carbon dioxide signal the respiratory center in the medulla oblongata to increase the depth and rate of respiration

c. ***Resting respiratory rate: 12-15 breaths per minute***

2. Cardiovascular System

a. Composed of heart, blood and blood vessels

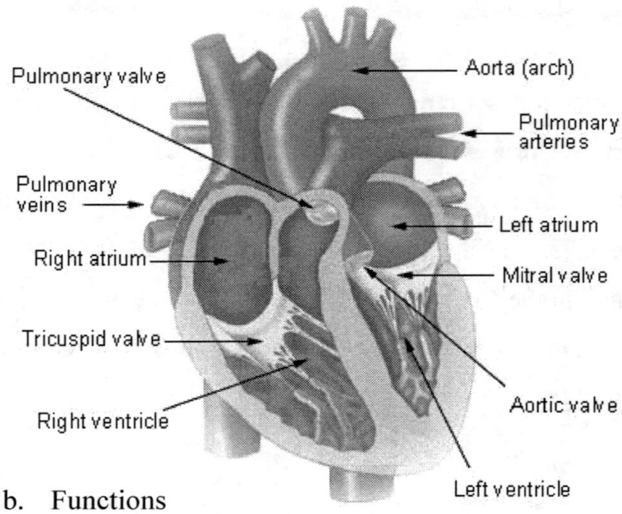

b. Functions

1) Heart contracts and relaxes rhythmically to circulate blood through the body
2) Cardiac cycle
   a) **Systole**: ventricles contract, ejecting blood from the left ventricle into the aorta and from the right ventricle into the pulmonary artery.
   b) **Diastole**: Ventricles dilate, drawing blood into the ventricles as the atria contract.
   c) Closure of valves produces heart sounds: mitral and tricuspid closure produces **S_1 (lubb)**; aortic and pulmonic closure produces **S_2 (dubb).** The aortic valve closes slightly before the pulmonic valve, and may be heard as 2 separate sounds, the split S_2.
   d) Ventricular filling in diastole may produce S_3.
   e) Atrial contraction may produce S_4 sound.
3) Electrical activity: an intrinsic conduction system and pace maker control heart rate
4) **Vascular system**
   a) ***Arteries lead from the heart; veins return blood to the heart***, circulating blood to and from the lungs and the rest of the body
   b) **Stroke volume (*amount of blood ejected from the heart per minute*) multiplied by the heart rate gives the cardiac output (*measure of the heart's ability to adapt to demands*): SV x HR = CO**
   c) Arteries are tough, tensile, less distensible; subjected to more pressure than veins
   d) Veins are less sturdy, more passive; valves keep blood flowing in one direction. If blood volume increases significantly, veins expand and act as repository for extra blood to diminish stress on the heart.
   e) Palpable and visible pulsations result from ventricular systole

f) Arterial blood pressure is the force exerted by the blood against the wall of an artery as the ventricles contract and relax.

(1) ***Systolic pressure (highest) is the force on the wall of the artery when the ventricles contract and is the result of cardiac output, blood volume, and arterial compliance.***

(2) ***Diastolic pressure (lowest) is the force against the arterial wall when the heart is filling or relaxed; it is the function of peripheral vascular resistance.***

(3) ***Pulse pressure is the difference between systolic and diastolic pressures.***

3. Breasts

a. Function

1) Produce milk to sustain the newborn.

b. Anatomy

1) Modified apocrine (sweat) glands located on anterior chest wall
2) Consists of: Glandular (mammary), fibrous (connective) & adipose (fat) tissue
3) ***15-20 lobes in each breast***
4) Alveolus with smaller lobes
   a) secretory acini
   b) contractile myoepithelial cells
5) Ducts extend from each lobe to lactiferous sinus
6) ***Montgomery glands on areola: for lubrication***
7) Infra-mammary ridge: ridge of fat on lower portion
8) ***Tail of Spence: glandular tissue that extends up to the axilla***
9) Cooper's Ligament: supports breast, runs vertically and attaches in the deep layer of subcutaneous tissue to the dermis.
10) Blood supply
   a) Internal and lateral thoracic arteries
   b) Internal mammary vein
11) Lymph nodes
   a) Axillary nodes
   b) Internal mammary nodes (along sternum)
   c) Supraclavicular

c. Breast Development

1) Mammary ridges at 5-6 weeks gestation
2) ***Thelarche (earliest sign of puberty) age 8-14, takes 4 years to complete.*** Signifies earliest development of hypothalamus-pituitary-ovarian axis. Estrogen has the greatest influence on breast growth at this time.
3) ***Tanner Staging***: Looks at breast and pubic hair development using a staging classification of I-V. Physical signs of breast development begin in stage I, prepubertal with elevation of papilla.

Stage	*Breast*	*Pubic Hair*
I (prepubertal)	Elevation of papilla only	No pubic hair
II	Elevation of breast and papilla as small mound; areola enlarged; Median age 9.8 yrs.	Sparse, long, along labia majora predominantly; Median age: 10.5 yrs
III	Further enlargement without separation of breast and areola; Median age 11.2 yrs.	Dark, coarse, curled hair sparsely spread over mons; Median age 11.4 yrs
IV	Secondary mound of areola and papilla above the breast; Median age: 12.1 yrs.	Adult-type hair abundant but limited to the mons; Median age: 12.0yrs.
V	Recession of areola of breast; Median age: 14.6 years	Adult type spread in quantity and distribution: Median age 13.7 yrs

d. Breast function

1) During each menstrual cycle, proliferation and active growth of duct tissue occurs during the follicular and ovulatory phases reaching a maximum in the late luteal phase and then regressing.
2) Complete development of mammary function occurs only in pregnancy
3) ***Premenstrual:***
   a) ***In puberty the major influence on breast growth is estrogen. Prolactin is needed to develop estrogen receptors. Estrogen stimulates gonadotropin releasing hormone (GnRH), which stimulates prolactin.***
   b) Estrogen primarily influences ductal growth whereas progesterone influences the growth of the alveolar components.
   c) Full development and differentiation of breast tissue occurs with both hormones but additional influences from insulin, cortisol, thyroxine, prolactin and growth hormone are needed.
   d) Glandular and nonglandular tissue reach maximal size in luteal phase.

4) Menopause: Lobules regress and are replaced with fat; easier to assess due to less nodularity

4. Gastrointestinal (GI) System

a. Composed of esophagus, stomach, small intestine, colon, gallbladder, liver

b. Functions

1) Primary: Digest food and drink
2) Secondary: Expel waste material (majority of expulsion of waste is done through lungs and urinary system)

c. Physiology of digestion

1) From midesophagus to anus smooth muscle surrounds alimentary canal
2) Responsible for active movement and segmentation of intestinal contents
3) Bands of longitudinal muscles are above the smooth muscles
4) Longitudinal muscles shorten the bowel, facilitating mixing of contents of intestines; primarily responsible for propulsive movement and segmentation
5) From stomach to colon repetitive spontaneous depolarizations occur
6) Waves of contractions cause a gradient of contractions with contents propelled distally

d. Liver

1) ***Important in metabolism of carbohydrates, fats, and proteins***
2) Stores glucose and converts as glycogen until stimulated by insulin level and hormones to reconvert and release it as glucose (gluconeogenesis).
3) Fats arrive at the liver as fatty acids, and are oxidized prior to entering the tricarboxylic acid cycle.
4) ***Cholesterol is used by the liver to form bile salts.***
5) Synthesis of fats from carbohydrates and proteins occurs in the liver.
6) Proteins are broken down to amino acids by hydrolysis, and waste products are converted to urea for excretion.
7) **Other liver functions**
    a) Storage of several vitamins and iron
    b) Detoxification of harmful substances
    c) ***Production of antibodies (immunoglobulins)***
    d) ***Conjugation and excretion of steroid hormones***
    e) ***Production of prothrombin, fibrinogen, and other coagulation factors***
    f) Production of most of the plasma proteins
    g) Synthesizes bile, secretes organic wastes into the bile, and converts fat-soluble wastes to water-soluble material for renal excretion

e. **Gallbladder functions**

1) ***Concentrates and stores bile from the liver***

2) In response to cholecystokinin (hormone from duodenum) it releases bile into the cystic duct; along with hepatic duct, it forms the common bile duct.

3) Bile maintains the acid pH of the small intestine to permit fat digestion.

5. **Musculoskeletal system**

a. Composed of bones, muscles, joints

1) **Joints are held together by ligaments**

2) **Bones are attached to muscles by tendons**

3) **Joints are cushioned by cartilage**

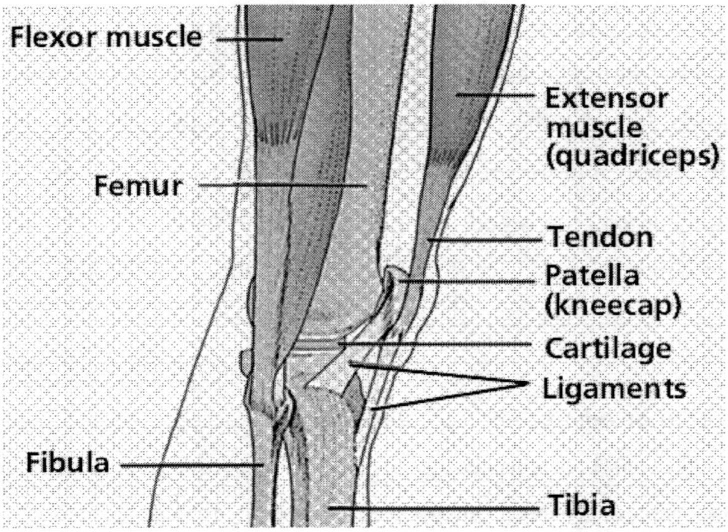

Muscles, tendons, ligaments, cartilage and their relation to bone in the knee joint

b. Functions

1) Provides stability and mobility for physical activity

2) Protects vital organs

3) Provides storage for minerals

4) Produces blood cells

5) Resorbs and reforms itself

6. **Neurologic system**

a. Components: Central and peripheral nervous systems

b. Functions: Maintains and controls all body functions by voluntary and autonomic responses.

1) **Central nervous system** (CNS): brain and spinal cord is the main network of coordination and control for body

2) **Peripheral nervous system**: motor and sensory nerves and ganglia outside the CNS; carries impulses to and from the CNS.

a) **Autonomic nervous system** ***regulates internal environment of the body; no voluntary control***

(1) **Sympathetic** division stimulates the body to action in times of physiologic and psychologic stress ("**fight or flight**")

(2) **Parasympathetic** division counters the sympathetic system by conserving body resources and maintaining **day to day functions such as digestion and elimination**

7. Integumentary system

a. Composed of skin and accessory structures, e.g., hair, nails, glands

b. Functions

1) Protects internal structures
2) Prevents loss of essential fluids
3) Protects against ultraviolet radiation
4) Regulates body temperature
5) Prevents invasion from microorganisms or toxins
6) Produces vitamin D
7) Detects stimuli such as touch, pain, temperature
8) Excretion (minor)

8. Immune System

a. Composed of lymph, lymphocytes, lymphatic vessels, lymph nodes, tonsils, spleen, thymus gland.

b. ***Function: Protection from viruses and other organisms and substances***

c. Lymphatic system

1) Fluid balance: removes extra fluid from interstitial (extravascular) spaces and returns it to the blood stream
2) Fat absorption from digestive tract
3) Defense: filters microbes from lymphatic fluid in lymph nodes and from blood in the spleen. Lymphocytes and other cells destroy microorganisms and other foreign substances.
4) Lymph nodes are throughout the body
5) Tonsils protect nose and mouth
6) Spleen responds to foreign substances in the blood, destroys aged erythrocytes, and acts as blood reservoir. Liver and other lymphatic structures can compensate for loss of the spleen.
7) Thymus gland produces lymphocytes, which move to other lymphatic tissues where they respond to foreign substances.

d. **Immunity**: ability of the body to resist damage from foreign substances, including microorganisms, chemicals, and toxins produced by microbes

1) **Innate immunity**: nonspecific; ability of body to recognize and destroy certain foreign substances. Ability does not improve each time the body is exposed.

a) **Mechanical mechanisms prevent entry** of substances or physically remove them; skin, mucus membranes.

b) **Chemical mediators promote phagocytosis and inflammation**; lysozyme, sebum, mucus, histamine, complement, kinins, interferon, prostaglandins, leukotrienes, pyrogens.

c) **Cells move to tissues that release attractant chemicals (chemotaxis).**

(1) Phagocytosis is ingestion and destruction of materials by neutrophils and macrophages.

(2) Basophils and mast cells release chemicals that promote inflammation (histamine, leukotrienes, prostaglandins, etc)

(3) Eosinophils release enzymes that reduce inflammation in allergic reactions and they destroy parasites

(4) Natural killer cells lyse tumor cells and those infected by viruses.

d) **Inflammation mobilizes the immune system and isolates invaders until they can be destroyed.**

(1) Vasodilation and increased vascular permeability

(2) Chemotaxis attracts phagocytes

(3) Local inflammation produces redness, heat, swelling, pain, and loss of function. Systemic inflammation produces increased numbers of neutrophils, fever, shock.

2) **Adaptive immunity**: specific; body's response to foreign substances improves with each exposure. Involves memory cells.

a) **Antigens** are large molecules that stimulate an adaptive immune system response; haptens are smaller molecules that combine with larger molecules to stimulate a response.

b) B cells and T cells are lymphocytes.

c) **B cells** provide **humoral (antibody-mediated) immunity**.

(1) **Antibodies** are proteins of the classes **IgA, IgD, IgE, IgG, IgM**. Also called gamma globulins or immunoglobulins. They bind to antigens and interfere with their activity; they cause the release of inflammatory chemicals when they combine with the antigen.

(2) Primary response results from first antigen exposure, and results in formation of antibodies and memory cells.

(3) Secondary response is from exposure to an antigen after the primary response; memory B cells quickly form plasma cells and additional memory cells.

d) **T cells** provide **cell-mediated immunity**.

(1) Antigens activate effector T cells and produce memory T cells.

(2) Cytotoxic T cells lyse virus-infected cells, tumor cells, and tissue transplants. They produce cytokines, which promote phagocytosis and inflammation.

e) **Acquired immunity**

(1) Active immunity: may be from natural exposure to an antigen (as with many ***childhood diseases such as varicella***) or artificial as a result of deliberate exposure to an antigen (as with ***vaccination*)**.

(2) **Passive immunity**: may be natural from transfer of antibodies from mother to fetus or baby (***as IgA with breast milk***) or artificial as in transfer of antibodies from immune person to nonimmune person (as with ***administration of Rh immune globulin to the Rh negative unsensitized mother***)

f) **Autoimmunity**: pathological condition in which the body produces antibodies against its own cells, resulting in the development of autoantibodies. May affect almost any cell or body tissue, e.g., multiple body tissues as in systemic lupus erythematosus, or single organs such as the thyroid gland in Hashimoto's Thyroiditis.

9. Endocrine System (also refer to Antepartum Chapter II and Gyn/Family Planning Chapter VI)

a. Composed of the pituitary gland and hypothalamus, thyroid gland, parathyroid glands, adrenal glands, pancreas, gonads, pineal body, thymus gland, and others.

b. **Function:** ***In concert with the neurological system, regulates virtually every other body system.***

1) **Autocrine hormones** are produced by and act on the same cell; paracrine hormones affect cells in close proximity without being transported by blood

a) Histamine, prostaglandins, prostacyclins, thromboxanes, leukotrienes (inflammatory)

b) Endorphins, enkephalins, dynorphins (analgesic)

2) **Neurohormones** are produced by neurons and act like hormones
    a) Oxytocin
    b) Antidiuretic hormone (vasopressin)
3) **Neurotransmitters** are produced by neurons and influence postsynaptic cells
    a) Acetylcholine
    b) Epinephrine
    c) Others
4) **Pheromones** are secreted into the environment to modify behavior and physiology of other individuals

c. Pituitary

1) ***Anterior pituitary*** produces prolactin (PRL), growth hormone (GH), thyroid stimulating hormone (TSH), adrenocorticotropic hormone (ACTH), melanocyte stimulating hormone (MSH), follicle stimulating hormone (FSH), and luteinizing hormone (LH).
2) ***Posterior pituitary*** stores and releases hormones produced in the hypothalamus – antidiuretic hormone (ADH, vasopressin) and oxytocin.

d. Thyroid

1) ***Function is to regulate triiodothyronine (T_3) and thyroxine (T_4) in circulating system and to produce calcitonin.***
2) Synthesis of thyroid hormones depends on the presence of iodide.
3) Thyroid hormones bind with receptor molecules to initiate new protein synthesis.
4) **Effects of thyroid hormones**
    a) Increase rate of glucose, fat, protein metabolism, increase body temperature
    b) Normal growth of body tissues
5) **Negative feedback** between thyroid gland and anterior pituitary: increased thyroid hormone production causes decreased production of TSH (hyperthyroidism). Decreased production of thyroid hormone causes TSH to increase (hypothyroidism).
6) **Calcitonin** decreases blood calcium and phosphate by inhibiting osteoclasts when blood calcium is high.

e. Parathyroid glands:

1) Produce parathyroid hormone (PTH), which increases blood calcium levels by stimulating osteoclasts.
2) Promotes calcium reabsorption by kidneys and formation of active vitamin D by kidneys, which increases calcium absorption by the intestine.
3) Decrease in blood calcium levels stimulates PTH secretion.

f. Adrenal glands

1) Medulla arises from neural crest cells and functions as part of the sympathetic nervous system; "fight or flight"
   a) Epinephrine increases blood glucose levels, glycogen and glucose use by skeletal muscles, and heart rate and force of contraction; causes vasoconstriction in skin and viscera and vasodilation in skeletal and cardiac muscle.
   b) Norepinephrine stimulates cardiac muscle and constricts most peripheral blood vessels.
   c) Hormones are released in response to emotions, injury, stress, exercise, low blood glucose levels.
2) Adrenal cortex is derived from mesoderm.
   a) Produces mineralocorticoids, especially aldosterone. Aldosterone acts on kidneys to increase sodium and decrease potassium and hydrogen ion levels in the blood.
   b) Produces glucocorticoids, especially cortisol. Cortisol increases fat and protein breakdown, increases glucose synthesis from amino acids, decreases the inflammatory response, and is necessary for normal development of some tissues (e.g., lungs).
   c) Some androgens are produced in the adrenal medulla, which stimulate axillary and pubic hair growth and sexual drive.

g. Pancreas

1) Exocrine function is to produce pancreatic digestive juices, e.g., amylase, in the acini.
2) Endocrine function is to produce glucagon in alpha cells, insulin in beta cells and somatostatin in delta cells.
   a) Insulin targets the liver, adipose tissue, muscle, and satiety center of hypothalamus. Nervous system is not targeted, but relies on blood glucose levels maintained by insulin.
      (1) Insulin increases uptake of glucose and amino acids by cells.
      (2) Glucose is used for energy or stored as glycogen.
      (3) Amino acids are used for energy or converted to glucose or proteins.
   b) Glucagon targets the liver, causing breakdown of glycogen and fats for energy.
3) Regulation of pancreatic hormones
   a) Insulin increases due to elevated blood glucose and amino acid levels, parasympathetic stimulation, gastrointestinal hormones. Sympathetic stimulation decreases insulin secretion (e.g., beta sympathomimetics such as terbutaline increase blood glucose levels).

b) Glucagon is stimulated by low blood glucose, certain amino acids, and sympathetic stimulation.

c) Somatostatin inhibits insulin and glucagon secretion.

4) Hormonal regulation of nutrients

a) After a meal

(1) Glucagon, cortisol, GH, and epinephrine are inhibited by high blood glucose; glucose release from tissues is reduced.

(2) Insulin levels increase as a result of high blood glucose level, increasing uptake of glucose, amino acids, and fats. Nutrients are either used for energy or stored.

(3) Some time following the meal, blood glucose levels drop. Glucagon, cortisol, GH, and epinephrine levels increase, insulin decreases, and glucose is released from tissues.

(4) Adipose tissue releases fatty acids, triacylglycerols, and ketones, which are used for energy by most tissues.

b) During exercise

(1) Sympathetic activity increases epinephrine and glucagon secretion, causing release of glucose into the blood

(2) Low blood glucose levels, from uptake of glucose by skeletal muscles, stimulate epinephrine, glucagon, GH, and cortisol secretion. This causes an increase in fatty acids, triacylglycerols, and ketones in the blood, which are used for energy.

10. Urinary system

a. Composed of kidneys, ureters, bladder, urethra

b. Eliminates wastes; regulates blood volume and blood pressure, ion concentration, and pH; red blood cell and vitamin D production.

c. Urine is produced by:

1) Filtration of blood; filtrate is plasma without blood cells and proteins. 99% of the filtrate is reabsorbed; reabsorption of filtrate in tubules; tubular secretion

2) Concentration is regulated by antidiuretic hormone (ADH, also called vasopressin); if ADH is present, water is absorbed and urine is concentrated.

d. Influences

1) Aldosterone

a) ***Decreased aldosterone*** results in less sodium reabsorption, decreased urine concentration and increase in urine volume; this results in a lowered blood volume.

b) ***Increased aldosterone*** results in greater sodium reabsorption, increase in urine concentration and decrease in urine volume. This results in raised blood volume.

c) "Water follows sodium".

2) Renin is produced by kidneys in response to lowered blood volume and decreased renal perfusion

   - Stimulates production of angiotensin I from angiotensinogen.

   a) Angiotensin-converting enzyme (ACE), produced by the lungs, converts angiotensin I to angiotensin II.

   b) Angiotensin II causes vasoconstriction and stimulates aldosterone secretion, leading to increased sodium retention, decreased urine production, and increased blood volume.

   c) Atrial natriuretic hormone is produced in the heart when the blood pressure increases. It inhibits ADH production and reduces the ability of the kidney to concentrate urine, thus increasing the output and lowering blood volume.

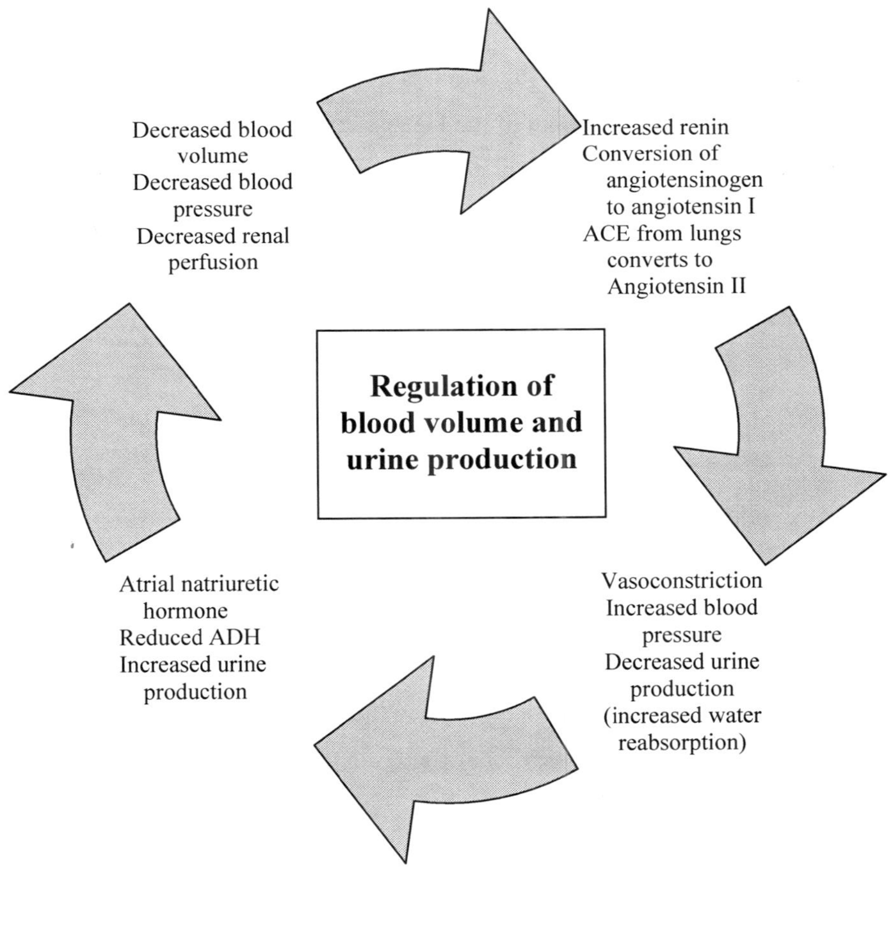

11. **Gonads and placental hormones**; see related chapters (II. Antepartum, VI. gynecology)

B. Pathophysiology

1. **Genetic**: if diseases such as cancer are included, approximately 90% of people will experience a disease with a genetic component in their lifetime. Birth defects may occur from genetic causes or environmental influences, and it may be difficult to differentiate the cause initially. A cluster of defects with the same cause may be a syndrome.

   a. Definitions

      1) **Gene**: the unit of inheritance which consists of a sequence of nucleotides within a deoxyribonucleic acid (DNA) molecule that occupies a specific locus on a chromosome and codes for a specific polypeptide chain.

      2) **Allele**: a version of a gene. It can be either dominant or recessive, which refers to how it behaves in combination with other alleles of the same locus (gene) on homologous chromosomes.

         a) *Dominant* allele: one which causes expression of a trait in the presence of a complementary allele with a different trait.

         b) *Recessive* allele: one which is expressed only when the complementary allele is the same, or in the absence of another allele (as in X linked recessive diseases).

      3) **Mutation:** a change in the DNA sequence of a gene that affects the expression of the gene. If it occurs in the germ cell, the mutation may be transmitted to future generations, i.e., it is heritable.

      4) **Genotype**: the combination of genetic factors in a particular individual.

      5) **Phenotype**: the observable characteristics of an individual, as determined by the genotype and environment.

      6) Genes code for structural parts of the cell/organism and for proteins that regulate other genes. DNA is transcribed into ribonucleic acid (RNA) and this RNA is translated into protein.

   b. **Mendelian genetics**

      1) Disorders result from mutations in single genes with large effects

      2) Variations in penetrance (how many people with the affected gene actually have a disorder) and expressivity (how the disorder presents in people with the mutant gene) are not fully understood or explained by Mendelian genetics

      3) Mendelian inheritance

         a) **Autosomal dominance**

            (1) When alleles on homologous chromosomes differ, the one which causes expression of the trait is dominant; only one copy of the gene (heterozygous) is needed for expression of the trait, i.e., offspring may inherit a trait from only one parent.

(2) Examples of autosomal dominant conditions

- Huntington disease
- Neurofibromatosis
- Polycystic kidney disease
- Familial polyposis coli
- Hereditary spherocytosis
- von Willebrand disease
- Marfan syndrome
- Osteogenesis imperfecta
- Achondroplasia
- Familial hypercholesterolemia
- Acute intermittent porphyria
- Antithrombin deficiency
- Factor V Leiden mutation
- Long QT syndrome

(3) Generally, at least one parent is affected with the disease as only one defective gene has to be inherited in order for the offspring to be affected.

(4) Males and females are affected equally

(5) EACH child of one affected (heterozygous) parent has a 50% chance of inheriting the disorder.

(6) If neither parent is affected, the disorder could be a new mutation.

(7) 2x2 table for calculating risk with one heterozygous parent Xx, one homozygous parent xx

	X	**x**
x	xX	xx
x	xX	xx

Risk of each conception for X is 50%

(8) **Co-dominance:** if alleles in a pair of genes are different and both are expressed in the phenotype, they are co-dominant. Examples are genes for hemoglobinopathies (both hemoglobins A and S, or S and C may be produced) and blood type (both A and B red blood cell antigens may be expressed in one person).

b) **Autosomal recessive**

(1) Both genes on homologous chromosomes must be the same (homozygous) for autosomal recessive traits to be expressed. If they are different, the dominant trait is expressed. If only one parent has the trait, the child is a carrier (heterozygous). Generally, in order to express the disorder, the person must be homozygous, i.e., inherit a copy of the defective gene from both parents.

(2) Examples of autosomal recessive conditions

- Sickle cell anemia
- Thalassemias
- Phenylketonuria
- Galactosemia
- Homocystinuria
- Lysosomal storage diseases
- Wilson disease
- Hemochromatosis
- Glycogen storage diseases
- Congenital adrenal hyperplasia
- Cystic fibrosis
- Albinism
- Tay-Sachs disease

(3) Most common type of Mendelian inheritance; males and females affected equally.

(4) EACH child has a 25% risk of being affected if both parents are carriers.

(5) Expressivity is more uniform and complete penetrance is more common than with autosomal dominant disorders.

(6) New mutations occur but are not usually detected clinically for several generations.

(7) Suspect consanguinity if the disorder is infrequent in a population.

(8) Calculate the risk of an autosomal recessive disorder for each conception in which one parent is homozygous for an autosomal recessive condition and the other parent is not a carrier for the condition. Using sickle cell anemia, where the allele controlling synthesis of normal β chain hemoglobin is A and the allele controlling synthesis of defective hemoglobin for the β chain is S:

	S	**S**
A	AS	AS
A	AS	AS

All children will inherit the trait (be carriers) for sickle cell anemia, but none would be homozygous for the disease. In other words, there is a 100% probability that each child will be heterozygous for sickle cell trait and 0% probability that each child will be homozygous for either the normal gene or the sickle cell gene.

(9) Calculate the risk of sickle cell anemia and carrier status in the case that both parents are sickle cell carriers (AS).

	A	**S**
A	AA	AS
S	AS	SS

In each conception there is a 25% risk that the child would have normal hemoglobin (homozygous for the normal gene) and a 25% risk that the child would have sickle cell anemia (homozygous for the defective gene). Each conception carries a 50% probability that the child is a sickle cell carrier (heterozygous for the sickle cell trait).

*Note that risks are probabilities for EACH conception.

Comparison of Autosomal Recessive and Autosomal Dominant Disorders	
Autosomal Recessive	**Autosomal Dominant**
Mutant gene is located on an autosome	Same
Males and females are affected similarly clinically and in equal numbers	Same
Both parents must contribute a defective gene	Only one parent is needed to contribute a defective gene
Family history may be negative for condition in previous generations but positive for siblings	Family history usually positive in previous generations, except in case of new mutation; if penetrance is incomplete, generations may be skipped
New gene mutation is rare	New gene mutation is frequent
Age of onset of disease is early in life	Adult onset of disease is frequent
Disease course is usually severe	Wide variability of expression
Often involves enzyme defect or deficiency	Often involves structural protein defects
Consanguinity is suspected if condition is rare in the population	Increased incidence as paternal age increases

Adapted from Blackburn T. (2003). Maternal. fetal and neonatal physiology: A clinical perspective. Elsevier.

c) **X linked** diseases may be dominant or recessive; most are recessive

(1) The male child of a maternal carrier of an X linked recessive gene is affected (e.g., hemophilia, color blindness) *if he inherits the X chromosome with the defective gene from her.*

(2) The gene is not expressed in the heterozygous maternal carrier due to its recessive nature, but it is expressed in the male who inherits it because he does not have a normal X gene for balance (he is hemizygous). In other words, the gene that is recessive in the mother acts as a dominant gene in the male offspring who inherits it.

(3) If X linked dominant (there are few of these diseases), or if the mother is homozygous for an X linked recessive gene, she is affected.

(4) Examples of X linked recessive disorders

- Duchenne and Becker muscular dystrophy
- Hemophilia A and B
- Glucose-6-phosphate-dehydrogenase (G6PD) deficiency
- Agammaglobulinemia
- Diabetes insipidus
- Fragile X syndrome
- Androgen insensitivity syndrome
- Color blindness

(5) Affected males do not transmit the disorder to sons, but all daughters are carriers. Sons of heterozygous women have a 50% chance of being affected.

(6) Random inactivation of one X chromosome in the female accounts for the possibility of full or (more commonly) partial expression of an X linked disorder in the heterozygous female. G6PD deficiency is an example: blood cells derived from marrow cells in which the normal X chromosome is randomly inactivated have the same risk of hemolysis as the red cells in the affected male. The proportion of abnormal cells depends on the random inactivation of the X chromosome, so a drug induced hemolytic reaction in the heterozygous female is almost always less severe than in the affected (hemizygous) male.

(7) Vitamin D-resistant rickets is an example of one of the few X linked dominant disorders. The son or daughter of an affected heterozygous female has a 50% chance of being affected; an affected father would transmit the disorder to all his daughters and none of his sons.

Comparison of sex chromosome linked genetic traits with autosomal traits	
Autosomal traits	**X-linked traits**
Affect males and females in equal numbers	Usually affect males; females usually are affected only if homozygous. i.e., receive a copy from the affected father and from a mother who is a carrier.
Heterozygous fathers will transmit the gene to 50% of their children, males and females in equal distribution	Affected fathers (heterozygous for a sex linked trait) transmit the gene to 100% of daughters, who become carriers. None of their male children are affected.
Recessive trait must be transmitted by both parents to be expressed	Recessive trait may be expressed with only one copy

c. Other forms of inheritance
   1) Mitochondrial inheritance
      a) Mitochondria have unique DNA (mtDNA) and genes, which code for different amino acids than nuclear DNA
      b) Present in cytoplasm of ovum (not sperm) thus solely inherited from mother
      c) Not consistent with Mendelian patterns of inheritance
      d) Relatively rare CNS, eye and muscle tissue diseases: Leber optic atrophy, mitochondrial myopathy, epilepsy and encephalomyopathy. All offspring of affected mother are affected.
   2) Germ line mosaicism
      a) Gene present only in germ cells of seemingly healthy individual
      b) Includes some instances of Duchenne muscular dystrophy & osteogenesis imperfecta
      c) Difficult to differentiate from autosomal dominant conditions
   3) Uniparental disomy
      a) Inherit pair of chromosomes from one parent, none from other
      b) More likely to have spontaneous abortions, birth defects and mental handicaps
      c) Examples: Beckwith-Wiedemann syndrome (2 paternal chromosome 11s), Silver-Russell syndrome (2 maternal chromosome 7s), transient neonatal diabetes mellitus (2 paternal chromosome 6s)
   4) Imprinting
      a) Sometimes called Parent of Origin: expression differs depending on which parent contributed the gene; not well understood.
      b) Example: deletion on long arm of chromosome 15. If inherited from father, condition is Prader-Willi syndrome, characterized by overeating and obesity, behavior problems and mild to moderate mental retardation; if deletion is on maternal chromosomes, condition is Angelman syndrome, characterized by mental retardation, seizures, absence of speech, frequent smiling, paroxysmal laughter.

d. Chromosomal disorders
   1) Most arise during gametogenesis, but may also occur during fertilization or after.
   2) May involve abnormalities in number or structure of chromosomes
      a) Numerical disorders
         (1) Polyploidy: multiples of 23 (haploid number of chromosomes); triploidy may occur from fertilization with 2 sperm or fertilization of ovum fused with polar body.

(2) Aneuploidy: abnormal number of chromosomes that is not a multiple of 23. Monosomy occurs when one of a pair of chromosomes is absent (rarely compatible with life). Turner syndrome is monosomy X (45, X). Trisomy is presence of extra chromosome. Down syndrome is trisomy 21; Patau syndrome is trisomy 13; Edward syndrome is trisomy 18; Klinefelter syndrome is male with extra X chromosome (47, XXY).

(a) Most trisomies occur as a result of meiotic nondisjunction

(b) The risk of nondisjunction increases with maternal age

(c) Only autosomal trisomies 13, 18, and 21 are seen in viable pregnancies; majority result in fetal loss before term.

(d) Trisomy 21 (Down syndrome) is the most common nonlethal trisomy; features are hypotonia, tongue protrusion, small head with flattened occiput, flat nasal bridge, and eipcanthal folds with upward slanting palpebral fissures. Often there is loose nuchal skin, short fingers, single palmar crease, inward curving of the little finger, and a gap between the big toe and the second toe. Major abnormalities include heart defects, gastrointestinal atresias, and mental retardation with IQs of 25-50. Social skills exceed mental age. There is a high incidence of leukemia and thyroid disease.

(e) Extra X chromosome, Klinefelter syndrome (47, XXY) in the male, is associated with lower IQ than controls and developmental problems. Males and females with extra X chromosomes tend to be tall. One extra X chromosome does not affect fertility in women, but males are likely to be infertile and may need testosterone replacement for normal genital development.

(f) Turner syndrome is absence of a sex chromosome (45, X) and is the only monosomy compatible with life. Many abort early in gestation. One third of fetuses with Turner syndrome are live born and may have characteristics such as short stature, broad chest with widely spaced nipples, congenital lymphedema with swollen fingers and toes, low hairline and webbed posterior neck, and bone and cartilage abnormalities. Cardiac defects may be present; intelligence is usually normal. Most have ovarian dysgenesis and require hormone replacement therapy. There is a wide range of phenotypes due to a high incidence of mosaicism.

b) Structural chromosome disorders

(1) More common than numerical disorders; deletions, duplications, inversions, translocations (balanced or unbalanced)

(2) May cause specific syndromes, mental retardation, infertility and spontaneous abortions.

(3) The person with a structural disorder may have a normal phenotype, but still transmit a chromosomal disorder to offspring. With certain translocations, the carrier will have a normal amount of chromosomal material but the karyotype is abnormal because of the arrangement of chromosomes. Depending on the genetic material contributed to an embryo, children could have a normal karyotype, be a carrier for a translocation, be monosomic or trisomic. Approximately 3-4% Down syndrome cases are due to translocations.

e. Multifactorial traits/disorders

1) Variations in traits may be caused by multiple genes in addition to effects of environment and lifestyle factors.

2) Examples are pyloric stenosis, infantile autism, neural tube defects, cleft lip and palate, some congenital heart disease, hypertension, coronary heart disease, stroke, diabetes mellitus and some cancers.

2. Infection

a. Microorganisms that inhabit specific portions of the human body without causing disease are normal flora. In the gut for example, they facilitate digestion, produce antibacterial substances, and manufacture beneficial metabolites, e.g., vitamin K. In the vagina, they produce hydrogen peroxide, which promotes defense against infection and overgrowth of organisms. When microorganisms are introduced into parts of the body where they are not normal flora, they may become pathogenic (e.g., when E. coli from the gut enter the urinary tract).

b. Stages of infection

1) Colonization: present in or on the body without tissue invasion; may become a source of infection for others (e.g., group B streptococcus)

2) Invasion: overcomes defense mechanisms in the body and attaches to host cells; may cause cell injury or death

3) Multiplication: reproduces utilizing host nutrients; causes tissue damage and disease symptoms

4) Spread: travels through the bloodstream or locally; causes local or systemic disease.

c. Factors that influence infection
   1) Mechanism of action
   2) Infectivity: ability to invade and reproduce
   3) Pathogenicity: ability to produce disease
   4) Virulence: potency of the pathogen, i.e., number of organisms needed to produce disease
   5) Immunogenicity: ability to evoke an immune response
   6) Toxigenicity: ability to produce toxins; affects virulence
   7) Portal of entry: how the pathogen enters the body, e.g., direct contact, inhalation, ingestion, injection (insect bite, for example)

d. Types of infectious organisms
   1) Virus: obligate intracellular organism that cannot reproduce without a host cell. They take over the cell's metabolic function and use it for their own survival and reproduction.
      a) Even smaller than viruses are prions, composed only of protein, e.g., bovine spongiform encephalopathy (mad cow disease).
   2) Chlamydiae, Rickettsiae, Mycoplasma and *Ureaplasma*
      a) Similar to bacteria in manner of reproduction and susceptibility to antibiotics; differ in structure and metabolic capabilities.
   5) Bacteria, spirochetes, mycobacteria
      a) *Bacteria need iron to multiply*; they injure cells by producing toxins.
      b) The immune response to toxins produces chemicals that cause fever and increase vascular permeability, which may lead to hypotension in septic shock with bacteremia.
      c) Common ways of identifying bacteria include their biochemical and morphologic characteristics, e.g., gram reaction, cellular shape and arrangement, aerobic or anaerobic growth, motility, catalase, benzidine, and oxidase, and other reactions. Examples are in the following chart

Identifying characteristics of bacteria and examples	
Gram negative rods	*Escherichia, Klebsiella, Serratia, Pseudomonas, Salmonella, Shigella*
Gram positive rods	*Lactobacillus, Bacillus, Clostridium*
Gram negative cocci	*Neisseria* (diplococci)
Gram positive cocci	*Staphylococcus, Enterococcus, Streptococcus*
Aerobic growth only	*Pseudomonas, Bacillus, Neisseria*
Anaerobic growth only	*Clostridium*
Aerobic or anaerobic	*Klebsiella, Shigella, Salmonella, Escherichia*, most other enteric genera
Oxidase positive	*Micrococcus, Pseudomonas, Neisseria*
Oxidase negative	*Staphylococcus, Streptococcus, Enterococcus, Lactobacillus, Clostridium*
Oxidase positive or negative	*Bacillus*
Nitrate reduction to nitrite	*Escherichia, Klebsiella, Serratia, Staphylococcus,*
Nitrite negative	*Pseudomonas*

6) Fungi: Relatively large microorganisms with rigid walls. Yeasts are singular ovoid or spherical cells; hyphae are branching filaments. Fungi that infect the skin are dermatophytes and usually produce mild disease.
   a) Fungi are usually life threatening pathogens only in immunocompromised individuals, as in AIDS.
7) Protozoa: single celled organisms with motility. They may be transmitted directly from person to person as with trichomoniasis, or they may require a vector, as with malaria and toxoplasmosis.
8) Helminths: Parasitic worms have complex life cycles, and the diseases they cause are often caused by an inflammatory response to the eggs or larvae (e.g., schistosomiasis).
9) Ectoparasites are arthropods (lice, ticks, mites, bedbugs, fleas) that attach to the skin. They may also serve as vectors for other pathogens.

Types of pathogenic organisms, examples, and diseases		
Type of pathogen	**Examples**	**Diseases caused**
Viruses: Obligate intracellular organisms	Rhinovirus, coronavirus	Colds and upper respiratory infection
	Influenza virus (types A, B, C)	Influenza ("flu"); A infects humans, pigs, horses, birds and is the usual cause of epidemics and pandemics. A single subtype of A predominates at a given time, and mutations occur periodically, leading to susceptibility to new strains even after infection with type A. Types B & C do not mutate, and infection in early childhood usually confers immunity.
	Adenovirus	Upper and lower respiratory tract infection, conjunctivitis, diarrhea
	Respiratory syncytial virus	Bronchiolitis, pneumonia
	Mumps virus	Mumps, pancreatitis, orchitis
	Rotavirus	Diarrhea
	Norwalk agent	Gastroenteritis
	Hepatitis A	Acute viral hepatitis
	Hepatitis B	Acute or chronic hepatitis
	Hepatitis C	Acute or chronic hepatitis
	Hepatitis D	Acute or chronic hepatitis (with HBV)
	Hepatitis E	Enterically transmitted hepatitis
	Measles virus	Measles (rubeola)
	Rubella virus	German measles (rubella, three day measles)
	Parvovirus	Erythema infectiosum (Slapped cheek syndrome, Fifth disease), aplastic anemia
	Vaccinia virus	Smallpox vaccine
	Varicella-zoster virus	Chickenpox, shingles
	Herpes simplex virus 1	Fever blister, cold sore, genital herpes
	Herpes simplex virus 2	(usually) genital herpes
	Cytomegalovirus	Cytomegalic inclusion disease
	Epstein-Barr virus	Infectious mononucleosis
	HIV 1, 2 (retrovirus)	Acquired immune deficiency syndrome (AIDS)
	Papillomavirus	Condyloma; cervical carcinoma
	Molluscum virus	Molluscum contagiosum
	Poliovirus	Poliomyelitis
	Rabiesvirus	Rabies
Chlamydiae: obligate intracellular organism	*Chlamydia trachomatis*	Genitourinary infections, conjunctivitis, respiratory infections of newborns, lymphogranuloma venereum
	Chlamydia pneumoniae	Mild pneumonia
Rickettsiae: obligate intracellular organisms; most transmitted by insect vectors	*Rickettsia prowazekii*	Typhus fever
	Rickettsia rickettsii	Rocky Mountain spotted fever
Mycoplasmas & (related) *Ureaplasma*: extracellular organisms	*Mycoplasma pneumoniae*	Atypical pneumonia ("walking pneumonia")
	Ureaplasma urealyticum	Urogenital infection

Type of pathogen	Examples	Diseases caused
Bacteria: cutaneous, mucosal, extracellular, facultative intracellular organisms	*Staphylococcus aureus, S. epidermidis*	Abscesses, cellulites, pneumonia, septicemia.
	Streptococcus pyogenes, β-hemolytic *streptococcus*	Upper & lower respiratory tract infection, erysipelas, scarlet fever, septicemia. Group B β-hemolytic *streptococcus* (GBS) : urinary tract infection, neonatal sepsis
	*Neisseria pneumoniae (*pneumococcus)	Lobar pneumonia, meningitis
	*Neisseria meningitides (*meningococcus)	Cerebrospinal meningitis
	Neisseria gonorrhoeae	Gonorrhea
	Escherichia coli, Klebsiella pneumoniae, Enterobacter aerogenes, Proteus spp. *(P. mirabilis, P. morgagni), Serratia marcescens, Pseudomonas* spp *(P. aeruginosa),*	Gram negative organisms causing urinary tract infection, wound infection, abscess, pneumonia, septicemia, endotoxemia, endocarditis. *E. coli* causes neonatal sepsis.
	Bacteroides sp (B fragilis)	Anaerobic infections
	Legionella pneumophila	Legionnaires disease
	Haemophilus ducreyi	Chancroid
	Calymmatobacterium donovani	Granuloma inguinale
	Haemophilus influenzae	Meningitis, upper & lower tract respiratory tract infections
	Bordetella pertussis	Whooping cough
	Corynebacterium diphtheriae	Diphtheria
	Enteropathogenic *E. coli, Shigella* sp, *Vibrio cholerae, Campylobacter fetus, C. jejuni, Yersinia enterocolitica, Salmonella* spp	Gastroenterocolitis, some with septicemia
	Helicobacter pylori	Gastritis, peptic ulcer disease
	Clostridium tetani	Tetanus
	Clostridium botulinum	Botulism
	Clostridium perfringens, C. septicum	Gas gangrene, necrotizing cellulites
	Clostridium difficile	Pseudomembranous colitis
	Bacillus anthracis	Anthrax, agent used for bioterrorism
	Listeria monocytogenes	*Listeria* meningitis, listeriosis
	Borrelia burgdorferi	Lyme disease
(Spirochetes)	*Treponema pallidum*	Syphilis
	Treponema pertenue	Yaws
(Mycobacteria)	*Mycobacterium tuberculosis, M. bovis*	Tuberculosis
	Actinomyces israelii	Actinomycosis
Fungi: cutaneous, mucosal extracellular, or facultative intracellular organisms	*Trichophyton* sp; *Microsporum & Epidermiphyton, Malassezia furfur*	Tineas (ringworm): capitis (scalp), pedis (athlete's foot), cruris (jock itch); tinea versicolor
	Candida spp., *C. albicans*	Thrush, vaginitis, systemic infection
	Histoplasma capsulatum, Coccidioides immitis	Histoplasmosis, coccidioidomycosis: fungal respiratory infections resembling tuberculosis
	Pneumocystis carinii	Pneumonia (opportunistic fungus-like organism)

Type of pathogen	Examples	Diseases caused
Protozoa: mucosal, extracellular, facultative intracellular, or obligate intracellular organisms	*Entamoeba histolytica*	Amebic dysentery, liver abscess
	Giardia lamblia	Diarrhea, malabsorption syndrome
	Trichomonas vaginalis	Urethritis, vaginitis
	Plasmodium vivax, P valariae, P. falciparum	Malaria
	Trypanosoma brudei, T. Rhodsiense, T. gambiense	African sleeping sickness
	Toxoplasmosis gondii	Toxoplasmosis
Helminths: mucosal, extracellular, or intracellular organisms	*Ancylosoma duodenale, Necator americanus*	Hookworms – anemia, malnourishment
	Taenia solium, Echinococcus granulosus	Tapeworms -- abdominal symptoms, convulsions, increased intracranial pressure, mental disturbances
	Schistosoma mansoni, S. japonicum, S mekongi, S. haematobium	Schistosomiasis – hepatic granulomas & fibrosis; granulomatous bladder disease with chronic obstructive uropathy
	Enterobius vermicularis	Pinworms
Ectoparasites: live on outside of body	*Pediculus humanus corporis & capitis; Phthirus pubis*	Lice; pediculosis (body pubic or head lice, "crabs")
	Sarcoptes scabiei; mites	Scabies; chiggers
	Ticks, bedbugs, fleas	Skin manifestations or may be vectors for other diseases

Adapted from Cotran, Kumar & Collins, Pathologic Basis of Disease (1999)

10) Methods of identifying pathogenic organisms include:

Gram staining:	Most bacteria
Acid-fast stain:	Mycobacteria (e.g., *Mycobacterium tuberculosis*)
Silver stains:	Fungi, legionellae, pneumocystis
Periodic acid-Schiff:	Fungi, amebae
Mucicarmine:	Cryptococci
Giemsa:	Campylobacteria, leishmaniae, malaria parasites
Antibody probes:	Viruses, Rickettsiae
Culture:	Organisms in all classes, though some are notoriously difficult to culture (e.g., *Treponema pallidum*)
DNA probes:	Viruses, bacteria, protozoa

3. Immune conditions

The immune system is in a constant balancing act defending the body from disease – it must be active enough to protect the body from infection and tumors, but not so sensitive that it destroys the body, as in an overactive allergic response or failing to detect self from non-self (as in autoimmune diseases).

a. Hypersensitivity reactions

1) Type I hypersensitivity reactions, i.e., anaphylaxis: a reaction develops rapidly, sometimes within minutes, when the body is exposed to an antigen to which antibodies already exist. This may be a systemic or local reaction. It is mediated by IgE antibodies attached to mast cells; mast cells produce histamine and adenosine.

Histamine causes bronchial smooth muscle contraction, vascular permeability, and increased nasal, bronchial, nasal, and gastric secretions. Adenosine potentiates mast cell production, causes bronchoconstriction, and inhibits platelet aggregation. Other substances include leukotrienes, which cause vascular permeability and bronchial smooth muscle contractions and which attract neutrophils, eosinophils, and monocytes; prostaglandins, which cause intense bronchospasm and mucus secretion; platelet-activating factor which reinforces the inflammatory reaction; and cytokines, which activate the inflammatory cells. Examples of cytokines are tumor necrosis factor (TNF-a), interleukins (IL).

a) The initial response, within a few minutes of exposure, involves vasodilation, vascular leakage, and smooth muscle spasm or secretions.
b) Another reaction may occur in a few hours and last for several days (e.g., allergic rhinitis, asthma); tissues are infiltrated with eosinophils, neutrophils, basophils, monocytes, and CD4+ T cells; may cause mucosal epithelial damage.
c) Systemic anaphylaxis may occur with the injection of even minute amounts of antigen, as with skin testing for allergies. Within a few minutes, itching, hives, and redness occur; then respiratory distress as the bronchioles contract; hoarseness from laryngeal edema; vomiting, abdominal cramps, diarrhea, and laryngeal obstruction follow. A person may go into shock and even die within an hour.
d) Local anaphylaxis (e.g., atopic allergy) occurs with reactions to inhaled, ingested, or otherwise exposed allergens such as pollen, animal dander, house dust, specific foods such as peanuts, etc. Atopic allergy is familial.

2) <u>Type II hypersensitivity</u> reactions are mediated by antibodies directed to antigens on cell surfaces or other tissues. The antigen may be a normal part of the cell membrane, as red cell antigens, or it may be exogenous, such as a drug metabolite. The reaction occurs in response to the binding of the antibodies to the antigens. Examples are transfusion reactions and erythroblastosis fetalis, both of which involve exposure of the red blood cell antigens to destructive antibodies. Other examples of Type II hypersensitivity reactions include thrombotic disorders with antiphospholipid antibodies, and acute rheumatic fever, with antibodies against streptococcal antigens cross reacting with heart muscle.
3) <u>Type III hypersensitivity</u> reactions are induced by antigen-antibody complexes that activate the complement system. The presence of antigen-antibody complexes does not constitute disease, just an immune response; factors causing pathogenicity are not well understood. Antigens may be exogenous, as with a microorganism, or

endogenous, as when a person produces antibodies to her own tissue. The reaction may be generalized or localized. Exogenous antigens causing Type III reactions include bacteria such as Streptococci (glomerulonephritis, endocarditis) and *Treponema pallidum* (glomerulonephritis); viruses such as Hepatitis B and cytomegalovirus (polyarteritis nodosa); parasites, and fungi. Drugs implicated in exogenous Type III reactions include quinidine and heroin. Endogenous antigens include nuclear antigens (systemic lupus erythematosus) and immunoglobulins (rheumatoid arthritis).

4) Type IV hypersensitivity reactions are cell-mediated reactions, initiated by specifically sensitized T lymphocytes. This is the typical response to a many intracellular microorganisms, viruses, fungi, protozoa, and parasites. Skin sensitivity to some chemical agents and graft rejection are also Type IV reactions. Granulomatous inflammation is characteristic of Type IV hypersensitivity reactions – a granuloma is an accumulation of macrophages that have been transformed into epithelioid cells, typically surrounded by lymphocytes (e.g., tuberculosis). Contact dermatitis is another example of a delayed type hypersensitivity reaction.

5) Transplant rejection involves both cell-mediated immunity and antibody production. Antigens that cause tissue rejection are those of the major histocompatibility antigen (HLA) system. As the transplant recipient's immune system recognizes grafted tissue as foreign (non-self), the immune response is initiated. The vasculature of the foreign tissue is the initial target of the antibodies.

b. Autoimmune conditions

1) Autoimmune diseases occur when the body mounts an immune reaction to its own tissue. There is probably a complicated interaction of immunologic, genetic and microbial factors that causes pathologic autoimmunity; the role of autoantibodies is not always clear as they may be found in healthy persons.

2) Diseases may be systemic, e.g., systemic lupus erythematosus: antibodies are produced against nucleic acids, red blood cells, coagulation proteins, phospholipids, lymphocytes, platelets. When the antigen-antibody complexes are deposited in the tissues containing these targeted substances, damage occurs to organs such as kidneys, brain, heart, spleen, lungs, gastrointestinal tract, skin and peritoneum. Transient lupus-like reactions may be caused by certain drugs (e.g., hydralazine) and some environmental factors such as ultraviolet light and infection. Clinical manifestations include arthralgias/arthritis, vasculitis, malar rash, rash from sun exposure, oral/nasopharyngeal ulcers, renal disease, hematologic abnormalities (hemolytic anemia, thrombocytopenia, leukopenia etc), neurologic disorders (seizure,

psychosis) and cardiovascular disease. There may be a false positive serologic syphilis test (e.g., RPR) and antiphospholipid (e.g., anticardiolipin) antibodies.

3) Diseases may be more localized, with autoantibodies against a single organ or tissue; such as Diabetes mellitus Type 1, in which autoantibodies are very specific for pancreatic islet β cells. They may occur as primary conditions or in association with other autoimmune diseases.

Examples of Autoimmune Diseases	
Systemic lupus erythematosus	Type 1 diabetes mellitus
Systemic sclerosus (scleroderma)	Multiple sclerosus
Sjogren's syndrome	Celiac disease
Inflammatory myopathies	Autoimmune thrombocytopenic purpura
Graves disease, Hashimoto disease	Myasthenia gravis
Post-gonococcal arthritis	Reiter syndrome
Rheumatoid arthritis	Dermatitis herpetiformis

c. Immune deficiency syndromes

1) Primary immunodeficiencies are genetic and may affect specific or nonspecific immune functions. Many are X linked recessive traits. They are usually diagnosed between 6 months and 2 years of age because of recurrent infections. An example is Isolated IgA deficiency, in which the individual cannot produce IgA, the primary immune globulin in external secretions (causing recurrent infections of the mucosa of the respiratory, gastrointestinal, and urogenital tracts). Other disorders are: common variable immunodeficiency, X-linked agammaglobulinemia of Bruton, Hyper IgM Syndrome, DiGeorge Syndrome, severe combined immunodeficiency diseases, and Wiskott-Aldrich syndrome (immunodeficiency with thrombocytopenia and eczema).

2) Acquired immunodeficiency syndrome (AIDS): infection with the retrovirus HIV-1 causes immunosuppression and leads to opportunistic infections, neoplasms, and neurologic symptoms. Transmission is by sexual contact, inoculation with contaminated needles or infected blood, or from an infected mother to her newborn during birth or breastfeeding. Immunosuppression primarily affects cell-mediated immunity, which results in a paucity of CD4+ T cells and malfunctioning helper T cells. Primary infection causes an acute illness with signs and symptoms such as fever, sore throat, myalgia, weight loss and fatigue, rash, cervical adenopathy, diarrhea, and vomiting; the acute phase develops within 3-6 weeks of infection and resolves spontaneously in 2-4 weeks. Subsequently there is a chronic phase during which the virus continues to replicate; infected persons may be asymptomatic or have

minor opportunistic infections such as thrush and herpes zoster (shingles), thrombocytopenia, and generalized lymphadenopathy. The middle phase is not truly latent, because the virus continues to replicate and infect new cells. The onset of constitutional symptoms such as fever, rash and fatigue occurs with the final or crisis phase. During the final phase, there is a dramatic increase in viral load; clinical disease progresses, with prolonged fever, fatigue, weight loss, diarrhea, and a CD4+ cell count <500 /microliter. Eventually (within 2-3 years for some and 7-10 years for most), serious opportunistic infections, cancers, and neurologic disease occur with AIDS.

a) Seroconversion (HIV+ lab test) occurs 3 to 7 weeks after exposure.

b) For reasons not completely understood, some persons who are HIV+ do not progress and remain asymptomatic. Factors involved may have to do with characteristics of the retrovirus itself or the individual's genetic constitution.

3) Immune deficiency may also be related to malnutrition, aging, intentional immunosuppression (as with an organ transplant), irradiation or chemotherapy for cancer, or other autoimmune diseases.

4) Adaptation in the maternal immune system relevant to pregnancy (which promotes tolerance of the products of conception) include delays in some immune reactions and increased susceptibility to some infectious organisms e.g., gram negative organisms and fungi. Transfer of immunoglobulins to the fetus during the third trimester renders the mother susceptible to colonization with organisms such as streptococci and staphylococci.

AIDS-defining infections and neoplasms in HIV+ persons

	Infection	**Condition**
Protozoa and helminthic	Cryptosporidiosis, isosporidiosis	Enteritis
	Pneumocytosis	Pneumonia, disseminated infection
	Toxoplasmosis	Pneumonia, CNS infection
Fungal	Candidiasis	Esophageal, tracheal, pulmonary
	Cryptococcosis	CNS infection
	Coccidioidomycosis	Disseminated infection
	Histoplasmosis	Disseminated infection
Bacterial	Mycobacteriosis	Pulmonary or extrapulmonary tuberculosis
	Nocardiosis	Pneumonia, meningitis, disseminated
	Salmonella infections	Disseminated
Viral	Cytomegalovirus	Pulmonary, intestinal, retinitis, CNS infection
	Herpes simplex virus	Localized or disseminated
	Varicella zoster virus	Localized or disseminated
	Progressive multifocal leukoencephalopathy	
Neoplasms	Kaposi sarcoma	Herpes virus cofactor (KSHV)
	B-cell non-Hodgkin lymphoma	Possibly, EBV
	Primary brain lymphoma	Epstein-Barr virus (EBV)
	Invasive cervical cancer	Human papilloma virus (HPV)

4. **Cancer** is the second leading cause of death in the U.S. (behind heart disease). Lung cancer has overtaken breast cancer as the leading cancer cause of death for women; colorectal cancer is the third most common cause of cancer death in women. Breast cancer occurs more often in women, but lung cancer causes more deaths.

   a. Definitions and explanations

      1) Neoplasia: literally, "new growth". Neoplasm is an abnormal mass of tissue, the new growth of which exceeds that of normal surrounding tissue. Tumor is synonymous with neoplasm. *Neoplasms may be malignant or benign.*

         a) Benign neoplasms usually grow slowly, are well defined and encapsulated, do not invade and cannot metastasize, are well-differentiated (cells are similar to the tissue from which they arise), and have a low mitotic index (few dividing cells).

            (1) Benign neoplasms of mesenchymal cells are designated by the suffix *-oma* attached to the cell of origin; there are exceptions to nomenclature rule. For example, a *fibroma* arises from fibroblastic cells; *chondroma* from cartilaginous cells; *osteoma* from osteoblasts. Epithelial cell neoplasms do not necessarily follow the same format, and may be named according to the cells of origin or microscopic or macroscopic appearance: *adenomas* form glandular patterns or arise from glandular tissue; *papillomas* form finger-like projections from epithelial surfaces; cystic masses are *cystadenomas*; a papillary growth protruding into a cystic space is a *papillary cystadenoma.*

         b) Malignant neoplasms generally grow rapidly, are not encapsulated, are poorly differentiated (i.e., may not resemble the tissue from which they arose), have the ability to invade, have a high mitotic index (i.e., many actively dividing cells), and may metastasize (i.e., spread to distant sites in the body, usually through the vascular or lymphatic systems)

            (1) Malignant neoplasms are also named for the cells from which they arose: tumors from mesenchymal tissue are *sarcomas* (e.g., fibrosarcoma, liposarcoma, leiomyosarcoma). If originating from epithelial cells of any germ layer, the tumor is called a carcinoma. A carcinoma with a glandular growth pattern is an adenocarcinoma; one with squamous cells is a squamous cell carcinoma. The organ of origin is usually included in the name (if known), e.g., uterine leiomyosarcoma, endometrial adenocarcinoma, placental choriocarcinoma.

            (2) If the cells of origin are not identifiable, the tumor may not be classifiable; the terms poorly differentiated or undifferentiated malignant tumor may be used.

(3) Examples of exceptions to the nomenclature rule are melanoma (cancer of melanocytes) and seminoma (cancer of testicular epithelium).

c) Polyp: a visible projection above a mucosal surface projecting into a lumen; usually benign unless referred to as polypoid cancer.

2) Cancer: Common term for malignant neoplasms.

3) Teratoma: tumor composed of a variety of cell types representing multiple germ layers. Usually they originate in the gonads from totipotential cells, and may produce any body tissue, e.g., skin, muscle, fat, gut, tooth, etc. May be benign (mature teratoma, dermoid cyst) or malignant (immature teratoma, teratocarcinoma).

4) Differentiation: extent to which the parenchymal cells resemble normal cells. Parenchymal cells are the functional cells of an organ; the stroma is connective, supporting tissue of the organ. Benign tumors are usually well differentiated; malignant tumors may be well differentiated or undifferentiated. Well differentiated tumors may function the same as the tissue from which they arise (i.e., produce the same hormones or other substance produced from original tissue). If undifferentiated, the cells may produce a variety of substances, including hormones not produced by the original tissue (e.g., human choriogonadotropin in testicular cancer) or fetal proteins not normally produced in the adult (alpha feto protein).

Characteristics of undifferentiated cells

- Pleomorphic (variation in size and shape)
- Hyperchromatic nuclei (abundant nuclear DNA stains dark)
- Disproportionately large nuclei
- Variable nuclear shapes with large nucleoli
- Large numbers of mitoses with atypical or bizarre figures
- Giant cells with single or multiple nuclei
- Disorganized growth pattern.

5) Dysplasia: disordered growth of cells, with loss of uniformity of cell size and orientation; pleomorphic cells, disproportionately large hyperchromatic nuclei, numerous mitotic figures, abnormal pattern of maturation from basement membrane to surface. Dysplasia usually precedes carcinoma (precancerous), but *dysplasia does not necessarily progress to cancer*.

6) C*arcinoma in situ:* dysplastic cells are marked and occupy the entire epithelial thickness, but do not invade the basement membrane.

7) Metastasis: tumor implants distant from the original tumor; only occurs with malignant tumors; benign neoplasms do not metastasize. Invasive cancerous neoplasms penetrate body cavities and blood and lymphatic vessels, allowing spread

of malignant cells. Almost all cancers have the ability to metastasize. Even cancers that usually do not metastasize (e.g., basal cell carcinoma of the skin) may be highly invasive.

8) Oncogenes: cancer-causing genes. Tumor suppressor genes control cell growth.

b. Carcinogens include ultraviolet light and ionizing radiation, some drugs (e.g., alkylating agents, griseofulvin), asbestos, arsenic, benzene, cadmium, ethylene oxide, nickel compounds, radon, vinyl chloride, polycyclic aromatic hydrocarbons (cigarette smoke and broiled or smoked meats), viruses and bacteria (e.g., HPV, Hepatitis B Virus, Human T-cell leukemia virus type 1 [HTLV-1], Helicobacter pylori), betel nuts, some food dyes, and nitrates (as in food preservatives).

c. Effect of age: each age group is predisposed to certain cancers, with ages 55-74 the most vulnerable.

d. Some cancers are hereditary, with an autosomal dominant pattern, while others are familial with no clear pattern of inheritance. Examples of inherited cancers: familial adenomatous polyposis, familial retinoblastoma, multiple endocrine neoplasia syndromes, neurofibromatosis types 1 & 2, some breast cancers, ovarian cancers, colon cancers; Xeroderma pigmentosum, Bloom syndrome, Fanconi anemia.

e. Tumor markers are biochemical indicators. They are not used for cancer screening, but are useful for supporting a diagnosis, determining response to therapy and to detect relapse. Examples of tumor markers are human chorionic gonadotropin (hCG), calcitonin, catecholamines, ectopic hormones, α-fetoprotein, prostatic acid phosphates, prostate-specific antigen (PSA), CA-125, and CA-15-3.

5. Substance abuse

a. Substance abuse and dependence are responsible for a wide variety of illnesses and conditions, and there is evidence that women suffer disproportionately more from drug abuse than men due to physiological and perhaps psychological differences. Women tend to become addicted more easily, and diseases resulting from abuse progress more rapidly among women than men.

b. Abuse occurs when one continues to use a substance despite social, occupational, psychological, or physical problems from its use.

c. Dependence or addiction occurs when tolerance develops (i.e., the dose of the drug must be increased to produce the effect originally achieved with smaller doses), and when physical dependence develops (i.e., manifested by a withdrawal, or abstinence syndrome). Heroin and alcohol produce strong physical dependence.

d. Psychological dependence occurs when there are feelings of satisfaction and a desire to repeat the drug experience or to avoid the discontent of not having it. Drugs that cause chiefly psychological dependence include cocaine, marijuana, amphetamine, and hallucinogens such as lysergic acid diethylamide (LSD), 3,4-methylenedioxymethamphetamine (MDMA), and peyote.

e. Tobacco use (smoked and smokeless) is associated with more mortality and morbidity than any other personal, environmental, or occupational exposure, causing almost 400,000 deaths per year in the U.S, and is associated with many more cases of chronic cardiovascular and pulmonary disease. Cancers associated with cigarette smoking include lung and larynx, esophagus, pancreas, bladder, and mouth. It is also associated with ischemic heart disease, cardiac arrest, cerebrovascular disease, arteriosclerosis, and chronic respiratory disease.

   1) Maternal smoking causes fetal hypoxia and is associated with low birth weight, prematurity, and spontaneous abortion; premature rupture of the membranes, placenta previa, and placental abruption. It is suggested to be associated with SIDS.
   2) Cigarette smoke is synergistic with other carcinogenic agents.
   3) Passive smoking is also associated with increased risks of lung cancer and heart disease in adults and respiratory and ear infections and asthma in children of smokers.

f. Alcohol abuse

   1) There are more than 15 million alcoholics in the U.S. A blood alcohol level of 80 to 100 milligrams per deciliter is the legal definition of drunk driving in the U.S. 200 mg/dL produces inebriation; coma, respiratory arrest and death occur at 300-400 mg/dL. Habitual drinkers may tolerate higher blood alcohol levels. Alcohol dependence has a genetic component.
   2) Alcohol use is implicated in many accidents.
   3) Ethanol is metabolized to acetaldehyde by alcohol dehydrogenase in the gastric mucosa and liver, and by cytochrome P-450 and catalase in the liver. Women have lower levels of gastric alcohol dehydrogenase than men, so similar amounts of alcohol result in higher blood alcohol levels in women than in men.
   4) Some of the deleterious effects of alcohol are caused by direct toxicity (e.g., to the liver, cardiovascular system, gastrointestinal tract and skeletal muscle) while others are caused by vitamin deficiencies, particularly thiamine (e.g., Wernicke syndrome, peripheral neuropathy).

5) Fetal alcohol syndrome is the leading cause of preventable mental retardation in the U.S. It is characterized by growth and developmental defects such as microcephaly, facial dysmorphology, malformation of the brain, cardiovascular system, and genitourinary system. The pathogenesis and amount of alcohol needed to produce fetal alcohol syndrome have not been established. Damage to the fetal central nervous system may be caused when acetaldehyde crosses the placenta.
6) Alcohol ingestion is associated with cancers of the oral cavity, pharynx, esophagus, liver, and possibly of the breast.

g. Other drugs of abuse

1) Central nervous system depressants include ethanol, barbiturates, and benzodiazepines.
2) Central nervous system stimulants include cocaine, crack cocaine and amphetamines. Cocaine is associated with hypertension, stroke and sudden death, and overdose causes seizures, cardiac arrhythmias and respiratory arrest. In pregnancy, cocaine is associated with spontaneous abortion, placental abruption, and preterm birth.
3) Narcotics cause sedation and altered mood, and include oxycodone, hydromorphone, heroin, morphine, and meperidine. Injecting drugs with shared needles places the user at risk for hepatitis B and HIV infection, endocarditis, and local infections.

6. Environmental exposures

Exposure to toxic substances may occur in the home, outdoors during work, recreation or travel, or as a result of occupation or hobbies.

1) Outdoor air pollution with ozone, nitrogen dioxide, sulfur dioxide, particulates, carbon monoxide and lead affect the respiratory systems of adults and children, particularly asthmatics.
2) Indoor air pollution occurs with carbon monoxide, nitrogen dioxide, wood smoke, formaldehyde, radon, asbestos, and bioaerosols. Carbon monoxide is a byproduct of burning a variety of substances, and if the level is high enough it can cause poisoning and death. Nitrogen dioxide and wood smoke are associated with respiratory infections. Radon is a decay product of uranium and may emanate from the earth under homes; it is associated with lung cancer. Aerosolization of microbes such as *Legionella* has caused pneumonia; allergens such as pet dander, dust mites, cockroaches, fungi and molds cause allergic rhinitis and exacerbate asthma.
3) Exposure to toxic substances occurs with industrial solvents and dry cleaning agents; manufacture of synthetic plastics, rubber and polymers; mining and manufacturing of metal products (including lead, arsenic, cobalt and tungsten carbide, cadmium, chromium, mercury and nickel). Fertilizers and pesticides used in the agricultural industry are hazards not only to the workers who mix and apply them and process the

crops, they may persist on the foods, the soil and water supply, and wildlife. Other environmental contaminants include hormones used in the dairy industry and antibiotics used in cattle industry which lead to resistant strains. Lead and mercury are discussed:

a) Lead may be in urban air due to use of leaded gasoline, soil contaminated with exterior lead paint, water from lead plumbing, and house dust in homes with interior lead paint. Ceramic glazes may contain lead. The absorption of ingested lead is enhanced by calcium, iron, or zinc deficiency, and children are at greatest risk of lead toxicity. Lead causes hypochromic anemia, renal toxicity, peripheral neuropathy, insomnia and fatigue, and cognitive deficits.

b) Mercury exposure may occur directly through industrial exposure, or it may be ingested by eating fish from contaminated water. Older, larger fish are likely to have higher mercury levels than smaller fish at the bottom of the food chain. Consumption of fish with high mercury levels by pregnant women has resulted in neurobehavioral deficits in their children. Therefore, women of childbearing age, pregnant and nursing women and young children are advised not to eat with the highest mercury levels and to consume only 12 ounces per week of fish with low mercury levels. Local guidelines should be sought, as there is variation in mercury levels in bodies of water. (Huffling, J Midwifery Womens Health 2006;51:19-25)

Fish with highest mercury levels (do not eat)

King mackerel
Shark
Swordfish
Tilefish

Fish with lower mercury levels (may eat 12 ounces/week)

Shrimp
Canned light tuna
Salmon
Pollock
Catfish

Up to 6 ounces of albacore ('white") tuna may be eaten per week

7. Food-borne and nutritional disease

a. Food-borne illness may be caused by bacteria, viruses, or parasites. Selected diseases are presented; the reader is directed to the source below for more complete information.

Organism	Source	Illness
Clostridium botulinum (children and adults)	Home canned foods	Vomiting, diarrhea, blurred vision, diplopia, descending muscle weakness
Clostridium botulinum (infants)	Honey, home canned fruits and vegetables, corn syrup	Lethargy, weakness, poor feeding, poor head control, constipation, poor suck
Enterohemorrhagic *E. coli* e.g., *E. coli* O157:H47	Undercooked beef, especially hamburger, raw milk and juice, raw fruits & vegetables, salami, contaminated water	Severe diarrhea, often bloody, abdominal pain, vomiting
Listeria monocytogenes	Fresh soft cheese, unpasteurized milk, ready to eat deli meats, hotdogs	Fever, muscle aches, nausea, diarrhea. Pregnant women may have flu like symptoms, stillbirth or premature birth.
Salmonella spp.	Diarrhea, fever, abdominal cramps, vomiting	Contaminated eggs, poultry, unpasteurized milk and juice, cheese, contaminated raw fruits and vegetables
Shigella spp.	Abdominal cramps, fever, diarrhea with blood and mucus	Food or water contaminated by human fecal material, person to person contact, ready to eat foods contaminated with an infected person, e.g., raw vegetables, salads, sandwiches
Staphylococcus	Sudden onset severe nausea, vomiting, abdominal cramps; diarrhea and fever are possible	Improperly refrigerated meats, potato and egg salads, cream pastries
Hepatitis A virus	Diarrhea, dark urine, jaundice, flu-like symptoms (fever, headache, nausea, abdominal pain)	Shellfish from contaminated waters, raw produce, contaminated drinking water, uncooked foods, cooked food not reheated after contact with infected handler
Noroviruses	Vomiting in children, diarrhea in adults, abdominal cramps, fever, myalgia, headache.	Shellfish, fecally contaminated foods, ready to eat foods handled by infected persons (salad, sandwiches, ice, cookies, fruit)
Giardia lamblia	Diarrhea, stomach cramps, gas	Uncooked food or food handled by an infected person, drinking water
Toxoplasma gondii	Usually asymptomatic – 20% have cervical lymphadenopathy +/or flu-like symptoms. In immunocompromised persons, CNS disease, myocarditis, pneumonitis. Fetus may be infected congenitally.	Accidental ingestion of contaminated substances (soil or fruit contaminated with cat feces), raw or partially cooked meat, especially pork, lamb or venison.
Others, including shellfish toxins and heavy metals	See source listed below for complete descriptions	

Centers for Disease Control. MMWR. April 16, 2004/53(RR04)1-33.

http://www.cdc.gov/mmwr/preview/mmwrhtml/rr5304a1.htm#tab1

b. Nutritional deficiencies may result from ignorance or poverty, chronic diseases, and self imposed dietary restriction; malabsorption syndromes (e.g., celiac disease), genetic diseases, and drug therapies.

1) Marasmus occurs when there is an absolute deprivation of food; kwashiorkor occurs when there is a deficit of protein but carbohydrate intake continues (e.g., as with infants in developing countries who are weaned to a high starch, low protein diet). In kwashiorkor, in contrast to marasmus, there is subcutaneous fat, hepatomegaly, and fatty liver. In marasmus there is insufficient caloric intake to support fat synthesis and storage. In long term starvation eventually death ensues from electrolyte imbalances and loss of renal, pulmonary, and cardiac function as the body exhausts muscle and visceral proteins for energy.

2) Anorexia nervosa primarily affects adolescent girls. It is characterized by refusal to maintain body weight in the normal range for height, intense fear of gaining weight or becoming fat, distorted body image, and amenorrhea. There are 2 types, one in which binge-eating and purging (bulimia nervosa) occurs and one in which it does not.

3) Vitamin and mineral deficiencies may occur because of reduced intake or reduced ability of the body to absorb or manufacture the substances. Fat soluble vitamins (A, D, E, K) may be stored in the body, whereas water soluble ones (B, C) are not.

Substance	Function	Source	Signs of deficiency
Fat Soluble Vitamins			
A	Visual pigment, maintenance of epithelia; resistance to infection	Animal sources: liver, fish, eggs, milk, butter; yellow and leafy green vegetables (carrots, squash, spinach) have carotenoids (e.g., beta carotene) which may be metabolized to active vitamin A in the body.	Night blindness, xerophthalmia (dry, lusterless cornea), blindness; squamous metaplasia; vulnerability to infection. Vitamin A toxicity may occur from acute or chronic excess.
D	Maintains normal calcium and phosphorus levels, leading to bone mineralization	Synthesized by precursors in skin when exposed to ultraviolet light in sunlight; or ingested from deep sea fish, plants and grains. Some foods are fortified with vitamin D	Rickets in growing children; osteomalacia in adults. The darker the skin, the more sun exposure is needed to produce vitamin D. *Breast milk may not contain adequate amounts of vitamin D. Breast fed babies, particularly African American breast fed babies need vitamin D supplementation starting at 2 months of age.*
E	Antioxidant: scavenges free radicals throughout the body	Vegetables, grains, nuts and their oils, dairy products, fish and meat	Spinocerebellar degeneration; uncommon except in association with diseases that impair fat absorption, premature infants, and rare genetic diseases affecting vitamin E metabolism
K	Cofactor in normal hemo-coagulation; may be involved in bone metabolism	Synthesized in gut by intestinal bacteria; widely available in Western diet	Bleeding diathesis – in adults, hematomas, hematuria, melena, ecchymoses, bleeding from gums; hemorrhagic disease of the newborn (including intracranial hemorrhage) – by 1 week gut is colonized and produces adequate vitamin K.

Substance	Function	Source	Signs of deficiency
Water Soluble Vitamins			
B_1 (thiamine)	Facilitates synthesis of adenosine triphosphate; maintains normal nerve conduction	Widely available except in refined foods	Affects 25% chronic alcoholics; *may result from hyperemesis gravidarum* or other causes of intractable vomiting or diarrhea. Causes polyneuropathy (dry beriberi), cardiovascular syndrome (wet beriberi), Wernicke-Korsakoff syndrome
B_2 (riboflavin)	Cofactor in enzymes affecting many metabolic processes	Meat, dairy products, vegetables	Occurs in alcoholics, chronic infections, advanced cancer, debilitating diseases. Deficiency causes cheilosis (changes at angles of mouth), glossitis, ocular and skin changes
Niacin	Metabolism of fat, carbohydrate, and amino acids	From diet or synthesized from tryptophan endogenously. In grains, legumes, seed oils, meats.	Pellagra (dermatitis, diarrhea, dementia) results from niacin or tryptophan deficiency. In pharmacologic doses, lowers plasma LDL.
B_6 (pyridoxine)	Cofactor in enzymes that metabolize lipids and amino acids and in immune response	Present in many foods, but processing may destroy.	Some drugs acts as pyridoxine antagonists: isoniazid, estrogens, penicillamine; acetaldehyde (e.g., in alcoholics) enhances degradation; pregnancy causes increased demand. Pyridoxine deficiency causes seborrheic dermatitis, cheilosis, glossitis, peripheral neuropathy, convulsions.
B_{12}	Required for normal folate metabolism and DNA synthesis; myelinization of spinal cord tracts.	Meat, eggs and dairy products	Megaloblastic pernicious anemia, degeneration of posterolateral spinal cord tract. Vegans must supplement diet as plant sources are probably inadequate. Absorption in stomach requires intrinsic factor.
C (Ascorbic acid)	Antioxidant, synergistic with vitamin E; collagen synthesis	Cannot be synthesized endogenously, so it must be ingested. Present in milk and some animal products (liver, fish), fruits and vegetables.	Scurvy: bone disease in children and hemorrhage and healing defects in children and adults.
Folate	DNA synthesis	Whole wheat flour, beans, nuts, liver, green leafy vegetables. Heat labile; destroyed in food processing.	Megaloblastic anemia, neural tube defects. Requirement in pregnancy increased. Oral contraceptives, anticonvulsants, ethanol, cigarette smoking, chronic malabsorption syndromes and metastatic cancer interfere with absorption,
Minerals			
Iron	Component of hemoglobin and some enzymes and proteins	Heme iron in animal foods that originally contained hemoglobin, such as red meats, fish, and poultry. Iron in plant foods such as lentils and beans is nonheme iron (the form of iron added to iron-enriched and iron-fortified foods). Heme iron is absorbed better than nonheme iron.	Hypochromic, microcytic anemia. Meat proteins and vitamin C improve the absorption of nonheme iron. Tannins (in tea), calcium, polyphenols, and phytates (in legumes and whole grains) can decrease absorption of nonheme iron. Some proteins found in soybeans also inhibit nonheme iron absorption. Iron absorption increases when body stores are low.
Zinc	Component of many enzymes	Meats, fish, shellfish, whole grain cereals, legumes.	Rare genetic conditions or total parenteral nutrition. Symptoms are rash around eyes, nose, mouth, and anus; anorexia and diarrhea; hypogonadism; impaired wound healing; impaired night vision; depressed mental function; congenital malformations in infant of zinc-deficient mothers.

Substance	Function	Source	Signs of deficiency
Selen-ium	Component of antioxidant proteins	Plants, meats, seafoods, some nuts (esp. Brail nuts). Plant content depends on soil in which it was grown, and meat content depends on grains it was fed.	Rare in U.S. in absence of absorption disorders. Common in some parts of China with low soil selenium levels: heart disease, osteoarthropathy, hypothyroidism
Cal-cium	99% supports structure of bones and teeth. 1% in blood, muscle, and interstitial fluid throughout the body, essential to neuromuscular functions.	Primarily dairy products; Chinese cabbage, kale, broccoli have lower amounts and less absorbable form; fortified drinks. Foods high in oxalic acid (spinach, collard greens, sweet potatoes, rhubarb, and beans) phytic acid (whole grain bread, beans, seeds, nuts, grains, and soy isolates), and fiber may inhibit calcium absorption. Vitamin D potentiates absorption	Osteoporosis, osteopenia
Mag-nesium	Muscle and nerve function, blood sugar regulation, immune system function, bone metabolism	Green vegetables (e.g., spinach); some legumes (beans and peas), nuts and seeds, and whole, unrefined grains. Tap water (if "hard", i.e., contains more minerals than "soft" water); amount varies according to water supply.	Anorexia, nausea, vomiting, fatigue, and weakness; progressing to numbness, tingling, muscle contractions and cramps, seizures, personality changes, abnormal heart rhythms, and coronary spasms. Hypocalcemia and hypokalemia if severe.
Copper	Component of many enzymes	Oysters and other shellfish, whole grains, beans, nuts, potatoes, and organ meats; dark leafy greens, dried fruits, cocoa, black pepper, and yeast	Muscle weakness, neurologic defects, hypopigmentation, abnormal collagen, anemia, neutropenia, bone abnormalities. Occurs in malabsorption syndromes, bottle fed infants. Wilson's disease is abnormal copper storage in the body, resulting in deposits in the brain, liver, and other organs.
Iodine	Component of thyroid hormone	Seafood and produce from coastal regions; iodized salt	Goiter, hypothyroidism

http://ods.od.nih.gov/index.aspx

c. Excessive intake of nutrients causing overweight and obesity is epidemic in the U.S., with 30% of adults over the age of 20 classified as obese. Conditions associated with obesity include:

- Hypertension
- Dyslipidemia (for example, high total cholesterol or high levels of triglycerides)
- Type 2 diabetes
- Coronary heart disease
- Stroke
- Gallbladder disease
- Osteoarthritis
- Sleep apnea and respiratory problems
- Some cancers (endometrial, breast, and colon)

A goal of Healthy People 2010 is to reduce the incidence of obesity in the population, but according to the CDC, the trend is towards INCREASING rates of obesity. There are a variety of methods of assessing weight:

1) Definition
   a) **Body mass index** (BMI) which calculates one's weight in relation to height (weight in kg/height in m^2 or weight in lb/height in $inches^2$ x 703).
      (1) 25 kg/ m^2 is normal, with an excess of 20% (BMI >27 kg/m^2) associated with increased mortality (BMI <20 kg/ m^2 is also associated with increased mortality).
      (2) BMI $\geq$30 defines obesity; BMI $\geq$40 defines extreme obesity
      (3) A caveat is that persons with large muscle mass (e.g., athletes) may have high BMI without excess body fat

   b) **Skinfold** measurements – not as widely used as in the past because of limitations (not all body fat is accessible to the calipers, such as intra-abdominal and intramuscular fat, and the distribution of subcutaneous fat can vary significantly over the human body; results are not generally reproducible).
   c) **Body circumferences**
      (1) Waist >40 inches (102 cm) is high risk for men, >35 inches (88 cm) high risk for women
      (2) Effects of obesity are related not only to the total body weight, but also to the distribution of weight. Central (visceral) obesity is associated with higher risks for some conditions that diffuse accumulations of fat. Such conditions as diabetes, hypertension, hypertriglyceridemia, low HDL cholesterol, and coronary artery disease are associated with central obesity. The precise pathophysiologic mechanisms are not completely understood.
2) Etiology: more energy is taken in than is expended, causing excess calories to be stored as triglycerides in adipose tissue.

C. Pharmacology (includes alternative/complementary therapies)

1. While not within the scope of this workbook to survey a complete list of drugs, the CNM/CM should be familiar with the following classifications of drugs
   a. analgesics, local anesthetics
   b. antibiotics, anti-infectives, antivirals
   c. antihypertensives, including diuretics
   d. anti-inflammatories, including steroidal and nonsteroidal
   e. hormones

f. vaccines

g. immune globulins

h. antihistamines, including H_1 blockers

i. vitamins, minerals

j. dermatologic agents

k. cholesterol-lowering drugs

l. psychiatric drugs – antidepressants, anxiolytics, antipsychotics, tranquilizers, hypnotics

m. anticonvulsants

n. hypoglycemics

o. asthma drugs

p. gastrointestinal preparations, including antiemetics, antidiarrheal, antispasmodics, laxatives, H_2 blockers, proton pump inhibitors, etc

q. sympathomimetics

r. anti and pro clotting drugs

2. Alternative/complementary therapies

a. Vitamin and herb regulation: The main problem with herbal remedies is that they are not standardized.

1) Guidelines for counseling on herbal therapies for the health care provider:

a) Routinely inquire about the consumption/use of herbal products. Herbal medicines are made from a plant, parts of a plant, or combinations of plants.

b) Acknowledge lack of standardization and variability in herb content

c) Terms used frequently in herbal therapy

Decoction	Liquid based preparation made by boiling plant parts in water
Demulcent	Herb to sooth mucous membranes
Extract	Concentrated form of herb derived from mixing plant with a solvent and distilling or evaporating. May be liquid or solid
Galactagogue	Promote lactation
Herb	Plant used for medicinal purposes; differs from biological definition, which refers to a plant with no woody aboveground parts.
Infusion	Liquid preparation made by steeping a plant in water below boiling point; tea
Oil, essential	Aromatic volatile oils extracted from an herb, usually diluted
Oil, infused	Mixture of volatile oils of an herb with another oil. The carrier oil extracts the volatile oils by soaking for a specified period of time.
Poultice	Plant material wrapped in soft cloth, moistened, and applied topically
Powder	Product of distilled herb which is then dried and ground
Tincture	Extract made by soaking plant in liquid (water, alcohol, vinegar, glycerin) and straining out plant material. Remaining liquid is used therapeutically.
Tonic	Focused on treating one particular body system

ALTERNATIVE THERAPIES

Safety and effectiveness

The product or practice should not cause any harm and should provide benefit when used as intended. Specific information about the safety and effectiveness of any alternative or complementary therapy should be readily available.

The practitioner's expertise

Closely examine the training, qualifications, and competence of any potential health care practitioner, whether a practitioner of conventional care or alternative care.

Quality of service delivery

Determine if the delivery of service adheres to standards for safety and care. Feel free to contact state or local regulatory agencies or health care consumer organizations; visit the practitioner's office, clinic, or hospital; and talk to people who have used the services.

Costs

Many alternative therapies are not covered by health insurance, so compare the costs with those of other practitioners or through professional associations.

If you combine conventional and alternative care, let all practitioners know

Adopted From JAMA Home Page, 1999

National Center for Complementary and Alternative Medicine web site: http://nccam.nih.gov
Office of Dietary Supplement web site: http://ods.od.nih.gov/

D. Assessment of the well woman

Midwifery management process
(based on ACNM Core Competencies, 2002)

- *Collect information*, e.g., history and physical, laboratory studies
- *Identify problems* and formulate diagnosis in collaboration with the client
- *Educate clients* and support them to make informed decisions and assume primary responsibility for their own health
- *Develop a comprehensive plan* of care with the client
- *Implement* individualized plans
- *Consult, collaborate, or refer/transfer* the care of the client as appropriate
- *Initiate management of emergencies*
- *Evaluate* with the client the effectiveness of care and modify the plan as appropriate

← Documentation formats (examples) →

C collection of information	or	**S** subjective
A analyze and assess information		**O** objective
D develop a plan		**A** assessment
I implement the plan		**P** plan
E evaluate		

1. History and review of systems

a. Purpose of the visit: Detection, diagnosis, treatment, screening, general health maintenance

b. Components: Systems: menstrual, medical/surgical, family, obstetric, contraceptive, sexual, social/cultural, nutritional, occupational, activity, nutritional, exposures

c. The interview: Establishing a relationship, setting the tone, collecting information and establishing the reason for the visit

d. **Menstrual history:** Menarche, last menstrual period (LMP), cycle length and frequency, pain, regularity, amount, premenstrual symptoms, tampon use, deodorant tampons/pads

e. **Gynecologic history:** Vaginitis, sexually transmitted diseases (STD), infertility, diseases of the reproductive tract; frequency of breast self exam (BSE); date and results of last Pap smear and pelvic exam

f. **Sexual history:** Number and gender of partners, age at first intercourse, sexual practices, frequency of intercourse, risk factors, satisfaction, information gaps

g. **OB history:** Gravida (G) and parity* using 4 digit system (TPAL)

G = number of pregnancies

T = term deliveries (≥37 weeks)

P = preterm deliveries (20-36 weeks)

A = spontaneous or induced abortion <20 weeks

L = number of living children

*Multiple gestation does not increase parity, it is evident in the number of living children

Outcomes with dates and current status, complications. Future pregnancy plans and need for preconception counseling.

h. **Contraceptive history:** Current and past use, satisfaction, problems with methods used

i. **Medical history:** Infectious or childhood diseases, chronic diseases including psychiatric, allergies, blood transfusions, vaccination status, medications taken on a regular basis (prescription and over the counter); substance use/abuse/dependence (alcohol, tobacco, illicit drugs – some consider this social history)

j. **Surgical history**

k. **Family history:** Endometriosis & osteoporosis, cancer, DES exposure; cardiovascular (age at onset, death), endocrine, psychiatric, congenital or genetic disorders, etc

l. **Social & cultural:** Status and quality of primary relationship, social support system, history or potential of domestic or sexual abuse, adequacy of housing. Relevant cultural practices. Expectations regarding health care.

m. **Occupational history:** Job title, industry, specific hazards to which the worker is exposed (e.g. heavy lifting, shift work, video display terminal, repetitive motion, chemicals). Include hobbies.

n. **Nutritional history:** 24 hour recall, dietary stimulants, changes in weight, dietary restrictions, satisfaction with weight, pica

o. **Exercise/activity:** Type, frequency, satisfaction

p. Review of systems

Symptom Analysis

- Onset
- Interval history
- Current Status
- Pain-related
    - Type
    - Location
    - Severity
    - Duration
    - Influencing factors (precipitating, relieving)
    - Associated symptoms

1) *Head, Eyes, Ears, Nose, Throat (HEENT), Neck*
    a) Head-headache, pain, head injury, dizziness
    b) Eyes-vision, corrective lenses, previous eye exam, pain, photophobia, redness, tearing, diplopia, blurred vision, scotomata, glaucoma, cataract
    c) Ears-hearing impairment, tinnitus, vertigo, earaches, ear pain, infection, discharge, dizziness
    d) Nose and sinuses-frequent colds, congestion, nasal obstruction, discharge or itching, hay fever, nosebleeds, sinus problems
    e) Mouth and throat-condition of teeth, gums, previous dental exam, dentures, crowns, braces, sore tongue, dry mouth, sore throats, postnasal drip, hoarseness
    f) Neck-goiter, lumps, pain, stiffness, swollen glands, thyroid problem
2) *Heart and lungs*
    a) Heart – chest pain or distress (include symptom analysis), dyspnea, orthopnea, edema, claudication, hypertension, previous myocardial infarction, exercise tolerance, past electrocardiogram or other test
    b) Lungs – dyspnea, chest pain, cyanosis, wheezing, cough, sputum, hemoptysis, night sweats, exposure to tuberculosis, date and result of last chest X-ray, TB skin test
    c) Hematologic – anemia, bruising, thromboses, thrombophlebitis, abnormality of blood cells, transfusions
3) *Breasts* – development, pain, tenderness, discharge, lumps, galactorrhea, mammograms and results, frequency of BSE
4) *Abdomen/CVAT/Urinary*
    a) GI - appetite, digestion, food intolerance, dysphagia, heartburn, nausea, vomiting, hematemesis, bowel regularity, constipation, diarrhea, change in stool, flatulence, hemorrhoids, hepatitis, jaundice, urine color; ulcer, gallstones, polyps, tumor; previous diagnostic studies; vaginal discharge, LMP

b) CVAT, urinary – dysuria, flank or suprapubic pain, urgency, frequency, nocturia, hematuria, polyuria, hesitancy, incontinence, stones, edema.

5) *Pelvis/gyn*

a) Menses – onset, regularity, duration, amount of flow, dysmenorrhea, last period, intermenstrual discharge or bleeding, itching, date of last Pap smear, age at menopause

b) Vulva -- Vaginal discharge, vulvar itching, pain, lesions

c) Sexual -- libido, frequency of intercourse, dyspareunia, sexual difficulties or questions, satisfaction, infertility

6) *Skin, extremities*

a) Skin – rash, lesions, itching, pigmentation or texture changes, excessive sweating, abnormal hair or nail growth

b) Extremities –Joint stiffness, pain, restriction of motion, swelling, redness, heat, bony deformity

7) *Neurologic, psychiatric*

a) Neurologic – syncope, seizures, weakness or paralysis, paresthesias, lack of coordination, tremors, loss of memory

b) Psychiatric – depression, mood changes, difficulty concentrating, nervousness, tension, suicidal thoughts, irritability, sleep disturbances

8) *Endocrine* – thyroid enlargement or tenderness, heat or cold intolerance, unexplained weight change, diabetes, polydipsia, polyuria, distribution and changes in facial or body hair, increased hat or glove size, skin striae

2. Physical examination

Preparation and Procedure for Physical Examination

- Meet woman dressed first
- Assemble equipment
- Involve woman; e.g., offer mirror
- Explain procedure
- Provide for privacy
- Gown and drape appropriately
- Be gentle, but accurate
- Be thorough
- Adequate exposure
- Comfortable positioning
- Warm hands and instruments
- Appropriate room temperature
- Adequate lighting
- Use standard precautions (wash hands, wear gloves etc)
- Be systematic
- Have adequate assistance

I. Primary Care (5%-10%)

a. HEENT

1) Inspection, palpation, auscultation

   a) Head

      (1) Texture, quantity, distribution of hair

      (2) Lumps, lesions, tenderness, scales, dandruff, infection, parasites

      (3) Size and contour of skull

      (4) Shape and symmetry of face, tremors (cranial nerve V)

      (5) Turn head to each side against resistance (cranial nerve XI)

   b) Eyes

      (1) Eyebrows, eyelashes, eyelids-condition, symmetry, distribution

      (2) Swelling, discharge, or lesions

      (3) Position and placement

      (4) Conjunctiva, sclera, pupil, iris for color, shape, inflammation

      (5) Six cardinal positions of gaze (cranial nerves III, IV, VI)

      (6) Visual acuity (cranial nerve II)

      (7) Opthalmoscopic exam - red reflex, optic disc, retinal vessels, macula

   c) Ears

      (1) Size, position, symmetry and hygiene of auricles

      (2) Presence of discharge, lesions, foreign bodies

      (3) Nodules, swelling, or tenderness

      (4) Otoscopic exam

         (a) Cerumen, redness, swelling, drainage

         (b) Tympanic membrane for color, plaques, bulging

         (c) Light reflex

         (d) Shape, position, prominence of malleus

      (5) Hearing acuity assessment (cranial nerve VIII)

         (a) Whispered voice

         (b) Weber test (tuning fork in midline vertex testing for lateralization)

         (c) Rinne test (tuning fork on mastoid and then close to auditory canal, timing disappearance of sound; air conduction should be twice as long as bone conduction of sound)

   d) Nose

      (1) Size, shape, color, symmetry

      (2) Flaring, discharge, excoriation of nares

      (3) Displacement, tenderness, or masses of nasal bridge

      (4) Nasal patency

(5) Sense of smell (cranial nerve I)

(6) Rhinoscopy (otoscope)

(a) Exudate, lesions, perforations of mucosa

(b) Color, swelling, bleeding, exudate, polyps of turbinates

(c) Paranasal sinuses palpation for tenderness

(d) Maxillary sinuses palpation for tenderness

(e) Transillumination of frontal sinus, infraorbital sinus

e) Mouth and throat

(1) Symmetry, color, moisture, lesions, ulcers of lips

(2) Mobility and tenderness of temporomandibular joint

(3) Lesions, ulcers, patches, nodes of buccal mucosa

(4) Color and intactness of hard and soft palate

(5) Inflammation, bleeding or retraction of gums

(6) Movement, size of tongue (cranial nerve XII)

(7) Color, fissures, lesions, ulcerations, papillae of dorsal tongue

(8) Inflammation, swelling, exudate of uvula, tonsils, posterior wall of oropharynx; elicit gag reflex on each side (cranial nerves IX and X with gag reflex and rise of soft palate with "ah")

(9) Clench teeth and smile (cranial nerve VII) for occlusion

f) Neck

(1) Symmetry of muscles

(2) Masses or swelling

(3) Distention of or bounding pulses, visible lymph nodes, thyroid enlargement

(4) Range of motion

(5) Size, shape, consistency, mobility, tenderness of lymph nodes

(6) Rate, rhythm, equality, bruits of carotid pulses

(7) Size, consistency, presence of thyroid nodules

b. Heart and lungs

1) Heart

a) Inspection

(1) Height and weight measurement, body mass index (BMI)

(2) Fingers and nail beds for clubbing, cyanosis

(3) Distended neck veins

(4) Edema

(5) Visualize apical pulse

b) Palpation

(1) Heaves, thrills, or lifts

(2) Point of maximal impulse (PMI)

c) Auscultation

(1) S_1 and S_2 are caused by valve closings.

- S_1 is the sound of atrioventricular (tricuspid and mitral) valves closing at the beginning of systole (LUB); Heard best at apex
- S_2 is the sound of closure of the semilunar (pulmonic) and aortic valves at the end of systole (DUB). Heard best at the base
- Split S_2 (D-DUB) is often heard during inspiration, especially in young people; it is the closure of the pulmonic and aortic valves.

(2) S_3 and S_4 occur during diastole, as the ventricles fill. They should be quiet and difficult to hear. S_3 (ventricular gallop) is Ken-TUC-ky; S_4 (atrial gallop) is Tenn-es-SEE. Loud atrial gallops always suggest pathology.

(3)Auscultatory areas:

(a) Aortic valve area: second right intercostal space, right sternal border

(b) Pulmonic valve area: second left intercostal space, left sternal border

> **Remember**
> Sinus arrhythmia can be a normal finding in a young reproductive aged woman. Have her hold her breath and see if it resolves.

(c) Second pulmonic area: third left intercostal space, left sternal border

(d) Tricuspid area: fourth left intercostal space, lower left sternal border

(e) Mitral (apical) area: apex of heart in fifth left intercostal space, midclavicular line

(4) Characterization of heart sounds

(a) Splitting

(b) Gallop

(c) Rub

(d) Murmur: loudness, location, pitch quality, timing, radiation, pattern, grade

Grading heart murmurs I-VI

I	Barely audible in a quiet room
II	Quiet but clearly audible
III	Moderately loud
IV	Loud, associated with thrill
V	Very loud, thrill easily palpated
VI	Very loud, audible with stethoscope not in contact with chest, thrill palpable and visible

2) Lungs

a) Inspection
   (1) Skin color
   (2) Nasal flaring
   (3) Fingernails (clubbing, color)
   (4) Tracheal position
   (5) Chest shape, symmetry
   (6) Rate, rhythm, depth, and effort
   (7) Bulging of interspaces (asthma)

b) Palpation
   (1) Tenderness
   (2) Abnormal movements
   (3) Tactile fremitus

c) Percussion tones
   (1) Flat
   (2) Dull
   (3) Resonant
   (4) Hyperresonant
   (5) Tympanic

d) Auscultation (using diaphragm of stethoscope) listening for normal and adventitious breath sounds

   (1) Normal breath sounds: Vesicular, bronchial, broncho-vesicular
   - ➢ **Vesicular** are heard over the periphery of the lung field (low pitch)
   - ➢ **Bronchial** are normally heard over the trachea and larynx (medium pitch)
   - ➢ **Bronchovesicular** are heard on both sides of the sternum in the first and second intercostal spaces, between the scapula and over the lung apices (high pitched). Bronchovesicular sounds can be heard over all lung fields in very thin people and in children; otherwise abnormal in peripheral lung fields.

   (2) Adventitious breath sounds
   - ➢ **Crackles** (formerly called rales) in pneumonia, bronchitis, asthma. Not cleared by cough
   - ➢ **Wheezes** in asthma, bronchitis, congestive heart failure; continuous. Sibilant wheeze; high pitched squeak.

- **Rhonchi in bronchitis**. Sonorous wheeze; low pitched; coughing may clear
- **Pleural friction rub:** dry, rubbing, grating.

c. Breast

1) Inspection: sitting with arms at the side, arms over the head, hands pressed against hips (or palms pressed together), and leaning forward from the waist
   a) Size, symmetry, contour, skin color and texture, venous patterns, lesions, dimpling
   b) Nipple and areola: 5 Ds
      (1) Discharge
      (2) Depression (inversion)
      (3) Discoloration
      (4) Dermatologic changes (peau d'orange)
      (5) Deviation (symmetry)
   c) Supernumerary nipples, accessory breast tissue along mammary line
   d) Palpation: breasts, axillae, supraclavicular region
      (1) Finger pads more sensitive than tips
      (2) Systematic: top to bottom vertically, concentric circles, wedges
         - Include Tail of Spence
         - Nipples: if compressed, should be gentle.
         - Lymph nodes in axillae and supraclavicular area
      (3) Note lumps or nodules
         - Location: quadrant, distance from nipple; illustrate
         - Size: length, width, thickness in centimeters
         - Shape: round, discoid, lobular, stellate; regular or irregular
         - Consistency: firm, soft, hard
         - Tenderness: degree
         - Mobility: mobile in which direction, fixed to skin or fascia
         - Borders: discrete, poorly defined
         - Retraction: dimpling, altered contour
         - ***All new solitary or dominant masses should be investigated***
      (4) Nipple discharge: color, origin; fix specimen on slide.

> **Remember**
> Mammograms are more accurate for menopausal/ postmenopausal women because the breast tissue is less dense.

d. Abdomen/Costovertebral angle tenderness (CVAT)

1) Inspection

   a) Skin color, lesions, SCARS

   b) Contour, symmetry, surface motion

   c) Umbilicus

   d) Distention: Fs

      - Fat
      - Fluid (ascites)
      - Feces
      - Fetus
      - Flatus
      - Fibroid
      - Full bladder
      - False pregnancy
      - Fatal tumor

   e) Movement: respiration, peristalsis, pulsation

2) **Auscultation**

   a) Bowel sounds all 4 quadrants

      (1) Normal frequency 5-35 per minute

      (2) Borborygmi (hyperperistalsis-loud, prolonged sounds “growling”)

      (3) Must listen for 5 minutes to establish absence

   b) Vascular sounds

      (1) Aorta, renal, femoral, iliac artery bruits

      (2) Friction rubs over liver or spleen

      (3) Venous hum at the umbilicus (hepatic cirrhosis)

3) **Percussion**: tympany to dullness is preferable

   a) Liver, stomach, spleen, kidneys (for tenderness)

4) **Palpation**: for organs, masses, muscle spasm, fluid, tenderness; all 4 quadrants

   a) Light palpation for muscular resistance or tenderness, large mass

   b) Moderate palpation to identify spleen and liver

   c) Deep palpation to delineate abdominal organs and detect subtle masses

   d) Evaluate liver, gallbladder, spleen, kidneys, aorta, bladder, abdominal reflexes

   e) Characterize abdominal findings

      (1) Involuntary tenderness or rigidity –peritoneal inflammation

      (2) **Rebound tenderness** (peritonitis; appendicitis for rebound pain at McBurney’s point): some consider the maneuver unnecessarily painful

      (3) **Guarding (**nervous state or may be perforated viscus)

      (4) **Hyperesthesia** (affected peripheral nerve)

(5) **Iliopsoas sign (retroperitoneal irritation; appendicitis):** lower quadrant pain on lifting leg against pressure

(6) **Obturator sign (possible ruptured appendix or pelvic abscess):** hypogastric pain on rotation of flexed right leg

(7) **Rovsing's sign (appendicitis):** right lower quadrant pain intensified by left lower quadrant palpation

(8) **Murphy sign (cholecystitis):** abrupt cessation of inspiration on gallbladder palpation

5) Costovertebral angle tenderness (CVAT)

a) Client sitting: Palm over CVA and strike with fist of opposite hand, or gently pound down each side of the woman's back with the ulnar side of fist from mid-scapula to mid-buttock

b) Pain at CVA may indicate renal disease

6) Rectal exam

7) Bimanual abdominopelvic exam may be indicated with abdominal symptoms, as pelvic conditions can cause referred abdominal pain

e. Pelvic examination (bimanual/speculum), including external genitalia

1) External genitalia: inspect and palpate with gloves on

a) Mons pubis, labia minora and majora, clitoris, urethral meatus, introitus, perineum and perirectal area, anus

(1) Hair distribution, skin

(2) Swelling, redness, tenderness: symmetry

(3) Excoriation, rash, lesions, nevi

(4) Discoloration, varicosities, trauma, scarring

(5) Shaving, tattoos, piercings, etc

b) Vaginal tone

2) Speculum exam: choose the correct speculum, not necessarily the smallest speculum (see box)

a) Inspect cervix and vagina

(1) Cervix: color, position, size, surface characteristics, discharge, lesions, size and shape of os

(2) Vagina: color, discharge, lesions, rugae

(3) Obtain Pap smear, cultures, and wet prep specimens if needed

(4) Note characteristics and odor of any secretions on blades when removed

3) Bimanual exam
    a) Palpate vagina
    b) Palpate cervix for texture, nodules, size, length, consistency, patency, mobility and tenderness
    c) Palpate uterus for position, size, shape, contour, consistency, mobility, tenderness.
        (1) Anteversion is forward inclination of the fundus toward the pubis
        (2) Anteflexion is the acute folding of the uterus forward toward the pubis
        (3) Retroversion is backward tilting of the uterus toward the sacrum
        (4) Retroflexion is the acute folding of the uterus backward toward the sacrum
    d) Palpate the adnexal area and ovaries.
        (1) Note size of ovaries if palpable (3cm x 2cm x 1cm is normal if not menopausal), tenderness, enlargement, nodularity.
        (2) Adnexal structures other than ovaries are not usually palpable, except round ligament
        (3) If mass is found, note size, shape, location, consistency, tenderness
4) Rectal, rectovaginal exam
    a) Assess tone of anal sphincter
    b) Palpate rectal walls and rectovaginal septum, rotating rectal finger
        (1) Explore for polyps, masses, nodules, strictures, irregularities, tenderness
        (2) Assess uterus and adnexae, especially if you were unable to do it with vaginal examination; particularly useful in assessing retroverted uterus
        (3) As fingers are withdrawn, evaluate posterior rectal wall
    c) Note stool or any blood or secretions on rectal glove; obtain specimen for occult blood if indicated
5) Following pelvic and rectal exam, assist the woman to a sitting position; share findings and elicit her response to the examination; or allow her to dress first

Selecting the Appropriate Vaginal Speculum

Type	**Characteristics**	**Appropriate Population**
Pediatric, Virginal	Smallest Narrow, short, flat blades	Young girls Women with little or no coitus
Graves	Standard (most common) Large (same but bigger)	Sexually active women Multiparity (especially higher order) Collapsing vaginal walls Very obese
Pederson	Long as Graves but narrower blades Flat blades	Sexually active but tight or nullipara Postmenopausal women

f. Skin/extremities

1) Skin

a) Inspection

(1) General survey-moisture, texture, thickness, mobility, turgor, vascularity, bleeding, bruising, scarring, burns

(2) Awareness of ethnic variability

(3) Skin color-hypopigmentation, hyperpigmentation, erythema, cyanosis, jaundice, pallor

(4) Lesions, discolorations, abnormalities: describe

- Macules, papules, vesicles, pustules, bullae, hives, warts, moles, ulcers, scars, keloids, petechiae, lipomas, flakes, blackheads, chancres: note type and anatomic location

(5) Nails-color, curvature, adhesion, pitting, hypertrophy

(6) Hair-alopecia, hirsutism, tinea capitis, pattern baldness

(7) Tattoos, piercings etc

b) Palpation

(1) Skin temperature

(2) Excessive moisture

(3) Dryness

(4) Turgor

(5) Nails for texture

(6) Scalp to assess hair distribution, texture and quantity

(7) Skin/lesion for blanching

(8) Lesions palpated for shape, density, mobility, tenderness, size

<u>Consider need for gloves before palpating a skin lesion!</u>

2) Extremities

a) Inspection

(1) Posture, skin, discoloration, swelling, masses, symmetry, alignment, size, deformity, contour, muscle wasting

(2) Range of motion

b) Palpation

(1) Bones, joints, muscles for heat, tenderness, swelling, crepitus

(2) Evaluate muscle strength

(3) Assess edema

(4) Measure and compare matching extremities if indicated

g. **Neurologic**

- ❖ Fundamental goal in primary care setting: Rule out neurologic abnormalities and refer as needed

1) Observe gait, muscle tone and coordination
2) Cortical function-intellectual
    a) Short and long term memory
    b) Speech and understanding speech
    c) Affect
3) Cranial nerves testing
    a) Olfactory (smell)
    b) Optic (vision)
    c) Oculomotor (lifts upper eyelid; turns eyeball upward, downward and medially; constricts pupil; accommodates eyes)
    d) Trochlear (assists in turning eyeball downward and laterally)
    e) Trigeminal (jaw muscles, sensory facial)
    f) Abducens (turns eyeball laterally)
    g) Facial (sensory-taste; motor - face, cheek, and scalp muscles; some salivary glands, lacrimal gland)
    h) Acoustic: vestibular and cochlear (hearing, position and movement of head)
    i) Glossopharyngeal (sensory – sensation and taste posterior third of tongue, motor – swallowing; parotid salivary gland)
    j) Vagus (motor – pharynx and larynx, involuntary muscle of trachea and bronchi, heart, alimentary tract from pharynx to splenic flexure of colon, liver and pancreas; sensory – taste from epiglottis and vallecula, afferent fibers from structures listed earlier)
    k) Accessory: cranial and spinal (cranial: muscles of soft palate, pharynx and larynx; spinal: sternocleidomastoid and trapezius muscles)
    l) Hypoglossal (muscles that control shape and movement of the tongue)
4) Motor function: Assess strength in each major muscle group
5) Sensory function: Light touch and pin-prick sensation in each of the dermatomes
6) Deep tendon reflexes
    a) Biceps, triceps, patella, and ankle jerk
        - Somewhat diminished 1+
        - Normal reaction 2+
        - Brisk 3+
        - Hyperactive 4+
    b) Plantar response (Babinski response indicates upper motor neuron disease)

h. Vital signs

1) Temperature: Oral, rectal, axillary, or tympanic membrane; variety of instruments are available
2) Pulse: Palpation of radial pulse is usually used for screening; note rate (beats per minute), rhythm, and amplitude
3) Respirations: Count cycles per minute; evaluate by inspection, observing rise and fall of chest and ease of breathing; note depth and use of accessory muscles
4) Blood pressure
   a) Choose correct size cuff: 1/3-1/2 circumference of limb; bladder should be 80% of limb circumference
      (1) Cuff that is too wide will give lower reading
      (2) Cuff that is too narrow will give higher reading
   b) Auscultate over artery (usually brachial) for Korotkoff sounds
      (1) First beat heard is Korotkoff 1 and is recorded as systolic pressure
      (2) Muffling is heard at Korotkoff 4
      (3) Disappearance of sounds is Korotkoff 5 and is recorded as diastolic pressure
   c) Difference between systolic and diastolic is pulse pressure, usually 30-50 mm Hg
   d) Classification of blood pressure

Normal

- Systolic ≤119 mm Hg
- Diastolic ≤79 mm Hg
- Treatment: Lifestyle modifications if indicated

Prehypertension

- Systolic 120–139 mm Hg
- Diastolic 80–89 mm Hg
  - ➢ Treatment: Lifestyle modifications
  - ➢ No antihypertensive drug

Stage 1 hypertension:

- Systolic 140–159 mm Hg
- Diastolic 90–99 mm Hg
  - ➢ **Treatment**:
  - ➢ Lifestyle Modifications
  - ➢ Thiazide – type diuretics for most
  - ➢ May consider ACEI, ARB, BB, CCB, or combination

Stage 2 hypertension:

- Systolic 160 mm Hg or higher
- Diastolic 100 mm Hg or higher
  - **Treatment:**
  - Lifestyle Modifications
  - 2 drug combination for most. Usually ACEI, ARB, BB, CCB

The Seventh Report of the Joint National Committee on Prevention, Detection, Evaluation and Treatment of High Blood Pressure (JNC 7), 2003; JAMA 289:2650-2573.

See section on hypertension for further discussion.

3. **Cultural factors**

   a. Health care providers wish to deliver care in a culturally sensitive and appropriate manner. In spite of such a desire, sometimes the provider's own culture or lack of knowledge about others impairs delivery of such care. In 1999, the ACNM released a position statement on *Ethnic and Cultural Diversity:*

"It is the position of the American College of Nurse-Midwives that every individual has the right to safe, satisfying health care with respect for human dignity as well as ethnic and cultural variations.

Midwifery care is focused on the needs of the individual and family for physical care, emotional and social support, active involvement of significant others according to cultural values and personal preferences. The profession of midwifery assumes the responsibility for ensuring that certified nurse-midwives (CNMs) and certified midwives (CMs) are provided with excellence in educational preparation which includes experiences that promote cultural competency and proficiency, and that they demonstrate professional standards of practice in keeping with these stated beliefs.

The American College of Nurse-Midwives seeks to promote educational preparation for its membership, which will develop respect for ethnic and cultural variations. The American College of Nurse-midwives also recognizes the richness that ethnic and cultural diversity brings to its membership. Therefore, the American College of Nurse-Midwives actively seeks to recruit and retain persons for ethnic and cultural minorities into educational programs, and the general membership. Furthermore the American College of Nurse-Midwives seeks to encourage diverse representation at all levels."

Source: Midwives of Color Committee

Approved by the ACNM Board of Directors: April, 1992

Revised: August 1997, June 1999 with Title Change

1) Cultural competency in the context of health care provision consists of:
    a) Awareness and acceptance of cultural differences
    b) Awareness of one's own cultural values
    c) Recognition that people of different cultures have different ways of communicating, behaving, interpreting, and problem-solving
    d) Recognition that cultural beliefs impact health beliefs, help-seeking activities, interactions with health care professionals, health care practices, and health care outcomes, including adherence to prescribed regimens.
    e) An ability and willingness to adapt the way one works to fit the patient's cultural or ethnic background in order to provide optimal care for the patient.

Levels of Cultural Competence in Health Care (Culhane-Pera et al)	
Level 1	No insight about the influence of culture on medical care
Level 2	Minimal emphasis on culture in medical setting
Level 3	Acceptance of the role of cultural beliefs, values, and behaviors on health disease, and treatment
Level 4	Incorporation of cultural awareness into daily medical practice
Level 5	Integration of attention to culture into all areas of professional life

2) Associated with the acceptance of the role of cultural beliefs, values, and behaviors on health, disease, and treatment (Level 3) are the knowledge, attitudes and skills objectives listed below (adapted from Culhane-Pera, et al)
    a) Knowledge
        (1) Define culture and list various factors that influence culture
        (2) Describe cultural beliefs, values and behaviors of a cultural group different than one in which you belong
        (3) Discuss important cultural influences of particular patients
        (4) Describe three traditional healing practices of specific ethnic groups in the local area
    b) Skills
        (1) Inquire about beliefs, practices and values for patients and families as pertinent to medical problems.
        (2) Obtain a medical history, considering cultural information
        (3) Consider cultural information in making diagnostic and therapeutic plans
        (4) Work with interpreters in an effective manner
        (5) Apply general cultural information as hypotheses and not as stereotypes

c) Attitudes

(1) Respect patients' and families' behaviors and values

(2) Be aware of the influence of sociocultural factors on patients, providers, the clinical encounter and interpersonal relationships

(3) Appreciate the heterogeneity that exists within and across all cultural groups and the need to avoid overgeneralization and negative stereotyping

(4) Be aware of own cultural beliefs, values, and practices that influence self as a cultural person.

d) Culture and the individual: Steps toward practicing culturally competent health care

(1) Examine your own cultural attitudes and knowledge

(2) Use of culturally sensitive interviewing tools

(3) Foster an open, sensitive approach to patient health care beliefs

http://www.musc.edu/fm_ruralclerkship/culture.html

E. Health promotion and disease prevention

1. Behavioral screening and counseling

a. Sexually transmitted infection

1) Healthy People 2010 (HP2K) goals:

a) Complete abstinence from sexual (vagina, oral or anal) intercourse during adolescence, reverting to abstinence after having had intercourse in the past, or use condoms consistently and correctly if sexually active

b) Routine hepatitis B immunization

c) Routine screening for asymptomatic *Chlamydia trachomatis* (CT) for all sexually active female age 25 or younger and other women at risk for CT

source: http://www.healthypeople.gov/Document/HTML/Volume2/25STDs.htm#

2) Monogamy

3) Use water based lubricants; nonoxynol 9 may not prevent transmission of AIDS, and may increase transmission of other STDs (CDC, 2003)

4) Give alternatives for safe and safer sexual activity

5) Explicitly describe unsafe sexual activity

b. Breast Self Examination (BSE)

1) Less than 50% of women perform SBE according to the American Cancer Society

2) Fifty percent of palpable breast cancers have metastasized at time of discovery

3) **Characteristic to look for in performing BSE:** new lumps, puckering, dimpling, thickening, hardening, retraction of nipples, bleeding or discharge from nipples

4) ***Do BSE one week after menses; postmenopausal women perform BSE at the same time each month***

5) Clinical Breast Exam (CBE): Sensitivity (true positives) about 45%; When mammograms are combined with CBE the sensitivity goes up to 88%.

6) Documentation:

   a) When the mass was first detected

   b) Size, location, shape, regularity, mobility, consistency, presence of nipple discharge, skin changes

   c) Use a diagram

   d) Health information & plan of care. How you respond may well affect her psychological state and her future adherence to breast screening

c. **Substance abuse:** Smoking, alcohol (ETOH), street drugs

1) Tobacco

   a) HP2K goal: Cigarette smoking is single most preventable cause of disease and death in US. Results in more deaths each year in the US than AIDS, alcohol, cocaine, heroin, homicide, suicide, motor vehicle crashes, and fires—combined.

   b) According to the surgeon general's office:

      (1) Tobacco dependence is a chronic condition that often requires repeated intervention. Effective treatments exist that can produce long-term or even permanent abstinence.

      (2) Every patient who uses tobacco should be offered at least one of these treatments:

      Patients *willing* to try to quit: effective treatments and "5 A's"

      - Ask (Systematically identify all tobacco users at every visit)
      - Advise (Strongly urge all tobacco users to quit)
      - Assess (Determine willingness to make a quit attempt)
      - Assist (Aid the patient in quitting, e.g., prescribe drugs)
      - Arrange (Schedule follow up contact)

      Patients *unwilling* to try to quit: brief intervention to increase their motivation – the "5 R's"

      - Relevance (Encourage woman to indicate why quitting is personally relevant)
      - Risks (ask woman to identify negative consequences of tobacco use)
      - Rewards (ask woman to identify benefits of stopping tobacco use)
      - Roadblocks (ask woman to identify barriers or impediments to quitting and note elements of treatment, e.g., problem solving, pharmacotherapy, that could address barriers)
      - Repetition (motivational intervention should be repeated every time an unmotivated patient visits the clinic setting)

c) Brief tobacco dependence treatment is effective, and every patient who uses tobacco should be offered at least brief treatment.

d) There is a strong dose-response relationship between the intensity of tobacco dependence counseling and its effectiveness. Treatments involving person-to-person contact are consistently effective, and effectiveness increases with treatment intensity.

e) Three types of counseling that are especially effective should be used with all patients who are attempting tobacco cessation:

- Provision of practical counseling (problem solving/skills training).
- Provision of social support as part of treatment.
- Help in securing social support outside of treatment.

f) Effective pharmacotherapies for smoking cessation exist. Except in the presence of contraindications, these should be used with all patients who are attempting to quit smoking.

(1) FDA approved medications include bupropion SR, nicotine gum, inhaler, nasal spray, and patch. Medications that are not FDA approved but may be used as second line treatments are clonidine and nortiptyline.

(2) Over-the-counter nicotine patches are effective relative to placebo, and their use should be encouraged.

g) Patients who have recently quit using tobacco should be provided relapse prevention treatment.

Reference: Fiore MC, Bailey WC, Cohen SJ, et. al. Treating Tobacco Use and Dependence. Quick Reference Guide for Clinicians. Rockville, MD: U.S. Department of Health and Human Services. Public Health Service. October 2000. accessed at http://www.surgeongeneral.gov/tobacco/tobaqrg.htm

2) Alcohol (ETOH) and illicit drug use

a) HP2K: Alcohol and illicit drug use are associated with many of this country's most serious problems -- violence, injury, HIV infection.

(1) Alcohol is the drug most frequently used by adolescents.

(2) Binge drinking is consuming five or more drinks on one occasion

(3) Drugs used: marijuana, cocaine, crack, heroin, acid, inhalants, and methamphetamines; abuse of prescription drugs and other "street" drugs.

(4) The younger a person becomes a habitual user of illicit drugs, the stronger the addiction becomes and the more difficult it is to stop.

(5) Long-term heavy drinking can lead to heart disease, cancer, alcohol-related liver disease, and pancreatitis.

(6) Alcohol use during pregnancy causes fetal alcohol syndrome, a leading cause of preventable mental retardation.

http://www.healthypeople.gov/Document/html/uih/uih_bw/uih_4.htm#subsabuse

b) Recommend:

(1) Drink alcoholic beverages sensibly and in moderation—up to one drink per day for women and up to two drinks per day for men.

(2) Alcohol should not be consumed by those who cannot restrict their alcohol intake; women who may become pregnant; pregnant and lactating women; children and adolescents; individuals taking medications that can interact with alcohol; and those with specific medical conditions.

(3) Alcoholic beverages should be avoided if engaged in activities that require attention, skill, or coordination, such as driving or operating machinery.

(4) Do not use illegal (street) drugs of any kind, at any time.

http://www.health.gov/dietaryguidelines/dga2005/recommendations.htm

c) Assessment – choose a system and use it for every client

(1) CAGE

C Have you ever felt that you should **C**ut down on your drinking?
A Have people **A**nnoyed you by criticizing your drinking?
G Have you ever felt bad or **G**uilty about drinking or something you did when you were drinking?
E Have you ever had a drink first thing in the morning (**E**ye opener) to steady your nerves or to get rid of a hangover?

(2) CRAFFT (use with adolescents)

C Have you ever ridden in a **C**ar with someone who is high on alcohol or other drugs?
R Do you drink or take drugs to **R**elax, feel better about yourself, or fit in?
A Do you ever drink or take drugs while you are **A**lone?
F Do you ever **F**orget things you did while using alcohol or drugs?
F Does a **F**amily member or **F**riend tell you to cut down on drinking or taking drugs?
T Have you ever gotten into **T**rouble from drinking or taking drugs?

d. Domestic violence

1) Cycle of abuse characterized by a pattern of control, coercion, and assaults that an adult or adolescent, most frequently male, uses to dominate or force compliance from a partner or spouse.

2) Violence against women: any act or crime that violates, humiliates, degrades or otherwise threatens or compromises the safety, health or wellness of women. It includes battering, rape, harassment, medical exploitation, and pornography.

3) Care consists of being able and willing to:

a) Ask the question in a sensitive manner

b) Respond in an empowering and respectful manner

c) Assess the level of danger in the situation

d) Provide accurate and forensically sound documentation

e) Provide safety planning
f) Offer information in a manner which may be acceptable to the survivor and empower her to make healthier choices for her life.

4) Dynamics and demographics of abuse
   a) 20-30% of all US women experience physical abuse from partners at some time
   b) 7-20% of pregnant women abused
   c) 1 in 3 women seeking ER care indicates history of partner violence
   d) Annually, 2000 women are murdered by a current or former partner
   e) Most likely time for the abuser to become homicidal is when woman leaves
   f) Occurs equally among all racial, ethnic, socio-economic, & sexual orientation groups. Occurs in absence of poverty, substance abuse, or other problems
5) **VIOLENCE AGAINST WOMEN IS THE NUMBER ONE PRIMARY HEALTH CARE PROBLEM FOR WOMEN IN THE U.S.**
6) Woman's unwillingness to leave is not a sign of acceptance
7) 25% of women seen in psychiatric ER have history of abuse
8) 25% of female suicide attempts have history of abuse
9) Abused women are constantly striving to stay alive—neither victims nor helpless
10) Substance abuse and battering are two different problems
11) 45-60% of children in households of female abuse are also abused
12) Using one's physical strength to control another is never acceptable behavior
13) No data to support that abusive women will repeat the relationship
14) The Cycle of Violence
    a) Tension building
    b) Battering
    c) Honeymoon
15) A more linear, progressively violent model also occurs
16) **Barriers to leaving are many including:**
    - Fear (leaving is the most deadly time)
    - Financial
    - Family
    - Failure
    - Faith
    - Father (fear of emotional damage to children without a father)
    - Face (culture says it's OK for men to abuse women)
    - Full (no room at a shelter)
    - Fantasy
    - Fix (she can fix it if she tries harder)
    - Familiarity (can't conceive of another way of living)
    - Fatigue (emotional exhaustion)

17) **Cultural barriers**

   a) Religion and culture

   b) Fear of deportation

   c) Power and control factors

18) **Everyone at risk;** age, drug abuse and unintended pregnancy may increase risk

   a) Ask the question: assessment screen

      - Always ask in complete privacy
      - Avoid "yes" or "no" questions
      - Avoid terms like "battered" or "abusive"
      - Lead in with statement that it's routine question due to widespread violence
      - Suggest as part of social history
      - Specific (e.g. "How do you and your partner resolve conflict?")

   b) Responding to the answer

      - Validate ("I believe...")
      - Empathize ("I'm sorry this happened. It's not your fault....")
      - Generalize ("Happens to many women and we often feel alone...")
      - Empower ("I can give you a number....I believe you know what is best....Whatever decision you make right now is right for you")

   c) Intervention

      - Danger assessment
      - Safety planning
      - Stage-based planning
      - Documentation

   d) Advocacy

      (1) Goal is to facilitate the process of personal empowerment, help women to set their own goals and make informed and safe personal decisions about their lives.

      (2) Self-care: Maintain safety and support, prevent burn-out

> ***"Violence in pregnancy affects more women than hypertension, gestational diabetes, or any other antepartum complication." (Boh, Parker 1993)***

e. Exercise/nutrition

1) Exercise

a) HP2K: Regular physical activity throughout life is important for maintaining a healthy body, enhancing psychological well-being, and preventing premature death.

b) Regular physical activity is associated with lower death rates for adults of any age; even when only moderate levels of physical activity are performed, decreasing risk of: death from heart disease, diabetes, and colon cancer. Helps prevent high blood pressure and reduce blood pressure in persons with elevated levels.

http://www.healthypeople.gov/Document/html/uih/uih_bw/uih_4.htm#physactiv

b) Recommendations

(1) To prevent chronic disease later in life: engage in at least 30 minutes of moderate-intensity physical activity, above usual activity on most days of the week.

- Most people have greater health benefits by engaging in physical activity of more vigorous intensity or longer duration.

(2) To help manage body weight and prevent gradual, unhealthy body weight gain in adulthood: Engage in approximately 60 minutes of moderate- to vigorous-intensity activity on most days of the week while not exceeding caloric intake requirements.

(3) To sustain weight loss in adulthood: Participate in at least 60 to 90 minutes of daily moderate-intensity physical activity while not exceeding caloric intake requirements.

(4) Achieve physical fitness by including cardiovascular conditioning, stretching exercises for flexibility, and resistance exercises or calisthenics for muscle strength and endurance.

http://www.health.gov/dietaryguidelines/dga2005/recommendations.htm

2) **Nutrition: USDA Dietary Guidelines for Americans 2005** www.MyPyramid.gov

➢ **Fats**

a) Keep total fat intake between 20 to 35 percent of calories, with most fats coming from sources of polyunsaturated and monounsaturated fatty acids, such as fish, nuts, and vegetable oils.

b) When selecting and preparing meat, poultry, dry beans, and milk or milk products, make choices that are lean, low-fat, or fat-free.

- **Carbohydrates**

a) Choose fiber-rich fruits, vegetables, and whole grains often.

b) Choose and prepare foods and beverages with little added sugars or caloric sweeteners.

c) Reduce the incidence of dental caries by practicing good oral hygiene and consuming sugar- and starch-containing foods and beverages less frequently.

- **Sodium and potassium**

a) Consume less than 2,300 mg (approximately 1 teaspoon of salt) of sodium per day.

- **Folic Acid: 0.4 mg/day. With history of previous child with neural tube defect, recommend 4 mg/day of folic acid.**

- **Food safety:** To avoid microbial food borne illness:

a) Clean hands, food contact surfaces, and fruits and vegetables. Meat and poultry should not be washed or rinsed.

b) Separate raw, cooked, and ready-to-eat foods while shopping, preparing, or storing foods.

c) Cook foods to a safe temperature to kill microorganisms.

d) Chill (refrigerate) perishable food promptly and defrost foods properly.

e) Avoid raw (unpasteurized) milk or any products made from unpasteurized milk, raw or partially cooked eggs or foods containing raw eggs, raw or undercooked meat and poultry, unpasteurized juices, and raw sprouts.

Calcium Intake varies by age:

Population Group	*Recommended Daily Intake*
Preteens and teens 9 to 18 years of age	1,300 mg
Adults 19 to 50 years	1,000 mg
Adults 51 and older	1,500 mg
Postmenopausal and on estrogen	1,000
Pregnant or Nursing Women	1200-1500

Note: The Dietary Guidelines for Americans 2005 contains additional recommendations for specific populations. The full document is available at www.healthierus.gov/dietaryguidelines, *http://osteoed.org/faq/prevention/calcium_intake.html*

f. **Injury Prevention**

1) Use smoke detectors in the home. Check batteries every month. Change batteries every year.

2) If there is a gun in the home, lock it and the ammunition up separately and keep them out of children's reach.

3) To help prevent falls:
   a) Make sure that hallways and stairwells are well lit.
   b) Remove or repair tripping hazards such as loose rugs, electrical cords, toys.
   c) Put handrails and traction strips on stairways and in bathtubs.
4) Away from home:
   a) Always wear seat belts while in the car.
   b) Never drive after drinking alcohol.
   c) Always wear a safety helmet while riding a motorcycle or bicycle.
   d) Be alert for hazards in the workplace and follow all safety rules.

g. **Depression:**

- The DSM IV criteria for major depression include 5 or more of the following symptoms, present for a 2 week period and representing a change from prior function. Either of the first 2 criteria must be present.
  - **Depressed mood nearly every day for most of the day either by self-report or observation**
  - **Diminished or absent pleasure in all or most activities, most of the day, most days.**
  - Significant weight loss or gain, or decreased appetite every day.
  - Insomnia or hypersomnia
  - Psychomotor agitation/retardation
  - Fatigue or loss of energy
  - Feelings of worthlessness, or inappropriate or excessive guilt, possibly delusional
  - Decreased ability to concentrate clearly, indecisiveness
  - Recurrent thoughts of death, suicidal ideation, suicidal plan or attempt

2. Laboratory tests and procedures

a. **Pap smears, STD testing**

Pap Smear:

- Yearly beginning 3 years after woman has sexual debut or at 21 years old
- ACOG says every 3 years after 3 normal annual Paps
- USPSTF recommends against routinely screening women older than age 65 for cervical cancer if they have had adequate recent screening with normal Pap smears and are not otherwise at high risk for cervical cancer

Chlamydia/Gonorrhea/AIDS/Syphilis

- Chlamydia through age 25

b. Mammogram

- Age >40, clinical breast exam q year
- Mammography q 1 year age ≥50

American Cancer Society:

- Age ≥40 need yearly mammogram
- Age 20-39, clinical breast exam q 3 years

1) For older women: American Geriatric Society (AGS) recommends annual mammograms age 65-75, and every 2-3 years for >75 with no risk factors.
2) Mammography is able to detect a mass up to 3 years before a mass is palpable. 5 to 10% of palpable breast lumps do not visualize on mammography. *95% of abnormal mammograms in women age 40-49 are false positives*
   a) Fewer false positives result in women with family histories
   b) Hispanic women have more false positives.
   c) Overall sensitivity of mammograms is 90-95% (i.e. 5-10% false negative rate)
   d) In premenopausal mammogram will miss 1/3 of the cancers.
   e) 25% invasive breast cancer is missed with mammogram in ages 40-49
   f) Hormone therapy may reduce the sensitivity of mammography screening

c. Bone density screening

Bone mineral density (BMD) ACOG advises BMD testing for the following:

- Postmenopausal women who have sustained a fracture
- Postmenopausal women under 65 years of age who have one or more risk factors, including personal history of fracture as an adult, Caucasian race, impaired eyesight despite adequate correction, and history of alcoholism
- Pre- or postmenopausal women with certain diseases or medical conditions associated with increased risk of osteoporosis: endometriosis, hemophilia, lymphoma/leukemia, eating and nutritional disorders, rheumatoid arthritis, multiple sclerosis. Use of certain drugs: e.g., **tobacco** in cigarettes, lithium, and heparin.
- In the absence of new risk factors, subsequent screening for osteoporosis should not be performed more frequently than every 2 years.
- The dual-energy X-ray absorptiometry (DEXA) is the "gold standard" for BMD testing, with advantages of high precision, minimal radiation exposure, and rapid scanning time.
- T-Score is the bone density compared to a healthy young adult
  - **Normal:** T-score above **–1**
  - **Osteopenia:** T-score between –1 and –2.5
  - **Osteoporosis:** T-score at or below –2.5

d. **Colon cancer screening**

1) **Fecal Occult Blood Test annually** >50 years old

2) **Sigmoidoscopy** every 5 years after age 50

e. **Lab tests, e.g., cholesterol, thyroid function**

1) Fasting lipid profile every 5 years beginning at age 20

USPSTF strongly recommends screening women ≥ 45 years for lipid disorders and treat abnormal lipids in persons who are at increased risk of coronary heart disease.

a) Total cholesterol and HDL can be non-fasting or fasting

b) Age to stop screening has not been established

http://www.guideline.gov/summary/summary.aspx?doc_id=5503&nbr=3746&string=cholesterol

ATP III Classification of LDL, Total, and HDL Cholesterol (mg/dL)

LDL Cholesterol – Primary Target of Therapy

<100	Optimal
100-129	Near Optimal/Above Optimal
130-159	Borderline High
160-189	High
≥190	Very High

HDL Cholesterol

<40	<40
≥60	≥60

Total Cholesterol

<200	Desirable
200-239	Borderline High
≥240	High

I. Primary Care (5%-10%)

LDL Cholesterol Goals and Cutpoints for Therapeutic Lifestyle Changes (TLC) and Drug Therapy in Different Risk Categories.

Risk Category	LDL Goal	LDL Level at Which to Initiate TLC	LDL Level at Which to Consider Drug Therapy
CHD or CHD Risk Equivalents (10-year risk >20%) *HIGH RISK*	<100 mg/dL	≥100 mg/dL	≥130 mg/dL (100-129 mg/dL: drug optional)
2+ Risk Factors (10-year risk ≤ 20%) *Moderate-moderately high risk*	<130 mg/dL	≥130 mg/dL	10-year risk 10-20%: ≥130 mg/dL 10-year risk <10%: ≥160 mg/dL
0-1 Risk Factor *Lower risk*	<160 mg/dL	≥160 mg/dL	≥190 mg/dL (160-189 mg/dL: LDL-lowering drug optional)

[1]Coronary heart disease (CHD) includes history of myocardial infarction, unstable angina, stable angina, coronary artery procedures (angioplasty or bypass surgery), or evidence of clinically significant myocardial ischemia.

[2]CHD risk equivalents include clinical manifestations of noncoronary forms of atherosclerotic disease (peripheral arterial disease, abdominal aortic aneurysm, and carotid artery disease [transient ischemic attacks or stroke of carotid origin or >50% obstruction of a carotid artery]), diabetes, and 2+ risk factors with 10-year risk for hard CHD >20%.

[3]Risk factors include cigarette smoking, hypertension (BP ≥140/90 mm Hg or on antihypertensive medication), low high-density lipoprotein (HDL) cholesterol (<40 mg/dL), family history of premature CHD (CHD in male first-degree relative <55 years of age; CHD in female first-degree relative <65 years of age), and age (men ≥45 years; women ≥55 years).

[4]Electronic 10-year risk calculators are available at www.nhlbi.nih.gov/guidelines/cholesterol.

[5]Almost all people with zero or 1 risk factor have a 10-year risk <10%, and 10-year risk assessment in people with zero or 1 risk factor is thus not necessary.

[6]Very high risk favors the optional LDL-C goal of <70 mg/dL, and in patients with high triglycerides, non-HDL-C <100 mg/dL.

[7]Optional LDL-C goal <100 mg/dL.

[8]Any person at high risk or moderately high risk who has lifestyle-related risk factors (e.g., obesity, physical inactivity, elevated triglyceride, low HDL-C, or metabolic syndrome) is a candidate for therapeutic lifestyle changes to modify these risk factors regardless of LDL-C level.

[9]When LDL-lowering drug therapy is employed, it is advised that intensity of therapy be sufficient to achieve at least a 30% to 40% reduction in LDL-C levels.

[10]If baseline LDL-C is <100 mg/dL, institution of an LDL-lowering drug is a therapeutic option on the basis of available clinical trial results. If a high-risk person has high triglycerides or low HDL-C, combining a fibrate or nicotinic acid with an LDL-lowering drug can be considered.

[11]For moderately high-risk persons, when LDL-C level is 100 to 129 mg/dL, at baseline or on lifestyle therapy, initiation of an LDL-lowering drug to achieve an LDL-C level <100 mg/dL is a therapeutic option on the basis of available clinical trial results.

2) **Plasma Glucose e**very 3 years after age 45 (according to the American Diabetic Association)

3) **Rubella serology or vaccination**
   - Must know history when of childbearing age

4) **Thyroid Stimulating Hormone (TSH)**
   - At age 45, then every 2 years until 60 and then yearly for the asymptomatic woman (conflicting recommendations)

http://www.ahrq.gov/clinic/uspstfix.htm

http://www.nhlbi.nih.gov/guidelines/cholesterol/atp_iii.htm

http://www.aafp.org/x7661.xml

3. Assessments indicated by status of woman

a. Ages 11-24: High risk groups

1) Hemoglobin
2) Bacteriuria testing
3) STD testing
4) HIV testing
5) Genetic counseling
6) TB skin test
7) Fasting glucose

b. Age 25-64: High risk groups

-Same as above and add the following:

1) Genetic testing/counseling
2) Thyroid-stimulating hormone
3) Colonoscopy
4) Osteoporosis $\geq$ age 60

c. Ages $\geq$65: High risk groups

1) Hemoglobin
2) Fasting glucose
3) STD testing
4) HIV testing
5) TB skin test
6) Thyroid stimulating hormone
7) Colonoscopy
8) Osteoporosis

d. Hormonal (endocrine)

1) Fasting plasma glucose every 3 years for women >45 (American Diabetes Association)
2) Some recommend thyroid screening at age 50, but USPSTF does not have a recommendation for screening with thyroid stimulating hormone (TSH) level
3) If no hormone replacement therapy (HRT), estrogen replacement therapy (ERT), or oral contraceptives (OC), ***follicle stimulating hormone (FSH) ≥ 40 mIU/mL is diagnostic of menopause***
    a) Progestin only therapy does not affect FSH levels
    b) By mid 50s assumption is made even if on hormonal therapy that menopause has occurred

4. Immunizations

CDC (2005 -- http://www.cdc.gov/omh/AMH/factsheets/immunization.htm) reports cultural and ethnic disparities in immunization rates, with older adults (>65) at risk for influenza and pneumonia related deaths. Older Hispanic and African-American adults are much less likely to be vaccinated against influenza and pneumococcal disease than their white counterparts. Poor children have lower immunization rates than those not living in poverty. Disparities in rates of immunization are of concern in large urban areas with underserved populations because of the potential for outbreaks of vaccine-preventable diseases. Healthcare providers can (and must) assist in getting children vaccinated by telling parents about the Vaccines for Children Program, which provides funding for all recommended vaccines for eligible children. Barriers to adult immunization include not knowing immunizations are needed, misconceptions about vaccines, *and lack of recommendations from health care providers*. Every opportunity should be taken to immunize adults during visits in offices, clinics or hospitals. Providers should address fears of adverse reactions to vaccines, provide information about the severity of influenza and pneumococcal disease, and inform women about other vaccine preventable diseases such as hepatitis B.

a. Adult immunization (http://www.cdc.gov/mmwr/preview/mmwrhtml/mm5440-Immunizationa1.htm

I. Primary Care (5%-10%)

FIGURE 1. Recommended adult immunization schedule, by vaccine and age group — United States, October 2005–September 2006

	Age group (yrs)		
Vaccine	**19–49**	**50–64**	**≥65**
Tetanus, diphtheria (Td)[1]*	1-dose booster every 10 yrs		
Measles, mumps, rubella (MMR)[2]*	1 or 2 doses	1 dose	
Varicella[3]*	2 doses (0, 4–8 wks)	2 doses (0, 4–8 wks)	
- - - Vaccines below broken line are for selected populations - - -			
Influenza[4]*	1 dose annually	1 dose annually	
Pneumococcal (polysaccharide)[5,6]	1–2 doses		1 dose
Hepatitis A[7]*	2 doses (0, 6–12 mos, or 0, 6–18 mos)		
Hepatitis B[8]*	3 doses (0, 1–2, 4–6 mos)		
Meningococcal[9]	1 or more doses		

For all persons in this category who meet the age requirements and who lack evidence of immunity (e.g., lack documentation of vaccination or have no evidence of prior infection)

Recommended if some other risk factor is present (e.g., on the basis of medical, occupational, lifestyle, or other indications)

* Covered by the Vaccine Injury Compensation Program.

FIGURE 2. Recommended adult immunization schedule, by vaccine and medical and other indications — United States, October 2005–September 2006

	Indication						
Vaccine	**Pregnancy**	**Congenital immunodeficiency, leukemia,[10] lymphoma, generalized malignancy, therapy with alkylating agents, antimetabolites, cerebrospinal fluid leaks, radiation, or large amounts of corticosteroids**	**Diabetes, heart disease, chronic pulmonary disease, or chronic liver disease, including chronic alcoholism**	**Asplenia[10] (including elective splenectomy and terminal complement component deficiencies)**	**Kidney failure, end-stage renal disease, or recipients of hemodialysis or clotting factor concentrates**	**Human immunodeficiency virus (HIV) infection 2,10**	**Health-care workers**
Tetanus, diphtheria (Td)[1]*	1-dose booster every 10 yrs						
Measles, mumps, rubella (MMR)[2]*	Contraindicated		1 or 2 doses				
Varicella[3]*	Contraindicated		2 doses (0, 4–8 wks)			Contraindicated	2 doses
Influenza[4]*	1 dose annually			1 dose annually	1 dose annually		
Pneumococcal (polysaccharide)[5,6]	1–2 doses	1–2 doses					1–2 doses
Hepatitis A[7]*	2 doses (0, 6–12 mos, or 0, 6–18 mos)						
Hepatitis B[8]*	3 doses (0, 1–2, 4–6 mos)				3 doses (0, 1–2, 4–6 mos)		
Meningococcal[9]	1 dose			1 dose	1 dose		

For all persons in this category who meet the age requirements and who lack evidence of immunity (e.g., lack documentation of vaccination or have no evidence of prior infection)

Recommended if some other risk factor is present (e.g., on the basis of medical, occupational, lifestyle, or other indications)

Contraindicated

* Covered by the Vaccine Injury Compensation Program.

1) **Influenza vaccine**

Adult immunizations have been noted as being a major public health problem. Could be good area for primary care questions.

a) *Medical indications*: chronic cardiovascular or pulmonary disorders, including asthma; chronic metabolic diseases, including diabetes mellitus, renal dysfunction, hemoglobinopathies, or immunosuppression; any condition (e.g., cognitive dysfunction, spinal cord injury, seizure disorder, or other neuromuscular disorder) that compromises respiratory function or that can increase the risk for aspiration; and *pregnancy during the influenza season.*

b) *Occupational indications*: health-care workers and employees of long-term--care and assisted living facilities.

c) *Other indications*: residents of long-term care facilities; persons likely to transmit influenza to persons at high risk (i.e., household contacts and caregivers of children aged 0--23 months, or persons of all ages with high-risk conditions), and anyone who wishes to be vaccinated.

d) For healthy, *nonpregnant* persons aged 5--49 years without high-risk conditions who are not contacts of severely immunocompromised persons in special care units, intranasally administered influenza vaccine (FluMist®) may be given instead of inactivated vaccine.

3) **Pneumococcal vaccine**

a) *Medical indications*: chronic disorders of the pulmonary system (excluding asthma); cardiovascular diseases; diabetes mellitus; chronic liver diseases, including liver disease as a result of alcohol abuse (e.g., cirrhosis); chronic renal failure or nephrotic syndrome; asplenia (e.g., sickle cell disease or splenectomy); immunosuppressive conditions; chemotherapy with alkylating agents, antimetabolites, or long-term systemic corticosteroids; and cochlear implants.

b) *Other indications*: Alaska Natives and certain American Indian populations; residents of nursing homes and other long-term--care facilities.

c) One-time revaccination is recommended after 5 years for certain high risk persons and those aged ≥65 years if they were vaccinated ≥5 years previously and were aged <65 years at the time of primary vaccination.

4) **Hepatitis B vaccine**

a) *Medical indications*: hemodialysis or clotting factor disorders.

b) *Occupational indications*: health-care workers and public-safety workers who have exposure to blood in the workplace and students of medicine, dentistry, nursing, laboratory technology, and other allied health professions.

c) *Behavioral indications*: injection-drug users; persons with more than one sex partner during the previous 6 months; persons with a recently acquired sexually transmitted disease (STD); men who have sex with men.

d) *Other indications*: household contacts and sex partners of persons with chronic hepatitis B virus (HBV) infection; clients and staff members of institutions for developmentally disabled persons; all clients of STD clinics; inmates of correctional facilities; and international travelers who will be in countries with high or intermediate prevalence of chronic HBV infection for more than 6 months.

5) **Measles, mumps, rubella (MMR) vaccination.**

a) *Measles component*: adults born before 1957 can be considered immune to measles. Adults born during or after 1957 should receive ≥1 dose of MMR unless they have a medical contraindication, documentation of ≥1 dose, history of measles based on health-care provider diagnosis, or laboratory evidence of immunity. A second dose of MMR is recommended for adults who 1) were recently exposed to measles or in an outbreak setting; 2) were previously vaccinated with killed measles vaccine; 3) were vaccinated with an unknown type of measles vaccine during 1963--1967; 4) are students in postsecondary educational institutions; 5) work in a health-care facility; or 6) plan to travel internationally. Withhold MMR from HIV-infected persons with severe immunosuppression.

b) *Mumps component*: 1 dose of MMR vaccine should be adequate for protection for those born during or after 1957 who lack a history of mumps based on health-care provider diagnosis or who lack laboratory evidence of immunity.

c) *Rubella component*: 1 dose of MMR vaccine to women whose rubella vaccination history is unreliable or who lack laboratory evidence of immunity. For women of childbearing age, regardless of birth year, routinely determine rubella immunity and counsel women regarding congenital rubella syndrome. Do not vaccinate women who are pregnant or who might become pregnant within 4 weeks of receiving vaccine. Women who do not have evidence of immunity should receive MMR vaccine upon completion or termination of pregnancy and before discharge from the health-care facility.

d) Persons allergic to eggs or neomycin should not receive MMR vaccination.

8) **Tetanus diphtheria (Td) vaccine**

a) Recommended for adults with uncertain histories of a complete primary vaccination series.

b) A primary series for adults is 3 doses; the first 2 doses at least 4 weeks apart and the third dose 6--12 months after the second. Administer 1 dose if the person received the primary series and if the last vaccination was received ≥10 years previously.

c) Second option for adults: a single Td booster at age 50 years for persons who have completed the full pediatric series, including the teenage/young adult booster.

d) A newly licensed tetanus-diphtheria-acellular--pertussis vaccine is available for adults.

9) Hepatitis A vaccine

a) *Medical indications*: clotting-factor disorders or chronic liver disease.

b) *Behavioral indications*: men who have sex with men or users of illegal drugs.

c) *Occupational indications*: Persons working with hepatitis A virus (HAV)--infected primates or with HAV in a research laboratory setting.

d) *Other indications*: persons traveling to or working in countries that have high or intermediate endemicity of hepatitis A or any person wishing to obtain immunity.

e) Administer a 2-dose series at either 0 and 6--12 months, or 0 and 6--18 months. If the combined hepatitis A and hepatitis B vaccine is used, administer 3 doses at 0, 1, and 6 months.

10) Varicella vaccine

a) Recommended for all adults without evidence of immunity to varicella, especially those who 1) have close contact with persons at high risk for severe disease (health-care workers and family contacts of immunocompromised persons) or 2) are at high risk for exposure or transmission (e.g., teachers of young children; child care employees; residents and staff members of institutional settings, including correctional institutions; college students; military personnel; adolescents and adults living in households with children; *nonpregnant women of childbearing age*; and international travelers). Evidence of immunity includes: 1) documented varicella vaccination; 2) U.S.-born before 1966 or history of varicella disease before 1966 for non-U.S.--born persons; 3) history of varicella; 4) history of herpes zoster; or 5) laboratory evidence of immunity.

b) *Do not vaccinate women who are pregnant or who might become pregnant within 4 weeks of receiving the vaccine.* Assess pregnant women for evidence of varicella immunity. Women who do not have evidence of immunity should receive dose 1 of varicella vaccine upon completion or termination of pregnancy and before discharge from the health-care facility. Dose 2 should be administered 4--8 weeks after dose 1.

11) **Meningococcal vaccine**

a) *Medical indications*: adults with asplenia or terminal complement component deficiencies.

b) *Other indications*: first-year college students living in dormitories; military recruits; and persons who travel to or reside in countries in which meningococcal disease is epidemic (e.g., sub-Saharan Africa during the dry season [December--June]), particularly if contact with local populations will be prolonged. Revaccination after 5 years might be indicated for adults previously vaccinated who remain at high risk for infection.

b. Travel recommendations

1) Individuals who travel to developing world should be immune to:
   - Measles, mumps, rubella, tetanus, diphtheria, pertussis, varicella
   - Travelers to Asia or Africa should also be immune to poliovirus
   - Influenza and pneumococcal vaccines should be administered
2) Additional immunizations are based on the diseases endemic to the area
   - Yellow fever, hepatitis A & B, typhoid, cholera, rabies, meningococcal disease, tuberculosis, tick-borne encephalitis
3) CDC updates weekly information regarding disease epidemics and immunization recommendations

c. Immunization in pregnancy

1) Ideally, women should be vaccinated prior to becoming pregnant
2) Indications for immunization during pregnancy
   a) Risk for exposure is high
   b) Infection poses a special risk to mother or fetus
   c) Vaccine not likely to cause harm
3) Live viral or bacterial vaccines should not be given during pregnancy unless exposure risk is high and disease poses a greater threat (e.g., MMR, varicella)
4) Only tetanus and diphtheria toxoids recommended for routine administration (especially important in situations where hygienic conditions during delivery cannot be maintained)

5) Hepatitis B vaccine series can be given to women who are at high risk and who test negative for Hepatitis B (HBV) infection
   a) Percutaneous use of drugs
   b) Acute episode of STD
   c) Multiple sex partners
   d) Health care workers
   e) Household contact with HBV carrier
   f) Receipt of clotting factors for bleeding disorders
6) MMR should be given at least 1 month prior to pregnancy or in immediate postpartum period
7) Yellow fever and polio vaccines should be given when traveling to areas where risk for exposure is high
8) Varicella-zoster immune globulin (VZIG) should be given to newborn if mother developed varicella within five days prior or 2 days after delivery
9) CDC recommends influenza vaccine be routinely offered to all pregnant women after lst trimester

d. Breastfeeding and immunization
   1) Not a contraindication for maternal immunization
   2) Not a substitute for pediatric immunization

e. Community health
   1) Public opinion can significantly affect vaccine uptake and consequently disease prevention.
   2) In developed countries, individual rights are highly valued.
   3) Reports of an association between vaccines and adverse effects get public attention. Example of consequences:
      - Early 1970's DPT uptake in U.K. was 81% and incidence of pertussis low. In 1974 a report ascribed neurological reactions to pertussis vaccine – the public lost confidence and uptake dropped to 31%; epidemic followed.

F. Deviations from normal: : Assessment, management and indications for consultation, co-management or referral

1. Cardiovascular/anemia

a. Hypertension: "Take home": <u>Hypertension</u> is still defined as BP $\geq$140/90!

Blood Pressure Classification in Adults (JNC 7)

BP Classification	SBP (mm Hg)	DBP (mm Hg)
Normal	< 120	and < 80
Prehypertension	120 – 139	or 80 – 89
Stage 1 Hypertension	140 – 159	or 90 – 99
Stage 2 Hypertension	≥ 160	or ≥ 100

1) Thiazide-type diuretics should be used in drug treatment for most patients with uncomplicated hypertension, either alone or combined with drugs from other classes.
2) Certain high-risk conditions are compelling indications for the initial use of other antihypertensive drug classes (angiotensin converting enzyme inhibitors [ACEIs], angiotensin receptor blockers [ARBs], beta-blockers, calcium channel blockers [CCBs]).
3) Most people with hypertension will require two or more antihypertensive medications to achieve goal blood pressure (less than 140/90 mm Hg, or less than 130/80 mm Hg for patients with diabetes or chronic kidney disease).
4) If blood pressure is greater than 20/10 mm Hg above goal blood pressure, therapy with two agents, one of which usually should be a thiazide-type diuretic, should be considered.
5) Compliance with therapy improves when patients trust and have positive experiences with their clinician. Empathy builds trust and is a potent motivator.

Compelling Indications for Individual Drug Classes

Compelling Indications	Recommended Drugs
Heart Failure	Diuretic, β-blocker, ACEI, ARB, aldosterone antagonist
Post-MI	β-blocker, ACEI, aldosterone antagonist
High coronary disease risk	Diuretic, β-blocker, ACEI, CCB
Diabetes	Diuretic, β-blocker, ACEI, ARB, CCB
Chronic kidney disease	ACEI, ARB
Recurrent stroke prevention	Diuretic, ACEI

6) **General cardiac symptoms**
    a) Angina is usually experienced by women before a myocardial infarction but it may be atypical (e.g upper abdominal pain, dyspnea, nausea and fatigue).

b) Chest pain is the most frequent presenting sign & symptom but its prognostic value is limited. Chest pain may be in one or both arms, in the neck or jaw or in the back and shoulders, pelvis or just vague discomfort. The classic picture of cardiovascular disease has not been identified in women.

c) Unrecognized or silent myocardial infarctions (MI) are more frequent in women; two-thirds of cardiac deaths in women are asymptomatic.

(1) Even though the incidence of MI is lower in women, the post-MI morbidity is higher (older, more CV risk factors).

b. Mitral valve prolapse

1) Incidence as high as 6% in women
2) Associated with autosomal dominant inheritance, Marfan's Syndrome, other connective tissue diseases
3) Symptomatology includes palpitations, dizziness, or chest pain
4) Physical Assessment: heard best at aortic area; late systolic apical murmur with a midsystolic click; widely spaced physiologic S_2
5) Differential diagnosis: thyrotoxicosis, MI, gastritis, esophageal reflux, pericarditis, angina
6) Diagnosis: Echocardiography
7) Antibiotic prophylaxis for endocarditis is recommended only for patients with valvular regurgitation or thickened leaflets, and for certain surgical procedures.

c. Hyperlipidemia (dyslipidemia): elevated or abnormal levels of plasma lipids. It is a risk factor for coronary artery disease.

Total cholesterol >200 mg/dL
HDL <35 mg/dL
LDL >130 mg/dL
VLDL>50% of total cholesterol
Triglycerides >160 mg/dL

1) Usually asymptomatic.
2) Physical examination may reveal carotid bruit, corneal arcus, xanthoma, hypertension.
3) Differentials: familial hypercholesterolemia, obstructive jaundice, biliary cirrhosis, hypothyroidism, von Gierke's disease, pregnancy, diabetes mellitus or other pancreatic disease, renal diseases, obesity, stress, high carbohydrate or high fat diet, inactivity, thiazide diuretic use or beta blocker use. \
4) Management is to reduce LDL and total cholesterol levels with lifestyle modifications for 3 to 6 months or drugs if necessary.

5) Pharmacologic therapy
   - Folic acid and pyridoxine (vitamin B6) reduce homocysteine levels
   - "Statins": 3-hydroxy-3-methylglutaryl coenzyme A (HMG-CoA) reductase inhibitors include fluvastatin (Lescol), lovastatin (Mevacor), pravastatin (Pravachol), simvastatin (Zocor), atorvastatin (Lipitor) reduce LDL levels without affecting homocysteine levels. Averse effects include liver damage and muscle weakness, and gastrointestinal distress.
   - Niacin and bile acid sequestrants may be added to statins to lower the LDL even more
   - Fibric acid derivatives – gemfibrozil (Lopid)
6) Educate the woman about diet and exercise, medication regimen and side effects. Followup includes ongoing support and reinforcement and monitoring liver function if on statins.

d. Anemias

Normal Hematocrit (hct): 36%-48%

Normal Hemoglobin (hgb): 12-16 g/dL

Anemia is defined as low hct & hgb

1) Symptoms: Dyspnea on exertion, palpitations, angina pectoris, light headedness, syncope, anorexia, tinnitus
2) Signs: pallor of mucous membranes and skin, mild tachycardia, peripheral edema, systolic ejection murmurs from increased flow
3) History: blood loss, alcohol abuse, diarrhea, jaundice, gallstones, chronic disease, drugs, familial causes (e.g., sickle cell, thalassemia)
4) **Laboratory evaluation**
   a) Complete blood count (CBC) contains red blood cell (RBC) indices
   b) Mean corpuscular volume (MCV): size
      (1) Microcytic: small: iron deficiency anemia and thalassemias
      (2) Macrocytic: Large: Megaloblastic Anemias
   c) Mean corpuscular hemoglobin concentration (MCHC): color
   d) Red cell distribution width (RDW): size variation
   e) Serum ferritin: reflects iron stores
   f) Reticulocyte count: immature non-nucleated red cell (RBC) containing reticular material (from dissolving nucleus); good way to monitor RBC production

(1) Reference range 0.5% - 1.5%

(2) Increased reticulocyte count indicates RBC production (erythropoiesis) has been accelerated

- Hemolytic anemias
- Sickle cell anemia
- 3-4 days after hemorrhage
- Cancer
- Post splenectomy
- Slight increase in pregnancy (due to increase in RBCs) and infants

(3) Decreased reticulocyte count indicates reduced RBC production by the bone marrow

- Iron deficiency anemia
- Pernicious anemia
- Aplastic anemia
- Chronic infection
- Radiation therapy

(4) Differentiate anemias due to bone marrow failure vs anemias resulting from hemorrhage or hemolysis

(5) Check effectiveness of treatment and recovery of bone marrow function

5) Iron deficiency anemia

a) Labs

(1) RBC indices change when hgb falls below 8-9g/dL

(2) Hypochromia (low MCHC) and microcytosis (low MCV) may appear.

(3) Total iron binding capacity (TIBC) increases and serum iron is decreased.

(4) ***Iron stores can be determined by serum ferritin levels*** (10-200 µg/ml)

1 mg ferritin = 8-10 mg stored Fe

b) Causes

(1) Blood loss

(2) Dietary deficiency

(3) Increased iron demand (pregnancy, lactation, adolescence)

c) Subjective data: blood loss or hemolysis, recent surgeries, rectal bleeding, medications, diet, smoking, alcohol use, previous anemia, splenectomy, family history of colon cancer

d) Objective data-physical examination

- Often no abnormalities
- Fatigue, tachypnea
- Vitals-Increased pulse and respirations, decreased BP on standing
- Skin-Pallor
- Mouth-Angular stomatitis, glossitis
- Cardiac-flow murmurs, tachycardia
- Abdomen-Splenomegaly, hepatomegaly, abdominal mass
- Pelvic exam-rule out masses
- Rectal exam-rule out masses, bleeding
- CNS-Altered mental state

e) Laboratory tests

(1) CBC with indices

(2) Confirm diagnosis with serum iron, TIBC, saturation, serum ferritin

(3) Follow up tests after treatment with iron supplements, iron rich foods

f) Treatment

(1) Ferrous sulfate 325mg po BID to TID. Better absorbed if taken between meals but better tolerated if taken with meals.

(2) Iron-rich diet

g) *If marrow does not respond to iron therapy, consider another cause of anemia such as inflammation, vitamin B_{12} or folate deficiency, continued bleeding

6) Megaloblastic anemia

a) Usually caused by folic acid deficiency or lack of vitamin B_{12} in diet

b) Labs: CBC with RBC indices

(1) Macrocytic: elevated MCV

(2) May be hypochromic (low MCH and MCHC) or normochromic (normal MCH and MCHC)

c) Pernicious anemia is lack of intrinsic factor that insures absorption of vitamin B_{12}. B_{12} must be given parenterally because it will not be absorbed from the GI tract.

7) Sickle cell anemia

a) Oxygen reduction triggers sickling

b) Incidence is 1/625 African American

c) Homozygous expression of S hemoglobin - SS (normal hemoglobin AA)

d) Most common clinical manifestation is vaso-occulsive crisis -probable result of impairment of blood flow from the irreversibly sickled cells.

e) Sickle cell trait AS - usually no clinical manifestations

f) *Diagnosis by hemoglobin electrophoresis*

8) Thalassemias: inherited disorder of hemoglobin synthesis; characterized by absent or diminished production of hemoglobin chains, alpha chains in alpha thalassemia and beta chains in beta thalassemia.

a) *Alpha thalassemia trait* may have mild microcytic, hypochromic anemia without clinical disease. Homozygous alpha thalassemia (alpha thalassemia major) is usually not compatible with life.

(1) Populations with high risk of alpha thalassemia are China, Philippines, Southeast Asia, India, Sri Lanka and Indonesia. Africans and African-Americans, Middle Easterners, and Native Americans may also have alpha thalassemia.

(2) Alpha thalassemia trait may be associated with beta chain hemoglobinopathies: sickle cell/alpha thalassemia trait, beta thalassemia, Hb C, Hb E, etc.

b) *Beta thalassemia minor* (trait) produces decreased beta globin chains, resulting in (usually mild) microcytic, hypochromic anemia. In pregnancy, the anemia may be severe because of hemodilution. In beta thalassemia major (Cooley's anemia), the person is homozygous, so production of both beta chains is abnormal; life expectancy is reduced. Pregnancy is unlikely and extremely dangerous for the mother and fetus. However, there are variations in severity of homozygous beta thalassemia.

(1) Populations at greatest risk are of Mediterranean descent (Greek and Italian), Southeast Asians, Pakistani and Indians, and North Africans; also to a lesser extent African, Caribbean, and Central Americans.

c) Diagnosis

Alpha thalassemia trait

- Hb normal or low
- RBC count normal or increased
- MCV 70-75 fL
- MCH <36 pg
- MCHC ~ 31 gm/dL
- Hemoglobin electrophoresis: Hb A,Hb A_2, Hb F normal (unless there is another hemoglobinopathy); Hb Constant Spring may be seen
- Blood smear shows microcytosis, hypochromia, anisocytosis, poikilocytosis
- Iron studies are normal unless there is also iron deficiency

Beta thalassemia trait

- Mild anemia (10-11 gm/dL in nonpregnant women)
- RBC count increased
- MCV 55-75 fL
- MCH < 26 pg
- Blood smear shows microcytosis, hypochromia, anisocytosis, poikilocytosis, targeting and basophilic stippling of RBCs
- Hemoglobin electrophoresis: Hb A_2 increased (3.5-7%), possibly elevated Hb F (2-5%), bone marrow has mild erythroid hyperplasia
- Iron studies normal unless there is also iron deficiency

d) Iron deficiency, if demonstrated, is treated as usual. Iron should not be given unless deficiency is demonstrated because of the risk of iron overload. Folic acid should be supplemented in pregnancy.

9) **Glucose-6-dehydrogenase (G6PD) deficiency**: X linked hereditary red blood cell enzyme deficiency. Usually found in blacks, Greeks, Sardinians, Sephardic Jews. Female carriers are usually asymptomatic, but ingestion of oxidant drugs (e.g., *sulfonamides, nitrofurantoin*, primaquine) or some foods (e.g., fava beans), or *exposure to viral or bacterial infections* can cause a mild hemolytic anemia.

a) There may be an increased incidence of urinary tract infections.

b) Fetal exposure (or through breast milk) to maternal ingestion of the oxidant drugs may cause fetal hemolysis, fetal hydrops, and fetal death.

c) Laboratory tests

- Decreased erythrocytes, hematocrit, hemoglobin with normal MCV unless there is also iron deficiency or hemoglobinopathy
- Iron studies normal (unless coexisting condition)
- G6PD levels decreased
- Hemoglobin electrophoresis: normal unless coexistent hemoglobinopathy
- Total bilirubin elevated during hemolysis
- Erlich stain shows $\geq$5 Heinz bodies in 40% of RBCs

Hemoglobin Electrophoresis*				
	Hb A	**Hb A_2**	**Hb F**	**Other**
Normal adult	>95%	1.5-3%	<2%	None
Sickle Cell Trait (HbAS)	60-70%			30-40% Hb S; If S is reduced, may have α thal trait
Sickle Cell Anemia (Hb SS)	Absent	Normal	0-20%	80-90% Hb S
Beta Thalassemia Trait	Normal	>3.5%	Elevated	
Alpha Thalassemia Trait	Normal	Normal	Normal	5-30% Hb H; Hb Bart's; any beta chain abnormality (β thal, Hb C, Hb E, Hb J Bangkok, Hb S); Hb Constant spring
G6PD deficiency	Normal	Normal	Normal	None

*There are other hemoglobinopathies, e.g., Hb C, Hb D, Hb E, Hb H, Hb SC

2. Dermatologic conditions

a. Carcinomas

1) Basal Cell Carcinoma

a) Most common type of skin cancer; 1 in 7 Americans

b) Risk factors

*Fair skin that burns easily

*Large amount of sun exposure

c) Markedly increases after age 40

d) Metastasis is uncommon (*invasion still occurs*); unpredictable course

e) Usually begins as small, shiny papule that enlarges over months and develops telangiectasias and a pearly border. After time, it develops a central ulcer that recurrently crusts and bleeds

f) Less common form appears as flat plaques

g) Use magnifying glass and good lighting to observe suspicious lesions.

h) Refer woman with suspicious lesions to dermatologist for skin biopsy

2) Squamous Cell Carcinoma

a) Second most common skin cancer. Most common skin cancer in African-Americans. Common in the oral cavity of women who smoke and drink, often on the posterior lateral borders of the tongue. Also arises in epithelium, usually in areas exposed to the sun: scalp, back of hand, and ear.

b) Precursor lesion is actinic keratosis (flat tan or brown spots with adherent scales and surrounding erythema) or leukoplakia, a white opaque patch found on the lips, oral mucosa, and vulva

c) Variable appearance, but usually begins as a reddish papule or plaque with a scaly or crusted surface. May mimic dermatitis. Later, may appear nodular or warty. Eventually, it ulcerates and invades underlying tissues

d) May be asymptomatic or have itching, irritation, bleeding, or change in skin

e) More likely to metastasize than basal cell carcinoma

f) Refer woman with suspicious lesion to dermatologist for diagnosis and management

3) Malignant melanoma

a) 2/3 of deaths from skin cancer due to melanoma; 1 in 90 will develop; leading cause of cancer death in women < 35 years

b) Risk factors:

- History of 6 or > sunburns
- Excessive sun exposure in first decade of life
- Indoor occupation with intermittent, intense sun exposure
- Large congenital hairy nevus
- Family history
- Immune dysfunction

c) Arises from melanocytes; 40-50% arise from pigmented moles

d) Lesion may be anywhere on the body

e) Early identification and prompt surgical excision offer only chance for cure.

f) Symptoms: change in skin lesion or nevus

- Enlargement
- Color change
- Pain (or itch)
- Bleeding

g) ABCDs on physical exam:

- Asymmetry
- Border: irregular, notched, or scalloped
- Color: haphazard shades of brown, red, blue, gray
- Diameter: >6mm (tip of pencil eraser)
- Surface or sensation: surface distortion may be subtle or obvious; sensation refers to itch, burn, or pain

h) Refer any suspicious lesion immediately to dermatologist

DIFFERENTIAL DIAGNOSIS OF SKIN CANCER	
Benign lesions:	Nevi, seborrheic keratosis, cysts, tags, dermatofibromas, keloids
Dermatoses:	Seborrhea, eczema, psoriasis, HPV, fungi
Pre-malignant:	Actinic keratosis, leukoplakia, dysplastic nevus syndrome
Skin cancers:	Basal cell, squamous cell (Bowen's, Paget's), Malignant melanoma, Mycosis fungoides (rare T-cell lymphoma that originates in skin)
Cutaneous metastasis:	3-5% of those with metastatic disease develop secondary skin cancer

b. Acne vulgaris

1) Sebaceous glands are stimulated by androgen; plugging of the follicle by sebum occurs. Bacteria, primarily *Propionibacterium acnes*, break down the sebum, disrupting follicle wall, and leading to inflammation.

2) Begins in adolescence and usually resolves by 20s (but may persist to 40s)

3) Severe cystic acne is more common in males.

4) Diagnosis is clinical, based on appearance and history. Inflammatory, open and closed comedones, papules and pustular nodules, cysts with scarring. Lesions occur on face, neck, upper back chest and shoulders.

5) Be aware of psychosocial implications – may lead to depression and social isolation.

6) Treatment aim is to prevent scarring.

- Avoid astringents
- For comedones: over the counter topical preparations with salicylic acid, resorcinol, and/or sulfur, benzoyl peroxide, alpha-hydroxyl acids may help. Topical tretinoin (Retin A) unplugs comedones and prevents new ones.
- Topical antibiotics, e.g., Clindamycin or erythromycin may be used in combination with tretinoin.
- If papules and pustules predominate, oral antibiotics are given, e.g., erythromycin, tetracycline, minocycline.
- If no response to above treatments, isotretinoin (Accutane) may be considered. Side effects may be serious and *it is teratogenic*. It is given only if there is a negative pregnancy test, started with menses, and 2 forms of contraception are advised.
- If oral contraceptives are prescribed, use a low androgen formulation (e.g., Ortho Tri-Cyclen)

7) No evidence that dietary restrictions, vigorous scrubbing or tanning are therapeutic. Pimples should not be squeezed. Use oil free makeup.

8) Refer severe or cystic acne to a dermatologist.

c. Rosacea

1) Chronic skin condition of middle age (30-50 years), more common in women. Four stages are (1) prerosacea, with transient flushing and erythema of face and neck; (2) vascular rosacea with persistent erythema and telangiectasia; (3) inflammatory rosacea, with inflammatory papules and pustules; (4) glandular hyperplastic rosacea, (usually in men), with lymphedema and hypertrophy of connective tissue.

2) Diagnosis is clinical, based on history and presentation.

3) Treatment is topical metronidazole gel or cream, with oral antibiotics if severe.

4) Triggers are excessive cold, wind, heat, alcohol, spicy foods.

5) Refer to dermatologist if severe.

d. Dermatoses

1) Mycotic infections with tinea (versicolor, corporis and capitis [ringworm], unguium [nail], and pedis [athlete's foot]) and candida. Treated with antifungal agents.

2) Atopic dermatosis (eczema): chronic disease with itching. Scratching may be to the point of excoriation. Flares occur with stress and fatigue. Serum IgE levels may be elevated, and client may also have asthma and seasonal rhinitis.

a) Diagnosis: weepy, inflamed, lichenified skin. Eczema is on face, sides of neck, flexural aspects of knees, elbows, wrists. Nummular eczema is on backs of hands, fingers, extensor aspects of forearms and legs. Differentiate from contact dermatitis and psoriasis (silvery).

b) Treatment: Topical steroid cream or ointments; oral prednisone taper if severe. Antibiotics if secondary infection occurs. Systemic antihistamines (e.g., hydroxyzine) may help with pruritus.

3) Seborrheic dermatitis: localized form of atopic dermatoses, usually on scalp, eyebrows, and forehead. Also may appear in groin, axillae, presternal chest.
   a) Diagnosis: greasy yellow or gray scales over red skin patches.
   b) Shampoo frequently with selenium sulfide or pyrithione zinc (Head and Shoulders®), left on hair for 10 minutes.
4) Contact dermatitis (irritant and allergic): exposure to irritants such as soap, solvents, detergents. Contact allergens include poison ivy and oak, nickel, latex, hair dyes, topical medications, cosmetics and perfumes, adhesive tape.
   a) Diagnosis: weeping, encrusted vesicles and bullae; may have linear streaking pattern. Distribution is asymmetric, and pattern may be diagnostic.
   b) Treatment: Remove substance causing the reaction (may involve lifestyle change). Medications used may be topical applications of Burow's solution or 1:10 vinegar: water solution for weeping lesions; topical steroids or even parenteral steroids if acute and severe reaction. Oral antihistamines (e.g., hydroxyzine) for pruritus.
   c) Refer to dermatologist if not responsive to treatment within 1 week.

e. Skin infections
   1) Impetigo: caused by *Staphylococcus aureus* or group A beta hemolytic *Streptococcus*. Lesions are varied in shape and size, but have in common a honey-colored crust. Treatment is empiric with broad spectrum antibiotic, e.g., dicloxacillin, erythromycin, or ciprofloxacin (unless pregnant). Highly contagious.
   2) Folliculitis: Infection or inflammation of hair follicle caused by various agents, e.g., *Staphylococcus aureus*, *Pseudomonas aeruginosa* (contaminated hot tubs or pedicure spas), fungal dermatophytes, oils or sweat. Bacterial folliculitis is common in diabetics. Treatment is according to causative agent. Bacterial cultures or KOH prep may be needed.
   3) Furuncles (boils, abscesses), carbuncles (furuncles that enlarge and coalesce): infection of hair follicle; deeper and more extensive than folliculitis. Usually caused by *Staphylococcus aureus*. Immunocompromised persons and nose/throat staph carriers are at risk. Treatment is incision and drainage with culture and sensitivity of exudate. Antibiotics such as dicloxacillin, azithromycin are given. Warm soaks are applied. Advise loose clothing and natural fibers to allow perspiration evaporation.

4) Cellulitis: infection of skin and subcutaneous tissue, without purulence. Usually caused by *Staphylococcus* or *Streptococcus*. Culture may not be helpful. Treat as for impetigo, with warm soaks and elevation of affected extremity. Mark area and evaluate within 1-2 days. Consult and refer promptly if there is fever, chills, evidence of systemic illness or no response to treatment.

5) Viral skin infections include warts caused by human papillomavirus, Molluscum contagiosum, herpes zoster, and herpes simplex virus (HSV) types 1 and 2. HSV is discussed in the gynecology chapter.

f. Skin infestations occur with scabies and lice, and these conditions are discussed in the gynecology chapter.

g. Diseases with dermatologic manifestations include systemic lupus erythematosus, syphilis, viral infections, celiac disease, and many others.

3. Endocrine disorders

a. Obesity: rising rates

1) Body Mass Index (BMI): measures weight and height; Calculate weight in kilograms divided by the square of the height in meters, or, calculate weight (pounds) X 703 divided by [height (in.)^2]

> **Calculating BMI:**
> Take the weight in kilograms (1 kilogram = 2.2 pounds)
> Measure height in meters (1 inch = 2.5 centimeters)
> Divide weight by height squared Kg / (m)^2
> Example: 68 kg / (1.6 m)^2 = 26

2) Body circumferences: waist to hip ratios: Not to exceed waist greater than 35 inches in women and 40 inches in men

a) High ratios are related to increased risk for chronic diseases

3) Optimum weights increase with age

BMI 19-25 between ages 25 to 35

BMI 21-27 after age 35

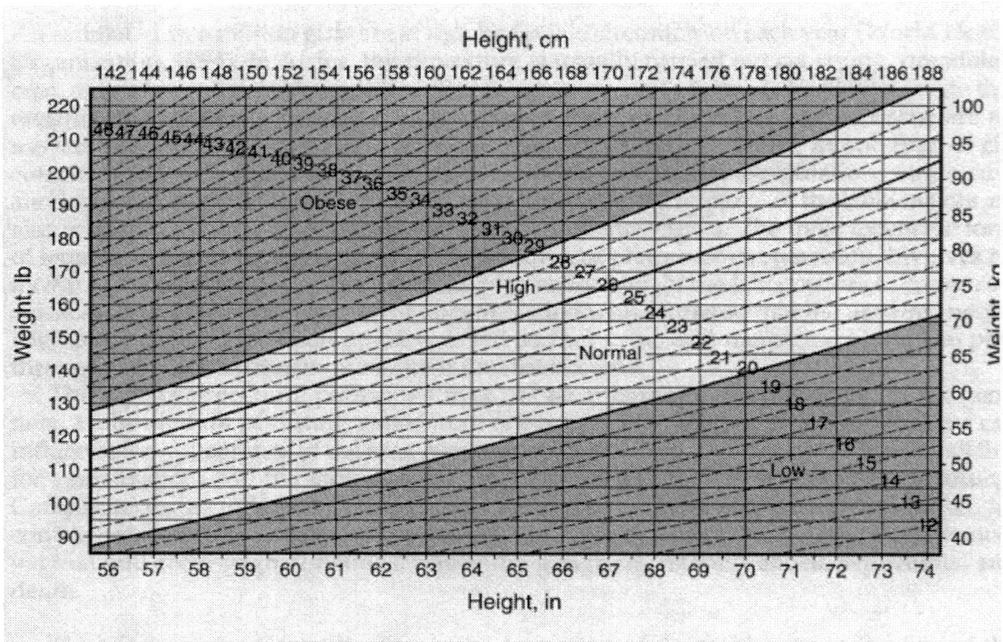

4) Incidence of chronic disease and relationship to BMI

   a) Type 2 Diabetes, hypertension, coronary heart disease and cholelithiasis, in both men and women are positively related to increasing BMI;

   b) Post-menopausal breast cancer, cancer of colon, kidney and endometrium, stroke, osteoarthritis and infertility are all positively correlated with increasing BMI

5) Weight guidelines

   a) Mortality clearly increases with BMI's greater than 25.

   b) BMI >25 but <30 is overweight.

   c) BMI > 30 is obese

   d) BMI >40 is extreme obesity (1995 Dietary Guidelines; American Institute of Nutrition (1993) and the WHO (1995)

6) Even within a weight and height classification, a gain of 11-22 lbs can result in an increased relative risk of 1.5 to 3 times for coronary heart disease, diabetes mellitus (DM) and hypertension.

b. Thyroid Disease

1) Screening (e.g., testing an asymptomatic person) is controversial

   a) TSH at age 45, then every 2 years until 60 and then yearly for the asymptomatic woman

2) ***Hypothyroidism: Thyroid hormone deficiency***

a) In the normal fetus the hypothalamic-pituitary-thyroid axis functions by the 11th week of gestation

b) Myxedema is severe hypothyroidism; characterized by edema of hand, face, feet and periorbital tissues. May lead to coma and death.

c) Women are ten times more likely than men to develop hypothyroidism

d) Linked to age -- 1:150 over the age of 20; 1:50 over age of 60

e) 95% of the time cause is primary failure of the gland itself

- ***Increased TSH with decreased Free T4 in Primary Hypothyroidism***
- ***Decreased TSH and Free T4 in Secondary Hypothyroidism***

Clinical Manifestations of Hypothyroidism	History
Lethargy, malaise, easy fatigability Cold intolerance Weight gain Muscle cramps Slowed reflexes Arthralgia Cool, pale, tough, dry skin with dry brittle nails Hoarse, husky voice and slurred speech Puffy face, myxedema Bradycardia, cardiomyopathy, pericardial effusions, cardiac enlargement Menorrhagia, amenorrhea Anemia Cerebellar ataxia Goiter (diffuse or nodular) Depression, irritability, apathy Reduced concentration and memory Constipation Thin, falling-out hair, including lateral third of the eyebrow	Previous radioactive iodine treatment Thyroid surgery Previous thyroid disease Previous pituitary disease Diabetes mellitus Adrenal insufficiency Hypoparathyroidism

3) Chronic autoimmune thyroiditis: Hashimoto's disease

a) Goitrous form

(1) May also be silent thyroiditis

(2) May be postpartum thyroiditis

b) Atrophic form called atrophic thyroiditis

c) Both characterized by thyroid antibodies in serum and by varying degrees of thyroid dysfunction

d) Differentiated by presence or absence of goiter

e) Average age of onset is 30-50 years

f) Four times more likely among women than men

4) ***Hyperthyroidism: overactive thyroid with excessive secretion of thyroid hormones***
   a) Typically, woman in her mid 20s or 30s
   b) Greater level of free thyroid in serum
   c) Often associated with autoimmune disease
   d) Graves Disease usually presents with a goiter and/or exophthalmos
   e) Accounts for approximately 60 to 90% of all hyperthyroidism
   f) Results when the body's tissues are exposed to excessive levels of thyroid hormone
      - ***Increased T3 and T4 and Decreased TSH***
5) Thyrotoxicosis is a clinical syndrome resulting from exposure of the peripheral tissues to excessive amounts of free thyroid hormone

CLINICAL PICTURE—HYPERTHYROIDISM	
Cardiovascular	Resting tachycardia Widened pulse pressure Palpitations Third heart sound Dyspnea Atrial fibrillation Increase in cardiac output & contractility Decrease in systemic vascular resistance
Muscular skeletal	Fine tremor of hands Weight loss Muscle Weakness Sweating
Ophthalmic	Exophthalmos Staring Gaze Lid Lag Diplopia
CNS	Nervousness Anxiety Chronic fatigue Brisk reflexes
Reproductive	Oligomenorrhea Amenorrhea Increased risk of spontaneous abortion Libido is maintained
Gastrointestinal	Frequent bowel movements
Thyroid gland	Thyromegaly Auscultation of thyroid bruit
Skin	Warm Smooth Heat Intolerance

6) ***Thyroid storm is a relatively rare, but life-threatening exaggeration of the clinical picture of hyperthyroidism***
   a) Usually occurs when a woman with Graves disease has another major illness or stress
   b) Generally requires hospitalization and management by endocrinologist

c) Typical signs include extreme anxiety, fever, tachycardia, nausea, vomiting, abdominal pain, and cardiac failure

7) Thyroid nodules

a) Relatively common finding (Estimated in England at almost 1% of men and more than 5% of women)

b) Solitary nodules often do not change (although can, of course enlarge or even disappear)

c) If solitary nodule, rule out cancer

(1) Fine needle aspiration

False negative 5-10%

False positive is rare

- If nodule disappears after aspiration, even if fluid is inadequate for evaluation, no further follow-up is needed
- If it does not, treatment of choice may be expectant—or consider unilateral thyroid lobectomy
- Thyroxine (to suppress secretion of thyrotropin)

(2) Thyroid scan

20% of cold nodules are malignant
< 1% of hot nodules are malignant

d) Multinodular goiters

(1) Usually caused by iodine deficiency

(2) First need to rule out hypo or hyperthyroidism

(3) Treatment is the same as above

8) Thyroid Cancer

Type of Cancer	% of Thyroid Cancer	10 Year Survival (local)	10 Year Survival (distant metastases)
Papillary	60	90	40
Follicular	25	90	40
Medullary	<10		60-70
Anaplastic	<10		<5

Measurement (Diagnosis) of Thyroid Function

Serum TSH	• Single best test ("gold standard") to demonstrate hypothyroidism produced by thyroid gland failure
	• Most specific for hypothyroidism
	• First finding in hypothyroidism
		• Normal range 0.1-5.0 (some sources say 0.3 to 6 mU/ml)
		• Hyperthyroidism is usually <0.1
		• Hypothyroidism
		  ○ Subclinical 6-16
		  ○ Overt primary 20-200
		  ○ Secondary 0.1-5.0

Diagnosis	Thyroid Stimulating Hormone (TSH)	T_3 Resin Uptake	Total Thyroxine (Total T_4)	Free Thyroxine (Free T_4)
Euthyroid	Normal	normal	normal	normal
Hypothyroid	High or Low*	low	low	low
Hyperthyroid	High* or Low	high	high	high
Pregnant	Normal	low	high	normal

*Depending on the cause. If primary, i.e., thyroid gland problem, TSH is high in hypothyroidism and low in hyperthyroidism. If secondary (e.g., pituitary tumor that secretes TSH or pituitary failure), TSH may be high in hyperthyroidism and low in hypothyroidism. Remember feedback mechanism of pituitary and thyroid glands. A high TSH with a normal T_4 usually indicates compensatory hypothyroidism. This condition usually leads to overt hypothyroidism in a relatively short period of time.

9) Treatment of hypothyroidism
   a) Goal: restore euthyroid state by replacing thyroid hormones
   b) Drug of choice is levothyroxine sodium
10) Treatment of hyperthyroidism/thyrotoxicosis
   a) Goal: To restore the woman to euthyroid state
   b) There currently is no therapy to reverse the underlying autoimmune defect causing Grave's disease
   c) Antithyroid drugs curb the activity of excess T_3 and T_4; also called thioamides
      (1) Propylthiouracil (*PTU®, Propacil®, Propyl-thyracil®*), a beta-adrenergic antagonist
      (2) Methimazole (*MMI®, Tapazole®*);More potent than *PTU*
      - Better suited for women who want once daily treatment and do not have severe symptoms
   d) Follow-up
      (1) Medications for 1-2 years (recurrence rate of 50-80% if medication is stopped)
      (2) Evaluate every 3 months
      (3) Need to keep serum at upper end of normal, and TSH at the lower end
      (4) Remember the drugs do not interrupt the release of stored hormone so clinical improvement usually is delayed for 2-3 weeks
      (5) Euthyroid state is usually in 4-6 weeks
   e) Note: Surgical removal of thyroid is another option, or treatment with radioactive iodine
      (1) Radioactive iodine is effective and relatively inexpensive although it is fairly common that a young woman then becomes hypothyroid. If chosen, a woman should be counseled to wait 6 months before attempting pregnancy.

(2) Any radioactive iodine agent is contraindicated in pregnancy as it is a teratogen and easily crossed the placenta and can concentrate in the fetal thyroid.

c. **Diabetes mellitus** (DM): group of diseases characterized by hyperglycemia, which may result from deficient insulin secretion, insulin resistance, or both. Most common endocrine disorder. Complications are cardiovascular and peripheral vascular disease, immune pathology, renal disease and ophthalmologic disorders. Tight control of blood glucose levels (with HgA1c levels maintained below 7.2%) decreases associated morbidity and mortality.

1) Type 1 DM

a) Severe insulin deficiency due to pancreatic beta cell destruction, usually from an autoimmune process in genetically susceptible individuals.

b) Classic symptoms due to hyperglycemia are polydipsia, polyuria, polyphagia, anorexia, and weight loss. Other associated symptoms are nocturnal enuresis, blurred vision, weakness and fatigue, nausea and abdominal pain, paresthesia, and candidal vulvovaginitis.

c) Diagnosis

~Random plasma glucose $\geq$200 mg/dL,

OR

~Fasting plasma glucose $\geq$126 mg/dL,

OR

~Plasma glucose $\geq$200 two hours following a 75 gram oral glucose load

*Confirm by repeat testing on a different day unless there is unequivocal hyperglycemia with acute metabolic decompensation.

d) Treatment is life-long adherence to diet, exercise, insulin therapy, and blood glucose monitoring. The therapeutic team consisting of an endocrinologist, primary care provider, diabetes educator, dietitian, the diabetic person, and her family. Diabetes management is probably beyond the scope of most CNM/CMs.

e) Diabetic ketoacidosis (DKA) brought on by illness, stress, or lack of insulin is an acute emergency. Features of DKA are blood glucose >350, plasma ketones >5mmol/L, and plasma bicarbonate <9 mEq/L. Symptoms are anorexia, thirst, nausea, vomiting, abdominal cramping, and polyuria. Kussmaul respirations follow, along with signs of severe dehydration, oliguria and altered consciousness. If untreated, coma, vascular collapse and renal shutdown occur with blood glucose levels reaching as high as 800 mg/dL. Treatment is administration of insulin, hydration, and correction of acidosis and electrolyte imbalances. DKA is more likely to occur in Type 1 DM than in Type 2.

f) Insulin preparations are administered parenterally

> *Rapid acting*: Insulin lispro, insulin aspart, and regular insulin

> *Intermediate acting*: NPH, Lente

> *Long acting*: Ultra lente, insulin glargine

> *Mixtures*: NPH and regular, Lispro protamine and lispro, aspart protamine and aspart

2) **Type 2 DM** is actually a group of diseases characterized by sufficient insulin production with resistance to the action of insulin and inadequate compensatory insulin secretion. 90% DM is Type 2. Previously known as Adult-onset DM or non-insulin dependent DM.

a) Asymptomatic in early stages, so diagnosis is often delayed for years.

b) Risk factors are genetic predisposition, generalized obesity, and central obesity. Americans of African, Hispanic, Native, Asian and Pacific Island descent are at risk. Risk increases with age, and women with a history of gestational DM or delivery of a macrosomic infant are at risk.

c) Symptoms are nonspecific, such as fatigue, pruritus, recurrent infections, visual changes, and paresthesias.

d) Diagnosis is similar to that of Type 1 DM.

e) Treatment goals are normal blood glucose levels and correction of any metabolic disorders.

(1) Diet and exercise are the mainstays of treatment of Type 2 DM, as insulin resistance decreases with weight loss and exercise.

(2) Usually oral hypoglycemic medication is needed to maintain normal blood glucose levels; the pancreas must be capable of secreting adequate amounts of insulin.

> *Sulfonylureas* (e.g., Diabeta®, Micronase® [glyburide], Diabinese® [chlorpropamid], Glucotrol XL® [glipizide]) augment beta cell insulin secretion

> *Biguanides* (e.g., Fortamet®, Glucophage ®, Riomet® [metformin]) inhibit hepatic glucose production and increase peripheral insulin sensitivity

> *α-Glucosidase inhibitors* (e.g., Glyset® [miglitol], Precose® [acarbose]) decrease postprandial hyperglycemia by delaying carbohydrate digestion and absorption.

> *Thiazolidinediones* (e.g., Actos® [ploglitazone], Avandia® [rosiglitazone] increase insulin sensitivity in adipose tissue

> *Amino acid derivatives* (e.g., Starlix® [nateglinide])

> *Combinations*, e.g., sulfonurea and biguanide (Metaglip®, Glucovance®), rosiglitazone and metformin (Avandamet®)

f) DKA is uncommon in DM Type 2, but Hyperglycemic Nonketotic Syndrome (nonketotic hyperosmolar syndrome) occurs. Severe hyperglycemia (>600 mg/dL) occurs in the absence of ketosis, with hyperosmolarity and profound dehydration. More common in older adults. Onset may be insidious, with decreased fluid intake, polyuria, polydipsia, and weakness for several days or weeks. Lethargy, confusion, and eventually coma ensue. Treatment is insulin, fluid replacement, and correction of electrolyte imbalances.

3) Gestational DM is diabetes that is diagnosed during pregnancy. It may have the onset during pregnancy or it may be pre-existing diabetes that is diagnosed during pregnancy. Treatment maybe with diet and exercise alone (A_1 GDM), with oral agents (e.g., glyburide), or insulin. If medications are needed to control blood glucose, it is classified A_2 GDM.. There is further discussion of GDM in the antepartum chapter.

d. **Metabolic syndrome** (Insulin Resistance Syndrome, or Syndrome X): conditions that increase the risk of cardiovascular disease and Type 2 DM. Includes 3 of the following:

> Waist circumference >40 inches in men or >35 inches in women.

> Plasma triglycerides ≥150 mg/dL

> Plasma HDL <40 mg/dL in men or <50 mg/dL in women

> Blood pressure ≥130/85 mmHg

> Fasting blood glucose ≥100 mg/dL

1) Individuals with metabolic syndrome should be screened regularly for diabetes

2) Lifestyle changes, the earlier they are instituted the better, reduce mortality from hypertension, diabetes, cardiovascular disease.

   a) Weight loss by reducing caloric intake

   b) Exercise

   c) Treat dyslipidemia

   d) Enhance insulin sensitivity

4. Eye, ear, nose and throat

a. Viral upper respiratory tract infections (URI)

1) The common cold

a) Causes: rhinovirus, adenovirus, echovirus, coxsackievirus, respiratory syncytial virus (RSV)

b) Presentation: congestion, sneezing, nasal discharge, dry sore throat, low-grade fever, cough

c) Physical exam: erythematous nasal and oropharyngeal mucosa

d) Management: Rest, hydration, decongestants (e.g. pseudoephedrine)

(1) Acetaminophen for analgesia, fever

(2) Antihistamines not beneficial

(3) Zinc gluconate lozenges q2 hours hastens cold resolution if started within 24 hours of symptoms

(4) Ipratropium (*Atrovent)* nasal spray 2 puffs BID or TID-symptomatic Rx

2) Influenza

a) Causes: orthomyxovirus types A, B, or C

b) Presentation: abrupt onset of high fever, chills, dry cough, headache, myalgia, malaise

c) Physical exam: usually unremarkable; chest x-ray usually normal

d) Management: self-limited, lasting 4-7 days. Rest, hydration

e) Acetaminophen for fever, discomfort

f) Antiviral medications:

(1) Amantadine hydrochloride 100mg po BID for 10 days may reduce symptoms and be used prophylactically or

(2) Rimantadine 100mg po BID for 10 days

b. Throat infections

1) Pharyngitis and tonsillitis

a) Causes: Streptococcus pyogenes, influenzavirus, Mycoplasma, Epstein-Barr virus, adenovirus and others

b) Presentation: sore throat, pain radiating to the ears and dysphagia, fever

c) Physical exam:

(1) Streptococcal infection: tonsillopharyngeal exudate, cervical lymphadenitis, pharyngeal erythema, fever

(2) Viral infection: concurrent URI symptoms, absent adenopathy, pharyngeal erythema

d) Management: Central question-viral or bacterial requiring antibiotics

(1) A reasonable approach in adults-treat all patients with fever, systemic symptoms, tonsillar exudate with antibiotics

- Penicillin (*Pen-Vee K*®) 500 mg po BID or TID
- Penicillin G Benzathine 1.2 million U IM
- Erythromycin 250-500 po q 6 hrs for 10 days

(2) Suspected viral throat infection-treat symptomatically with lozenges, over-the-counter (OTC) pain management

(3) Quick streptococcal test or culture can be done when the diagnosis is unclear

c. Allergic rhinitis

1) Presentation: Seasonal component or specific agent such as cats, dogs, dust

2) Physical exam: Excessive tearing (coryza), pale mucous membranes

3) Management:

a) Antihistamines may be helpful

- Chlorpheniramine (*ChlorTrimeton*®)
- Cetirizine (*Zyrtec*®)
- Loratadine (*Claritin, Alavert*®)

b) Nasal steroids (*Flonase*®, *Nasacort*®)

c) Ipratropium nasal spray

d. Vasomotor rhinitis

1) Nasal mucosal swelling engorgement without allergy or infection; due to recumbency, cold, humidity, pregnancy

2) Management: Oral or topical decongestants (Afrin)

a) Nasal steroids

b) Ipratropium nasal spray

5. Gastrointestinal

a. Hepatitis

1) Hepatitis B (HBV)

a) Most HBV infections in developed countries are from sexual activity, injection drug use, occupational exposure, or perinatal transmission.

b) Up to 30% cannot identify cause

c) Syndrome of acute, icteric liver inflammation, i.e., jaundice.

(1) Most HBV infections are asymptomatic.

(2) Symptoms may be erythematous rash, urticaria, polyarthralgias, arthritis; lassitude, anorexia, nausea, vomiting, headache, fever, dark urine, jaundice, hepatomegaly with tenderness.

d) Treatment of chronic HBV with antivirals alpha-interferon or lamivudine

e) May cause chronic illness, destruction of liver cells, cirrhosis, liver cancer, and death.

b. Gastroesophageal reflux (GERD)

1) Reflux of stomach secretions into the esophagus

2) Includes pyrosis (heartburn) and often noncardiac heart pain

3) Be suspicious if woman complains of frequent or difficult to control heartburn, dysphagia, nocturnal wheezing, atypical chest pain, chronic cough, sore throat, or even nocturnal regurgitation of fluid or food particles

4) Symptoms often aggravated by supine position, bending, or tight clothing

5) Usual treatment of GERD is dietary manipulation (avoidance of fried and fatty foods, oils, peppermint, acidic juices, heavy spices, onion, garlic, methylxanthines/xanthines, chocolate, alcohol; eat small meals; weight reduction) and avoidance of medications that many be involved (*B* adrenergic antagonists, calcium channel blockers and anticholinergics). Smoking cessation is also recommended.

6) Pharmaceutical treatment includes drugs for acid suppression – H2 blockers and proton pump inhibitors.

7) Prolonged GERD may cause hyperplasia of gastroesophageal junction, and precancerous (dysplastic) lesions (Barrett esophagus) and esophageal carcinoma. Refer for esophageal endoscopy and biopsy if symptoms are prolonged.

c. Peptic Ulcer Disease

1) Peptic ulcer disease is an inflammation of the stomach and/or duodenum

2) High risk clinical picture: Male, over 40, weight loss, abdominal/epigastric pain, occult blood as opposed to reflux found as major symptom in GERD

3) Some irritation of gastric lining is secondary to use of medications

4) Majority of ulcers involve a bacteria, *Helicobacter pylori* also known as *H. pylori*

a) Spiral, gram negative rod

b) Humans are the only known reservoir

c) Disease probably spreads by fecal oral route

d) Therefore, it is imperative that if an ulcer is suspected, the person should be referred and treated for *H. pylori* if for no other reason than to decrease the risk of stomach cancer. Usual treatments include antimicrobials like metronidazole and tetracycline as well as acid lowering drugs and bismuth.

d. Constipation

1) First consider the etiology of condition of constipation
2) Most common digestive complaint in America: accounts for 2.5 million ambulatory visits annually
3) Usually self limiting and nonpharmaceutical agents will be sufficient
4) Conditions associated with constipation include:
    a) Pregnancy
    b) Drug interactions
    c) Metabolic disorders
    d) Endocrine disorders
    e) Dietary variations
5) Average US citizen gets 15-20 grams of dietary fiber a day; 20-50 grams are estimated to be needed for normal bowel function
6) Ideal laxative is nonirritating, nontoxic, would act only on the descending and sigmoid colon and would produce a normally formed stool in a few hours after which its action would cease; it does not exist.
7) An estimated 20-30% of individuals over 65 years of age are dependent upon laxatives
8) Classification of laxatives generally based on mechanism of action
    a) All can result in bowel dependency
    b) Women who do develop bowel dependency need to be weaned gradually
    c) Elderly or chronically ill may have difficulty defecating due to weak abdominal muscles, thus sometimes elevating the feet on a step stool while on the commode may help
    d) Although laxatives have not been found to be effective weight loss agents, they are frequently abused for that reason
    e) Most of these agents are found over the counter
    f) Do not mix agents
    g) Essentially all agents benefit from and/or require water intake

e. Diarrhea

1) Etiology of diarrhea: usually self limiting
    a) Food related
    b) Infectious syndrome (Gastroenteritis)
        (1) Usually viral
        (2) Can be bacterial
    c) May be drug related

d) Less common is chronic diarrhea (usually over 2 weeks)

(1) Can be infectious or drug related, but should be suspicious of:

- Parasites
- Absorption defects (celiac sprue; lactase or pancreatic insufficiency)
- Cancer
- Alcoholism (Cirrhosis)
- Hyperthyroidism
- Diabetes Mellitus
- Inflammatory Bowel

Usual treatments for infectious diarrhea

Pathogen	Incubation	Characteristics	Recommended Adult Dosage
S. Aureus from food poisoning	1-8 hours	No antimicrobial recommended. Usually more vomiting than diarrhea. From meats, dairy and bakery. Restore fluids and support	
Salmonella	8-48 hours	Drugs not recommended usually. Often associated with bloody diarrhea.	TMP-SMZ 160/800 bid for 2 weeks if absolutely needed
Shigella	24-72 hours	Often bloody or purulent diarrhea.	TMP-SMZ 160/800 bid for 5-7 days
Campylobacter jejuni	2-10 days	Major clinical sign is massive diarrhea.	Erythromycin 500 mg q 6 hours for 5-10 days
C. Difficile	2-10 days	Major clinical sign is massive diarrhea., cholestyramine binds toxins	Metronidazole 125 mg q 6 h for 7 days Vancomycin 250 mg po q 8 h for 7 days Cholestyramine 4 grams q 6 hours
Giardiasis		Most common protozoal cause of diarrhea.	Atabrine-quinicrine 100 mg q 8 h for 7 days Metronidazole 250 mg q 8 h for 7 days
Amebiasis		Metronidazole for intraluminal phase	Iodoquinol 750 mg q 8 h for 10 days; 650 mg q 8 h for 20 days Pepto-Bismol 30- 60 mL q 6 hours daily
Traveler's Diarrhea**			TMP-SMZ 160/800 bid for 5 days Doxycycline 100 mg q 12 h for 5 days Ciprofloxacin 500 mg q 12 h for 5 days
Adapted from Rakel , R. (1996). Textbook of family medicine. Philadelphia: Saunders and Theoharides, T. (1992). Essentials of pharmacology. Boston: Little Brown and Company			

**When taken prophylactically, doxycycline, trimethoprim-sulfamethoxazole (TMP-SMZ) and ciprofloxacin consistently reduce the incidence of traveler's diarrhea by approximately 50 to 90%.

f. Irritable bowel syndrome (IBS)

1) An estimated 60% of visits to gastroenterologists are for IBS
2) More common among women than men
3) Characterized by alternating diarrhea and constipation
4) Often complain of bloating, but not necessarily gas
5) Diffuse gastrointestinal pain is almost pathognomonic

6) All symptoms are exacerbated by stress
7) No single agent has been found to be curative
8) Refer for workup by specialists; gastroenterologists usually rule out ulcerative colitis or Crohn's disease
9) Dietician to identify needed nutritional support
10) Supportive therapy to reduce stress
11) Do not empirically treat without appropriate workup
12) Usually pharmacologic treatments are bulk forming laxatives, stop all medications possible (reintroduce slowly and individually if needed), antispasmodics, antidiarrheals if needed.
13) Amitriptyline has been suggested for pain.
14) Plantago seed and husk (psyllium or plantain) and camomile tea have been suggested as herbal remedies.

g. Hemorrhoids

- ***Internal Hemorrhoids: Painless bright red bleeding with bowel movement***
- ***External Hemorrhoids: Pain/Itching with bowel movement***

1) Main therapeutic agents are anesthetics, vasoconstrictors, protectants, counterirritants, astringents, wound-healing agents, antiseptics, keratolytics and anticholinergics
2) Products with several agents may not be optimal due to potential interactions or suboptimal doses
3) Each agent works differently; must link agent with complaint
4) Increase bulk forming agents, fiber and water
5) Stool softener
6) If thrombosed hemorrhoid, refer

h. Vomiting

1) Vomiting is a complex sequence of events
    a) Usually begins with nausea
    b) Duodenal and jejunal tone is increased
    c) Peristalsis is slowed
    d) Reflux of duodenal contents into stomach
    e) Abdominal pressure causes reflux into stomach
    f) While trying to inspire, abdominal pressure may move contents into esophagus
    g) During actual vomiting, more contents are moved into esophagus and out of mouth

h) Events coordinated by emetic center; three sites usually involved (any single one of them; or all)

(1) Periphery

(2) Pharynx and gastrointestinal tract

(3) Chemoreceptor Trigger Zone (CTZ)

(4) Cortex

2) Two types of drugs involved in treating vomiting

a) Emetics (stimulate), e.g., Ipecac

b) Antiemetics (stop)

- Antihistamines (*Benadryl*®)
- Phenothiazines (*Compazine*®, *Phenergan*®)
- Antidopaminergic (*Reglan*®)
- Anticholinergic (*Scopolamine*®)
- Selective 5-HT3 receptor antagonists (*Anzemet*®, *Kytril*®, *Zofran*®)
- Corticosteroids are thought to affect the CTZ

c) Thorough history and physical to determine cause

i. Gallbladder disease: Inflammation (cholecystitis); obstruction (cholelithiasis)

1) Obstruction is caused by gallstones that form in bile that is supersaturated with cholesterol from the liver. Decreased motility enhances formation of stones that block the cystic or common bile ducts causing pain and inflammation.

2) Symptoms are epigastric and right upper quadrant pain that radiates to the upper back and intolerance of fatty foods. Other symptoms may be flatulence, heartburn, epigastric discomfort, pruritus, and jaundice. Pain may be intermittent or constant.

3) Abdominal tenderness and fever indicate cholecystitis

4) Jaundice indicates obstruction of the common bile duct

5) Diagnosis is by history, physical examination (positive Murphy sign), and radiographic evaluation

a) Oral or intravenous contrast X-rays

b) Abdominal ultrasound

6) Drugs may dissolve stones that are not causing obstruction (chenodeoxycholic acid or ursodeoxycholic acid)

7) For obstructions, surgery is the preferred alternative. Cholecystectomy may be by laparotomy or laparoscopy.

8) Refer women with acute gallbladder disease to a surgeon

6. Musculoskeletal

a. Osteoarthritis

1) Degenerative joint disease
2) Most common form of joint disease
3) Incidence increases with advancing age
4) Primarily affects weight bearing joints
5) Risk factors
   a) Obesity
   b) Female gender
   c) Genetic factors
6) Common sites: knees, hips, ankles, thumb, large toe
7) Chief complaints:
   a) Joint pain worsening following activity
   b) Stiffness, limited range of motion
   c) Swelling of joint; possible crepitus over joint
8) Does not usually respond well to anti-inflammatory drugs
9) Management
   a) Balance of rest and activity
      - Rest for acute painful phase
      - Gradual activity when acute symptoms abate
   b) Specific recommendations for various joint involvement
      - Shoulder: avoid aggravating positions
      - Hip: decrease amount of time spent sitting
      - Knees, ankles: avoid excessive standing
      - Feet, toes: comfortable, pliable shoes
   c) Nonsteroidal anti-inflammatory drugs (NSAIDs) may or may not help
   d) Referral to physical therapy for ROM and strengthening exercises
   e) Encourage weight loss
   f) Encourage swimming and water exercises
10) Refer to orthopedist for debilitating disease
11) Differentiate from rheumatoid arthritis (RA)
   a) RA is a chronic inflammatory disease of the joints with no known cause. It has systemic manifestations; involvement of peripheral joints in a symmetric distribution.
   b) Prodrome is fatigue, anorexia, weight loss, weakness, and mild musculoskeletal pain. Possible history of low grade fever.

c) Defining features of RA are morning stiffness lasting more than 1 hour and symmetric peripheral joint swelling and pain (3 or more joints).

d) There may be x ray findings suggestive of RA.

e) 70-90% people with RA test positive for rheumatoid factor (RF) and 25% healthy older people may test positive, so it is not diagnostic. Other diseases with similar presentations may cause positive RF: systemic lupus erythematosus (SLE, lupus), sarcoidosis, mononucleosis, HBV.

f) If RA is suspected, refer patient to rheumatologist

Osteoarthritis (OA) versus Rheumatoid Arthritis (RA)		
	OA	**RA**
Onset	Age 50-55	Age 20-60
Gender affected	Men=women	Women 2-3x> men
Constitutional s/s	None	Present
Joints affected	Hips, knees, spine, DIP, PIP, MTP	Wrists, MCP, PIP, MTP
Pattern	Asymmetrical, often only 1 weight bearing joint	Symmetrical, often multiple joints
Other signs	Crepitus Heberden's nodes Characteristic x ray findings	Deformities: swan's neck, boutonniere of fingers Rheumatoid nodules on bony prominence, especially elbows
Lab tests	None indicated	Elevated sedimentation rate + Rheumatoid factor (70-90%)

DIP: distal interphalangeal joint; PIP: proximal interphalangeal joint; MTP: metatarsophalangeal joint; MCP: metacarpophalangeal joint --- Adapted from Youngkin & Davis 2004, p. 764

b. Low back pain

1) Cause often multifactorial
2) Common conditions leading to low back pain
   a) Low back strain
   b) Degenerative disc disease
   c) Spondylolisthesis (dislocation of a vertebra)
   d) Spinal instability
   e) Herniated disc
3) May be accompanied by complaints of sciatica (pain radiating down leg)
4) Complete history and physical to evaluate symptoms
5) Evaluate to exclude fracture, neoplasm, infection
6) If serious medical causes ruled out, guidelines for management:
   a) Avoidance of activities that aggravate pain
   b) Cold packs or alternating cold and warm packs
   c) NSAIDS, acetaminophen for pain
   d) Gradual exercise

c. Carpal Tunnel Syndrome

1) Common nerve entrapment syndrome often caused by repetitive use of hands
2) Chief complaints: pain, tingling, numbness of thumb, index, and radial side of ring fingers that increases at night
3) Unilateral or bilateral
4) Increased incidence
    a) Diabetics
    b) Persons with thyroid disease
    c) Persons with rheumatoid arthritis
    d) Pregnant women
5) Physical examination
    a) Positive Tinel's sign: hand is "shocked" with tapping median nerve
    b) Positive Phalen's test: replication of symptoms with palmar flexion
    c) May have atrophy of muscles and decreased strength in thumb
6) Management
    a) Wrist splint: joint kept in neutral position
    b) Vitamin B_6: not evidence based
    c) NSAIDS not very effective
    d) Reduction in repetitive motions
    e) Frequent rest periods when must do motions
    f) Steroid injection if all other options ineffective
7) Refer to orthopedist if no improvement in 6-8 weeks

d. Osteoporosis

1) 41 million Americans by the year 2015 will have osteoporosis. After a hip fracture 12-20% die within 6 months, half go to a long term care facility.
2) Osteoporosis: bone mineral density (BMD) of the lumbar spine at least 2.5 SD below the mean value in premenopausal white women (T Score). The T-score is the number of standard deviations from the value at peak bone density of a young (25-30 year old) adult. The Z-score is the number of standard deviations from the value of ambulatory individuals of the same sex and age.
    - Normal bone T-score greater than -1
    - Osteopenia T-score between -1 and -2.5
    - Osteoporosis T-score less than -2.5

    Established osteoporosis includes the presence of a non-traumatic fracture

3) Etiologic factors
   a) Treatment with glucocorticosteroids, vitamin D deficiency, hyperparathyroidism, active peptic ulcer disease, abnormal renal function, abnormal hepatic function, malabsorption syndromes, estrogen loss (as in menopause). Contributing risk factors are race (whites have higher rates), smoking, family history, excessive exercise, eating disorders, hyperthyroidism, excessive alcohol consumption, slender body size.
   b) About ***80% of the peak bone mass is determined by inherited factors***, and all other life-style factors, including diet, account for the remaining 20%.
4) Diagnosis is ideally by dual-energy x-ray absorptiometry (DEXA), which measures small changes (1% loss) in BMD, whereas single or dual photon absorptiometry is imprecise
5) Management of osteoporosis (The midwife will usually consult for treatment of osteoporosis; screening and prevention are the midwife's role)
   a) Diet adequate in calories, protein (not excessive), vitamin D and calcium. If celiac disease is a factor causing malabsorption, a gluten free diet is prescribed.
   b) Exercise: Weight-bearing exercise such as walking at least 30 minutes 3 times a week.
6) Pharmacologic management of osteoporosis
   a) Alendronate (*Fosamax®*): Bisphosphonate; antiresorption agent used for prevention and treatment. (Etidronate, Risedronate and Pamidronate are other bisphosphonates)
      (1) Mechanism of action: decrease bone turn-over, inhibit osteoclast-mediated bone resorption, leads to greater formation of bone rather than resorption.
   b) Salmon Calcitonin Nasal Spray (*Miacalcin®*): hormone that inhibits bone resorption. Rhinitis is a side effect.
   c) Raloxifene (*Evista®)* and other selective estrogen receptor modulator (SERM). SERMs act like estrogen on skeletal and cardiovascular system but block estrogen's effect on breast and uterus. Has estrogen-antagonistic effect on breast and uterus. An estrogenic-agonist effect on bone and cholesterol. Builds bone and improves serum lipid profile, decreases LDL but does not increase HDL. Bone density shows small increases, which are less than seen with estrogen; Studies report no loss of BMD (with 60mg.day) and an increase of 1.2-1.6% over 2 years (hip, femoral neck and total body) in white, postmenopausal women.

d) Estrogen, estrogen/progestin: no longer first line treatment for prevention of osteoporosis, but may be useful for women who cannot tolerate other treatments, also need treatment for vasomotor symptoms, and have no contraindications to estrogen. Estrogen inhibits bone resorption.

e) Vitamin D: Metabolites increase the intestinal absorption of calcium. Recommendations are 800 IU vitamin D in a multivitamin plus 1200 mg of elemental calcium in the diet or as a supplement. Milk has approximately 100 IU of vitamin D per cup

f) Isoflavones (phytoestrogen): results of studies are contradictory; theoretically act as estrogen.

g) Thiazide diuretics for women who are also hypertensive may decrease bone loss by reducing urinary excretion of calcium.

7. Neurologic

a. Headache

1) ***Migraine without aura (common migraine)***

a) 2 of the following

- Unilateral location
- Pulsating quality
- Moderate or severe intensity
- Aggravated by routine physical activity

b) Plus 1 of the following

- Nausea or vomiting
- Photophobia and phonophobia

c) Neurologic exam, physical exam, and history do not reveal an organic cause

2) ***Migraine with aura (classical migraine)***

a) 3 of the following

- One or more fully reversible aura symptoms indicating cerebral cortical or brainstem dysfunction
- Aura symptom develops gradually over several minutes
- Aura lasts less than 60 minutes
- Headache follows aura within 60 minutes (or may occur concurrently)
- Headache usually lasts 4-72 hours

b) Neurologic exam, physical exam, and history do not reveal an organic cause

c) Treatment

(1) Non-pharmacologic

- Dietary changes
  - Avoid monosodium glutamate, nitrites, alcohol
  - Reduce caffeine
- Lifestyle changes
  - Regular eating, sleeping, exercise
  - Behavior therapies

(2) Biofeedback, stress management

- Acute therapy (at home)
  - o NSAIDs
  - o Butalbital, aspirin, and caffeine *(Fiorinal)*
  - o Ergotamine derivatives
  - o Abortive therapy
    - ✓ Isometheptine mucate (*Midrin*®)
    - ✓ Sumatriptan (*Imitrex*®) subcutaneously
    - ✓ Ergotamine tartrate, caffeine (*Cafergot*®)
    - ✓ Dihydroergotamine (*Migranal*®)
    - ✓ Prochlorperazine (*Compazine*®)
- Prophylaxis
  - o Amitriptyline (Tricyclic antidepressants)
  - o Propranolol (beta-blocker)
  - o Verapamil (calcium channel blocker)
  - o NSAIDS (menstrual cycle headaches)
  - o Ergotamine
  - o Anticonvulsants
  - o Fluoxetine (and other SSRIs)

3) Tension type headache

a) 2 of the following criteria

- Pressing or tightening quality
- Mild or moderate intensity
- Bilateral location
- No aggravation by routine physical activity

b) Neurologic exam, physical exam with in normal limits

c) Tension headache subtypes

(1) Episodic

- Lasting 30 minutes to 7 days
- No nausea or vomiting
- No photophobia or phonophobia, or one without the other
- History of 10 or more similar headaches
- Less than 15 headaches in a month

(2) Chronic

- Averages 15 headaches or more per month
- No vomiting
- No more than one of the following: nausea, photo-phobia, phonophobia

d) Treatment

(1) Symptomatic: simple analgesics, NSAIDs

4) Cluster headaches

a) Severe unilateral, orbital, supraorbital, or temporal pain

b) Lasts 15 minutes to 3 hours

c) Associated with at least one of the following:
   - Lacrimation
   - Nasal congestion
   - Forehead and facial sweating
   - Rhinorrhea
   - Miosis (small pupil)
   - Ptosis
   - Eyelid edema

d) Headache occurs from 1 to 8 times daily

e) At least 5 attacks occur as above

f) Treatment

(1) Acute therapy
   - Oxygen inhalation at flow rate of 6-8L/min for 15 minutes
   - Intranasal lidocaine on ipsilateral side
   - Sumatriptan
   - Parenteral therapy

(2) Preventive therapy
   - Low dose ergotamine
   - Verapamil
   - Prednisone

5) Secondary headaches for referral

a) Increased intracranial pressure

b) Tumor

c) Arteritis

d) Acute effects of substance abuse

e) Substance withdrawal

f) Meningitis

g) Drug rebound headache

h) Subarachnoid hemorrhage

b. Seizures

1) Definitions

a) Epilepsy-recurrent seizures than reflect aberrant electrical activity of cerebral cortical neurons

b) Convulsion-seizure in which motor manifestations predominate

2) Causes

a) Metabolic disorders

b) Hypoglycemia

c) Physical brain injury

3) Classifications
   a) Primary generalized seizures-bilateral, symmetric without focal onset-usually idiopathic
   b) Absence -- brief (2-10 seconds) lapse of consciousness
   c) Myoclonic -- quick paroxysmal contractions of part of a muscle, group of muscles
   d) Clonic tonic -- loss of consciousness with clonic tonic convulsion; postictal confusion
4) Treatment
   a) Single drug therapy to avoid impaired effectiveness
      (1) Carbamazepine, phenytoin
   b) Some antiseizure drugs reduce the effectiveness of oral contraceptives

8. Respiratory

a. Bronchitis (acute)

1) Caused by a variety of viruses; occasionally bacterial
2) Presentation includes productive cough with purulent sputum, rhonchi, sometimes fever
3) Physical exam is usually unremarkable; may ascultate rhonchi. Diagnosis made through exclusion of pneumonia, sinusitis or chronic respiratory disease
4) Management studies do not support antibiotic therapy
   a) Cough suppressants such as dextromethorphan (although no solid evidence of efficacy)
   b) Bronchodilators such as albuterol (metered dose inhaler or orally)
5) Consider a diagnosis of pertussis if cough lasts longer than 2 weeks

b. Pneumonia

1) Acute infection of the alveolar spaces or interstitial tissues (or both) of lung
2) Common pathogens: Streptococcus pneumoniae and Haemophilus influenzae
3) Subjective data
   a) Sudden onset of chills (rigor)
   b) Fever 101 degrees F or greater
   c) Rusty colored or purulent sputum
   d) Chest pain, shortness of breath
4) Objective data
   a) WBC count often higher than 12,000
   b) Chest x-ray may reveal lobar or segmental consolidation
   c) Sputum culture confirms diagnosis

5) Treatment
   a) Antibiotic therapy
      - Penicillin V
      - Erythromycin
   b) Prophylactic therapy: Pneumococcal vaccine for patients ≥50 years or immunocompromised

c. ***Tuberculosis (TB)***

1) Causative agent is mycobacterium tuberculosis
2) Acquisition is airborne transmission via droplet nuclei which incites a granulomatous pulmonary reaction
   a) Coughing, sneezing, singing, forceful speaking release infected particles into air
   b) Particles may remain suspended in normal air currents for extended periods
   c) Repeated exposures increase probability of infection; normally takes 2 months of exposure to acquire the disease
   d) Process of infection: three stages of infection of pulmonary TB
      (1) Primary or initial infection
      (2) Latent or dormant (asymptomatic) infection
      (3) Secondary or reactivation of infection
3) Primarily a pulmonary disease, but can plant in distant organ
4) ***Signs and symptoms of active TB***
   a) Chronic cough with minimal sputum production, possible hemoptysis
   b) Low grade fever
   c) Weight loss
   d) Night sweats
   e) May be asymptomatic
5) Physical exam: apical rales possible; lymphadenopathy with cervical node enlargement most common physical sign, often physical exam is unrevealing
6) Chest X-ray: Variety of infiltrative patterns; may be associated with cavitation or mediastinal lymphadenopathy
7) ***Sputum culture: gold standard for diagnosis***
8) Epidemiology
   a) TB has re-emerged as major public health concern
   b) Leading cause of death by infection worldwide
   c) 1/3 to ½ of world's population thought to be infected
   d) Most common opportunistic pathogen among HIV infected persons in less developed countries

e) Increase in TB related to: homelessness, poverty, inadequate access to health care, substance abuse, immigration of TB infected persons, overcrowded prisons

f) High risk groups

- Persons with HIV
- Close contacts with infected persons
- Persons with certain medical risk factors
- Foreign born persons from endemic countries
- Alcoholics and IV drug users
- Residents of long-term care facilities, prisons, nursing homes
- Emergency and medical personnel

9) Screening: Purified protein derivative (PPD)

10) Treatment of active TB per CDC guidelines: 4 drug regimen: INH, rifampin, pyrazinamide, and ethambutol or streptomycin

11) Preventive therapy for +PPD, no active disease: INH for 6 continuous months

d. Asthma

1) Definition/ Characteristics

a) Obstructive lung disease that is characterized by transient reversible attacks of

- Cough
- Wheeze
- Dyspnea
- Viscous mucus
- Always associated with widespread bronchospasm

b) Episodic in nature

c) Rapid increase in severity

d) May be complete absence of symptoms between attacks

2) Etiology

a) Airways hypersensitivity, hyperactivity of bronchial mucosa to irritating stimuli

b) Epithelial damage from inflammation

c) Desquamation bronchitis

d) Under-treatment and inappropriate therapy major factor in ↑ morbidity, mortality

e) “Urban disease”

3) Signs/symptoms of Asthma

a) History of transient attacks

b) Cough

(1) Tenacious mucus

(2) May be only symptom

c) Dyspnea

(1) ***Prolonged expiratory phase, accessory muscle use***

(2) Tachypnea, tachycardia, diaphoresis, cyanosis

d) Wheezing

(1) May be audible, expiratory and/or inspiratory

(2) Diminished when in distress (ominous sign)

e) Hyperresonant chest

(1) Usually reversible, may lead to barrel chest if frequent prolonged attacks

f) Possible dehydration due to hyperventilation, diaphoresis

4) Classification of Asthma by Symptoms

National Asthma Education and Prevention Program: Classification of Asthma Severity

Classification	Symptoms	Night symptoms	Pharmacologic Tx.
Step 1: mild intermittent asthma	Symptoms occur twice a week or less No symptoms and normal peak expiratory flow (PEF) between exacerbations Brief exacerbations (lasting a few hours to days) with variable intensity	Symptoms occur no more than twice a month	No daily meds, Short-acting Beta 2 agonist prn Course of systemic Corticosteroids for severe exacerbations
Step 2: mild persistent asthma	Symptoms occur more than twice a week Exacerbations may affect activity	Symptoms occur more than twice a month	Low-dose inhaled corticosteroids Short-acting Beta 2 agonist prn
Step 3: moderate persistent asthma	Daily symptoms Daily use of inhaled short-acting beta agonist Exacerbations affect activity Exacerbations occur more than twice a week and may last for days	Symptoms occurring more than once a week	Low-medium dose inhaled corticosteroids and long acting Beta 2 agonist Short-acting Beta 2 agonist prn
Step 4: severe persistent asthma	Continual symptoms Limited physical activity Frequent exacerbations	Frequent symptoms	High dose inhaled corticosteroids and long acting Beta 2 agonist; Oral corticosteroid if needed Short-acting Beta 2 agonist prn

5) **Asthma TRIGGERS:**
   a) Allergens
   b) Irritants
   c) Medical Conditions (e.g. URI)
   d) Drugs, additives
6) Precipitating factors for the different types
   a) Extrinsic: Specific antigens (bronchial) e.g. pollen, mold, cockroaches, dust mites, food, drugs
   b) Intrinsic: Generalized hypersensitivity to irritating stimuli; Preceded by primary respiratory infection, especially viral
   c) Mixed: Gradual development from extrinsic to intrinsic
   d) Significant overlap is common
7) **Diagnosis of asthma**
   a) Cough, wheeze related to triggers
   b) Family history
   c) Pulmonary Function Tests (PFTs)
      (1) Airway Challenge to confirm suspected asthma
      (2) Bronchial Provocation
   d) Other tests
      (1) RAST (measures IgE antibodies in serum (radio-allergosorbent)
      (2) Blood gases (to distinguish severity of attack)
8) **Status Asthmaticus**
   a) Prolonged attack refractory to bronchodilator therapy 12-24 hr.
   b) Life threatening
   c) 20-50% mortality
   d) Often secondary to infection or abuse of medication
   e) Characterized by
      (1) Intense mucus plugging
      (2) Atelectasis
      (3) Fatigue
   f) Ominous signs
      (1) No wheezing, diminished, barely audible breath sounds
      (2) Pulsus Paradoxus: systolic BP drops more than 10 mm with inspirations
      (3) Pulse > 120

9) Complications

a) Pneumothorax

b) Apnea - sudden onset

10) Treatment

a) Avoidance of precipitating factors

b) Close monitoring of peak expiratory flows (PEF)

c) Immunotherapy

d) Drug Therapy

(1) Corticosteroids

- Now recommended as first line treatment
- Aerosolized for maintenance
- Oral for more severe or persistent symptoms
- IV for acute attacks

(2) Bronchodilators

- PRN rescue inhalers
- Sympathomimetics

(3) Xanthines

(4) Parasympathetic blockers

(5) Cromolyn Na: prophylactic use only, pre-exercise

(6) Oxygen therapy

(7) Bronchial Hygiene

(8) Mucolytics - controversial

e) Nutrition - often stunted growth especially with steroids

11) Prognosis

a) Number of fatalities has increased in last decade (> 300%)

b) Asthma paradox: only "preventable" disease where morbidity and mortality rising even with increased use of Beta agonists.

c) Recent evidence suggests B_2 agonists may be contributing to irreversible aspects of disease.

9. Urinary

a. Urinary Tract Infection (UTI)

1) Pathology

a) 70%to 80% due to *E. coli*

b) Other enterobacteriaceae

c) Group B streptococcus

d) *S. saprophyticus*

e) Chlamydia (CT) & gonorrhea (GC) may cause urethritis

2) Risk factors
    a) Low socioeconomic status (SES)
    b) Sickle Cell trait
    c) Pregnancy: due to pooling and stasis secondary to dilation of renal calyces, pelves and ureters
    d) Birth with loss of sensation and overfilling (i.e. distention)
    e) Catheterization in labor: 15% incidence of bacteriuria
    f) Hypoestrogenic states
    g) Diabetes

3) *Signs & Symptoms of UTI*
    a) Cystitis
        (1) Frequency, urgency, dysuria
        (2) Microscopic hematuria and pyuria
    b) Pyelonephritis (incidence 1-2% in pregnancy)
        (1) Low grade fever with spikes or hypothermia
        (2) Chills
        (3) Dysuria, flank pain (i.e. CVA tenderness)
        (4) Usually unilateral and right-sided 50% of the time
        (5) Bilateral 25% of the time

4) Diagnosis
    a) Asymptomatic bacteriuria (ASB): Clean-voided specimen containing more than 100,000 organisms of a single uropathogen per mL
    b) Cystitis: Positive nitrites, WBCs on dipstick, microscopic urinalysis

5) *UTI Treatment*
    a) ASB
        (1) 5-6% incidence in pregnancy
        (2) Routinely screen only in pregnancy
        (3) Antibiotic therapy appears to be effective in reducing risk of pyelonephritis in pregnancy (OR 0.25) Treat empirically.
        (4) ***Without treatment approximately 25% will develop acute symptomatic infection***. LBW and prematurity were also decreased with treatment of ASB (OR 0.60), (Cochrane Review, 2000)
        (5) Sulfasoxizole: avoid third trimester to avoid competition for bilirubin binding sites
        (6) Nitrofurantoin, sulfonamides, salicylates: risk of G6PD deficiency in fetus at risk for hemolysis

b) Cystitis

(1) Antimicrobial therapy (optimal treatment controversial)

(2) ***Three-day therapy now recommended for acute uncomplicated cystitis in non-pregnant women***. Single dose with penicillin and cephalosporins give unacceptably low cure rates. Selective use of trimethoprim-sulfamethoxazole (TMP/SMZ, *Bactrim*) if single dose therapy is selected.

- TMP/SMZ (*Bactrim*®) 80/400 mg q 12h for 3 days = 95% cure rate OR
- TMP/SMZ (*Bactrim*®) 160/800 mg 2 tabs times one: 90% cure rate
- Trimethroprim 100mg q12h for 3 days
- Ciprofloxacin 250mg q.12h for 3 days

(3) ***Seven day therapy should be used in pregnancy.***

c) Acute pyelonephritis use 14 day course BID of TMP/SMZ (*Bactrim*®) 160/800 mg.

(1) 1-2 % of all pregnant women; two-thirds had pre-existing ASB. Pregnant women with pyelonephritis are usually treated in the hospital with parenteral antibiotics; consult.

(2) Ampicillin: not reliable; too many resistant *E.coli.*

(3) Aminoglycosides: use with caution due to renal impairment

(4) Cephalosporin (e.g. cephalexin/250-500mg/qid; or extended-spectrum PCN: good choices

(5) Recurrent cystitis in non-pregnant women: Antibiotic prophylaxis (either continuous or post-coital) using nitrofurantoin, a quinolone, or TMP/SMZ (*Bactrim*®) reduces infection rates.

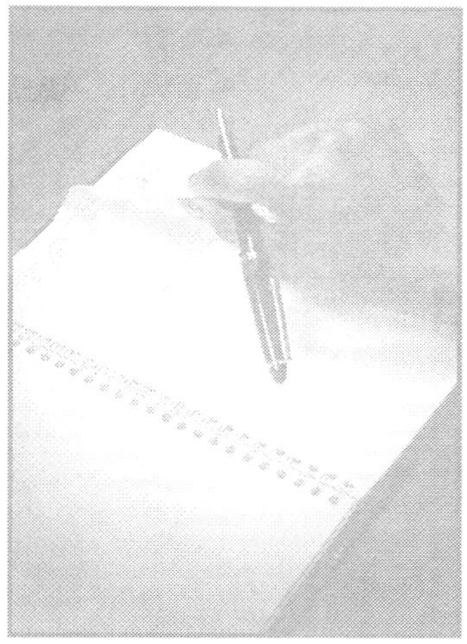

Chapter II

Antepartum Care

II. Antepartum Care (25-30%)

A. Physiology/Pathophysiology

1. Pregnancy
2. Genetics (see Chapter I, Primary Care), embryology, fetal development

B. Diagnosis of pregnancy

1. Presumptive, probable and positive indicators of pregnancy
2. Laboratory tests
3. Ultrasound
4. Counseling regarding pregnancy options

C. Collection of data base for pregnancy

1. **Historical data**
2. **Exposures and habits**
3. **Genetic risks, counseling and/or referral**
4. **Physical examination**
    a. Vital signs
    b. Pelvic examination
    c. Clinical pelvimetry

D. Calculation of current gestational age and estimated date of birth

E. Baseline laboratory tests (order/obtain/interpret)

1. Serum tests
2. Pap smear and cultures

F. Management of pregnancy

1. **Interval assessments to evaluate status of pregnancy**
    a. Vital signs/urine
    b. Weight gain patterns
    c. Auscultation of the fetal heart
    d. Assessment of fetal movement (includes fetal movement counts)
    e. Assessment of fundal height
    f. Leopold's maneuvers
2. **Laboratory tests (order/obtain/interpret)**
3. **Diagnostic tests and procedures**
    a. Nonstress testing
    b. Contraction stress testing (includes nipple stimulation)
    c. Ultrasound
    d. Amniotic fluid index/biophysical profile

4. **Counseling regarding normal pregnancy**
   a. Common discomforts, including use of alternative and complementary therapies
   b. Health promotion and disease prevention (includes exercise, hygiene, prenatal Rh immune globulin)
   c. Nutritional assessment and counseling
   d. Psychologic/emotional response to pregnancy (includes family relationships)
   e. Referral to community resources

G. Patient and family education to prepare for childbirth and parenthood

1. Informed childbirth methods/pain management options/birth plan/assisted delivery techniques
2. Counseling/preparation of women for external breech version
3. Counseling regarding vaginal birth after cesarean
4. Infant nutrition (includes breast and bottle feeding)/parenting skills

H. Assessment and management of deviations from normal pregnancy; indications for referral

1. Hypertensive disorders
2. Cytomegalovirus
3. Toxoplasmosis
4. Varicella
5. Human parvovirus B 19
6. Rubella
7. Thyroid disease
8. Multiple gestation
9. Sexually transmitted diseases
10. Bleeding in early pregnancy
11. Bleeding in late pregnancy
12. Postdates/post term pregnancy
13. Asthma
14. Gestational diabetes mellitus
15. Prelabor rupture of membranes

A. Physiology/Pathophysiology

In most instances, physiologic activity is increased. Only smooth muscle (e.g. urinary and G.I. tract) decreases its activity

> Of the three types of endogenous estrogens, estradiol and estrone increase 100 times in pregnancy, but estriol increases 1000 times!

1. Pregnancy

a. Endocrine System

1) Estrogen

a) Sites of production

(1) Syncytiotrophoblast (cells in the placenta)

(2) Ovaries (small amount produced first 2-4 weeks post-ovulation)

(3) Fetus (i.e. fetal adrenals) is source of 90% of the precursor of estriol formed in the placenta.

(4) The androgen compounds utilized for estrogen synthesis are derived in the early months of gestation from the maternal bloodstream. By the 20th week of pregnancy, the vast majority of estrogen excreted in the maternal urine is derived from fetal androgens.

(5) As early as the 7th week of gestation, >50% of estrogens entering maternal circulation are produced in the placenta.

b) Function/action of estrogen

(1) Promotes development of ductal system and mammary tissue growth in breast

(2) Increases myometrial activity

(3) Promotes myometrial vasodilation

(4) Increases sensitivity of uterus to progesterone in late pregnancy

(5) Softens fibers in cervical collagen tissue

(6) Increases pituitary secretion of prolactin (decreases sensitivity of receptors to prolactin)

(7) Decreases plasma proteins

(8) Increases serum binding protein and fibrinogen

2) Progesterone

a) Sites of production

(1) Corpus luteum (under the influence of hCG) during the first 5 weeks after fertilization

(2) Syncytiotrophoblast using cholesterol precursors from the mother after 5 weeks

(3) 250-300 mg/day produced in late pregnancy.

b) Functions/actions of progesterone

(1) The fetal adrenal lacks enzymes necessary for synthesis of some important corticosteroids. The fetus must utilize progesterone substrate from the placenta in order to accomplish this.

(2) Decreases myometrial activity and irritability, i.e. promotes uterine "quiescence"

(3) Constricts myometrial vessels

(4) Inhibits prolactin production

(5) Suppresses maternal immunologic response to fetal antigens

(6) Decreases sensitivity of maternal respiratory system to CO_2

(7) Relaxes smooth muscles in G.I. and urinary tract

(8) Increases sodium and chloride excretion.

3) Human Chorionic Gonadatropin (hCG): "The pregnancy hormone"

a) Site of production

(1) hCG is a glycoprotein with alpha and beta subunits—biologically similar to LH, FSH, and TSH. *Syncytiotrophoblast* produces hCG

(2) Generally detectable in maternal serum ~ 7 days after conception

(a) **Concentration in maternal serum doubles every 48 hours until it peaks at 60-90 days after conception**.

b) Functions/Actions of hCG

The primary function of hCG is to maintain the corpus luteum in early pregnancy

(1) "Rescues" and maintains the corpus luteum to provide for continued progesterone production.

(2) Stimulates the fetal testes and adrenals to enhance testosterone and corticosteroid secretion

(3) Stimulates production of placental progesterone and suppresses maternal lymphocyte responses, therefore preventing maternal rejection of the placenta

c) Persistent low levels of hCG may indicate an abnormal placenta, ectopic pregnancy, or impending spontaneous abortion.

d) Levels remain elevated in women with hydatidiform mole or choriocarcinoma.

4) **Human placental lactogen (hPL)**: Also called chorionic growth hormone, chorionic somatomammotropin)
   a) Site of production
      (1) Syncytiotrophoblast (starts 5-10 days after conception, rises, and then levels off by 34-36 gestational weeks)
      (2) hPL is similar in structure to human growth hormone (somatotropin) and prolactin.
      (3) Concentration of hPL is proportional to the placental mass. (e.g. moles have high hCG, but low hPL.
      (4) Synthesis of hPL is stimulated by insulin
      (5) HPL is present in maternal serum by 4 weeks post-conception (6 weeks gestational age); little is found in urine.

> Secretion of hPL is regulated by long-term changes in glucose. When glucose is low for an extended period, hPL is high and maternal lipolysis is increased. Short-term changes have no effect.

   b) Functions/actions of hPL
      (1) Promotes fetal growth by altering maternal protein, carbohydrate (CHO), and fat metabolism; it is secreted primarily into the maternal circulation and acts in maternal (not fetal) tissue.
      (2) 2 primary methods of action of hPL
         (a) Lipolysis and an increase in circulating free fatty acids (an energy source for maternal metabolism and fetal nutrition)
         (b) Anti-insulin action leads to increased maternal serum glucose levels, providing a constant source of nutrients for the fetus - important concept for understanding glucose intolerance in pregnancy, gestational diabetes, and the effect of pregnancy on preexisting diabetes

5) **Placenta:** Essential for transfer of nutrients and gases from the mother to the fetus and for removal of fetal waste products.
   a) Development
      (1) Day 6/7 post fertilization (or 20-21 days gestational age): trophoblast cells invade endometrium.
      (2) Fingerlike projections protrude between the cells of the endometrial epithelium into the endometrial stroma.
      (3) Day 7 (or 21 days from LMP), trophoblast begins to differentiate into 2 layers:

(a) ***Cytotrophoblast forms the chorionic villi and the amnion and new syncytial cells.*** A syncytium is a group of cells with no cell walls, i.e., the cytoplasm of adjoining cells is continuous; a giant multinucleate cell results.

Trophoblast is a layer of tissue that forms the wall of the blastocyst in early embryonic development. In the lower picture, the projections into the endometrium compose the syncytiotrophoblast.

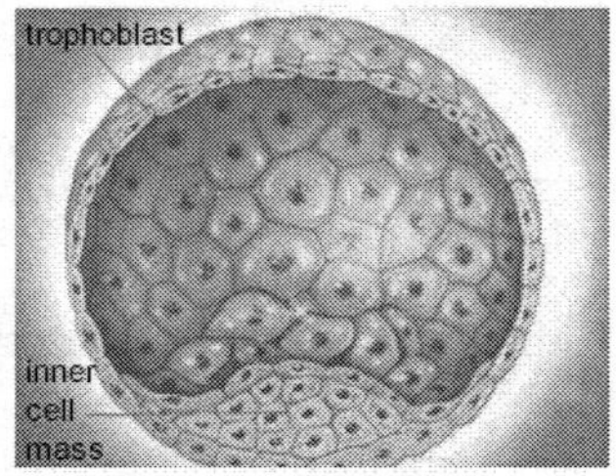

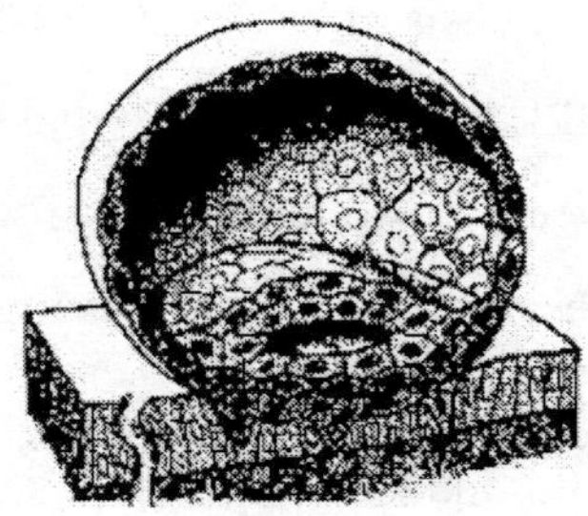

http://www.nurseminerva.co.uk/placenta.htm

(b) Syncytiotrophoblast puts out finger-like projections that invade the endometrial epithelium, engulfing uterine cells. It is able to digest cells of the endometrium, causing a small erosion on the uterine wall in which an embryo nidates (implants).

b) **The syncytiotrophoblast produces hCG, which maintains the corpus luteum during early pregnancy.** It is also thought to produce a protein that has immunosuppressive function. These substances appear in maternal blood about 7 days after ovulation.

c) ***Placenta is established by 8-10*** weeks post-conception or 12-14 gestational weeks

(1) There are no new lobules after 10-12 weeks post-conception

(2) Achieves full thickness by 4 months

d) Separating the villi of the placenta are lakes (lacunae) of blood. Maternal blood flows into these lakes surrounding the villi, allowing substances to pass into the fetal circulation.

e) The ***placenta is primarily a fetal structure with maternal and fetal components.***

(1) Functions

(a) Transport: movement of gases, nutrients, waste materials, drugs across the placenta

(b) Immunologic

- Protection of fetus from pathogens and prevention from rejection by mother
- Most bacteria are too large to cross placenta; placenta allows passage of maternal IgG antibodies to fetus late in pregnancy.
- The fibrinoid glycoprotein coating of the trophoblast acts as an antigen barrier and contains an alpha globulin of the IgG class.

> **Remember**
>
> ❖ **Conceptional age** refers to time elapsed from ovulation.
>
> ❖ **Menstrual age** (the usual reference for clinical dating and management) refers to time elapsed from the last menstrual period.
>
> ❖ **LMP dates** are 2 weeks later than conception dates, assuming a 28 day cycle.

(c) Endocrine production includes synthesis of hCG, hPL, estrogen, and progesterone plus other pregnancy associated proteins, glycoproteins, and growth factors.

6) **Thyroid**

a) Significant alterations occur in thyroid hormones. These are important in supporting the altered CHO, protein, and lipid metabolism of pregnancy.

b) Moderate diffuse enlargement of the thyroid is caused by hyperplasia of the glandular tissue and increased vascularity

c) Basal metabolic rate increases by 20-25% beginning at 4 months.

7) **Adrenal**

a) Little morphological change in adrenals but profound changes in secretion of cortical hormones.

b) By 15 weeks EGA, increased aldosterone secretion produced by the adrenal cortex regulates sodium and potassium balance in the blood

(1) Increases more if Na intake is restricted

c) At the same time, levels of renin and angiotensin II substrate are normally increased which act on the adrenals to increase aldosterone.

> "Natriuretic" refers to a substance that inhibits the resorption of Na ions from the glomerular filtrate in the kidneys, thus allowing more sodium to be excreted with the urine

d) The increased secretion is believed to protect the woman from the natriuretic effect of progesterone (see box)

Other anatomic and physiologic changes during pregnancy

b. Integumentary System

The basis for changes in skin, hair, and secretory glands is generally believed to be hormonal, particularly the effects of estrogen and adrenocortical steroids.

1) Pigmentation alterations
   a) Freckles, nevi, and recent scars darken—may increase in size
   b) Linea alba darkens and becomes linea nigra
   c) Chloasma (melasma; mask of pregnancy) is irregular, blotchy areas on face
   d) Pigmentary demarcation lines (esp. Japanese, Blacks, and Hispanics) appear as abrupt transitions between deeply pigmented skin and lighter skin; most common along the anterior brachial surface of the arms.

2) Connective tissue
   a) Striae gravidarum are linear tears in dermal collagen. Initially appear as irregular, pink, or purple wrinkled linear streaks that gradually become white.
      (1) Most prominent by 24-28 weeks gestation. Appear first on abdomen, then breast, thighs. Cause is a combination of hormonal changes and stretching.
      (2) Degree of distention is unrelated to striae formation.
      (3) May be more strongly correlated to adrenocortical activity than abdominal girth.

3) Cutaneous tissue and mucus membranes
   a) Epulis (lesion of the gums –pregnancy tumor)
   b) Gingivitis
   c) Changes in vagina and cervix (softening of cervix, increased mucosal transudate (leukorrhea of pregnancy), vasocongestion leading to blue or purplish coloration, changes in pH and microecology of vagina, etc.
   d) Skin tags (fibromata molle or moluscum fibrosum gravidarum): soft, flesh colored or pigmented skin tags which are small, pedunculated fibromas that appear during the 2nd half of pregnancy -- thought to be hormonal.

4) Vascularity
   a) Purpura or varicosities are induced elastic tissue fragility due to increased estrogen. Also, increased venous pressure in lower extremities from pressure of gravid uterus and familial tendency. Appear within first two trimesters.
   b) Hemangiomas are usually on head and neck at end of first trimester.
   c) Palmar erythema is redness of palms and fingertips, or diffuse mottling of entire palm.

d) Cutis marmorata is transient bluish mottling of legs on exposure to cold that arises from vasomotor instability secondary to increased estrogen

e) Non-pitting edema: increased vascular permeability and sodium retention due to the increased estrogen. In lower extremities, it is aggravated by pressure from growing uterus.

f) Spider nevi/angiomas are central dilated arterioles, flat or slightly raised with extensive radiating capillary branches. Most prominent in areas of skin drained by the superior vena cava (eyes, neck, throat, and arms). Due to increased estrogen (differential diagnosis is liver disorder).

5) Secretory glands

a) Increased secretory gland activity with a "greasy" feel to skin

b) Montgomery's tubercles on areola of breasts

c) Apocrine (large, deep glands in axilla, anal/genital, and mammary areas) sweat gland activity decreases, possibly result of hormonal changes

d) Eccrine (glands in skin that promote cooling by evaporation of their secretions) sweat gland activity gradually increases. Possibly due to increased thyroid activity along with increased body weight and metabolic activity. Important in thermoregulation; helps dissipate excess heat produced by increased metabolic activity. Can lead to prickly heat (miliaria) or dyshidrotic (abnormal sweating) eczema.

6) Hair and nails

a) Estrogen increases the length of the growth phase of hair follicles leading to increased hair loss postpartum.

b) Mild hirsutism in early pregnancy (upper lip, chin, cheeks, suprapubic midline)

c) Frontal hair loss sometimes in late pregnancy.

d) Nail changes are uncommon and of unknown etiology -- transverse grooves, increased brittleness, distal separation of nail bed (onycholysis).

c. Breast

1) Estrogen

a) Ductal system development

b) Glandular tissue (mammary) growth

2) Progesterone

a) Alveolar system development

b) Contributes to mammary growth

3) hPL-Stimulates mammary growth

4) Prolactin-Serum levels rise but estrogen suppresses its effect

5) Breast changes

a) Two-fold increase in blood flow to breast

b) Weight increases ~12 ounces

c) Externally, increased size and areolar pigmentation

d) First trimester

(1) Tenderness and tingling in early weeks due to increased blood flow

(2) Nodularity and enlargement due to hypertrophy of mammary alveoli

(3) Nipples more erectile

(4) Darkening of the nipple

(5) Montgomery's tubercles more prominent

(6) Skin over the breasts appears thinner; blood vessels more prominent

e) Second trimester

(1) Primary and secondary areola more deeply pigmented and broader

(2) Colostrum develops and can be expressed

(3) Striae may develop

d. Cardio-respiratory systems

1) Respiratory

a) Anatomic (structural) changes

(1) Diaphragm rises about 4 cm

(2) Subcostal angle widens and the transverse diameter of the thoracic cage increases about 2 cm.

(a) Result: Breathing is more diaphragmatic than costal.

(b) Thus, ***less air in lungs at end of expiration than at any other time.***

(c) With less residual air, mixing of inspired air during breathing is more efficient.

b) Physiologic (functional) changes

(1) ***Increased tidal volume*** (amount of air breathed with each breath)

(2) Tidal volume exceeds oxygen needs of pregnancy

(3) Amount of Hgb increases as does cardiac output which means the total oxygen-carrying capacity increases

(a) As a result, maternal arteriovenous oxygen difference is decreased

(b) ***Compensated respiratory alkalosis***

(4) Respiratory rate changes little (some sources say the respiratory rate does not change in pregnancy)

(5) Increased awareness of a desire to breathe is common—felt as dyspnea

(a) ***Physiologic dyspnea*** thought to be due to increased tidal volume that lowers the blood pCO_2 slightly, which paradoxically causes dyspnea

2) Hematologic

a) ***Blood volume increases***

(1) Starts during first trimester, expands most rapidly during the second trimester, and then rises at a much slower rate during the third trimester to plateau the last several weeks of pregnancy

(2) Meets demands of uterus with its greatly hypertrophied vascular system

(3) Protects mother and fetus from deleterious effects of impaired venous return in the supine and erect positions

(4) Safeguards mother against the adverse effects of blood loss during childbirth

b) ***Physiologic (dilution) anemia***

(1) Plasma volume increases more rapidly than the production of erythrocytes

(2) Erythrocytes increase ~33% but still not as much as plasma volume increases; therefore, Hemoglobin and Hematocrit decrease slightly

(3) Whole blood viscosity decreases as a result

(4) Hemoglobin (Hb) at term averages 12.5 g/dL when iron stores are sufficient

(a) <11g/dL is considered abnormal and usually due to iron deficiency

(b) CDC defines anemia in pregnancy as Hb <11 g/dL in first and third trimester and Hb <10.5 g/dL in second trimester. Some sources cite Hb < 11 g/dL as anemia.

(c) The dip in Hb in the second trimester is an important sign that the physiologic expansion of blood volume has occurred. The Hb then rises towards term, as the hemodilution abates.

(5) Hb production in the fetus is not impaired, as the placenta obtains iron from the mother in sufficient amounts for fetus

Factors that increase Hb concentration

Smoking ½ to 2 packs per day adds 0.3 to 0.7 g/dL
*Anemia: Hb < 11.3-11.7 g/dL
High altitude increases Hb
*Anemia: Hb < 11.2 g/dL at 3000 ft,
Hb < 11.5 g/dL at 5000 ft
Hb < 12.3 g/dL at 8000 ft

Source: Sinclair C. A Midwife's Handbook

c) Leukocyte changes

(1) Prepregnancy	4300-4500
(2) Pregnancy	5000-12,000
(3) Labor	14,000-16,000

d) Blood coagulation

(1) Fibrinogen concentration increases ~50%

(2) Fibrin split products (FSP), also called fibrin degradation products (FDP) are detected by tests that detect D dimers. If there is a consumptive coagulopathy, the D dimer is abnormally high.

(3) Prothrombin (PT) and partial thromboplastin times (PTT) may be prolonged in conditions of coagulopathy.

(4) Erythrocyte sedimentation rate (ESR) is increased in pregnancy, so its use in pregnancy is limited.

3) Cardiovascular

a) ***Pulse rate increases 10-15 beats*** per minutes (bpm)

b) As diaphragm becomes progressively elevated, heart is displaced to left and upward, while at same time it's rotated somewhat on its long axis.

(1) Result: Apex is moved somewhat laterally

c) Heart sounds

(1) Systolic murmur in 90% of pregnant women

(2) Soft diastolic, transient murmur in 20%

(3) Continuous murmurs arising in breast vasculature in 10%

(4) Exaggerated S_1: Splitting of the first heart sound with increased loudness of both components.

4) Cardiac output (CO)

a) ***Increases***

b) Very sensitive to body position changes—may increase by as much as 22% when moved from her back to her side

(1) CO = stroke volume x heart rate

c) By term, the heart rate increase accounts for much of the increase in CO

5) Blood pressure

a) Posture affects arterial BP

b) BP in brachial higher when sitting, lowest when lying in the lateral recumbent position, and intermittent when supine

c) Decreases to a nadir during 2nd trimester or early 3rd trimester and rises thereafter. It should NOT rise above the baseline (prepregnancy) blood pressure.

6) Circulation

a) Blood flow in legs is impeded except in a lateral recumbent position due to occlusion of pelvic veins and inferior vena cava by uterus. Elevated venous pressure returns to normal if woman lies on her side. Returns to normal after delivery.

(1) Contributes to dependent edema near term

(2) Contributes to development of varicose veins in legs, vulva, and rectum (hemorrhoids).

e. Gastrointestinal system

1) Gastrointestinal (GI) tract

a) Stomach and intestines are displaced, causing physical findings in certain diseases to be altered (e.g. appendix is usually displaced upward and laterally)

b) ***GI motility decreased (caused by progesterone)***

c) Gastric emptying slowed, which leads to a prolonged emptying time.

d) Pyrosis (heartburn) is caused by reflux of acidic secretions into lower esophagus. The altered position of the stomach, decreased lower esophageal sphincter tone, decreased esophageal peristalsis, lower amplitude of esophageal peristalsis, lower intra-esophageal pressures, and higher intragastric pressures all contribute to this.

e) Gums become hyperemic and softened-may bleed with brushing. Epulis may develop.

2) Liver and gallbladder

a) No significant increase in liver size.

(1) Total bilirubin, liver enzymes (AST, ALT), and bile salts should not be elevated in pregnancy

(2) Serum alkaline phosphatase may be elevated.

(3) While total serum albumin increases, the concentration decreases.

(4) There is an increase in globulins, causing a decreased albumin-to-globulin ratio

b) Sluggish gallbladder leads to stasis and thickened bile. Increased prevalence of cholesterol stones in women who have been pregnant.

f. Renal system

1) Kidneys

a) Increase slightly in size

b) Increased glomerular filtration rate (GFR) ~50% early in pregnancy (estimated by the creatinine clearance)

c) Increased renal plasma flow (RPF) ~25-50%

d) Loss of nutrients in urine rises (protein, amino acids, and water-soluble vitamins), probably due to increased GFR and increased RPF

2) Ureters

a) Hydronephrosis and hydroureter (hydronephrosis = distention by urine that cannot flow because of an obstruction)

(1) Presumably an effect of progesterone

(2) When uterus rises out of the pelvis, it rests on the ureters, compressing them at the pelvic brim.

(a) Results in ureteral dilation

(b) Hydronephrosis is greater on the right side of 86% of pregnant women (because the sigmoid colon on the left cushions the uterus)

3) Bladder

a) Decreased bladder capacity: hyperemia and hyperplasia of muscle and connective tissue together with the increased size of the uterus elevates the bladder trigone and causes thickening of its posterior margin. Leads to deepening and widening of trigone with result of less capacity.

b) Edema: pressure of the presenting part impairs blood and lymph drainage, often resulting in an edematous lower bladder which is easily traumatized

4) ***Increased UTI risk***

a) **Urinary stasis:** Dilation of the urinary tract along with partial obstruction of the ureters from ureteral compression at the pelvic brim results in urinary stasis. Large amounts of urine may stay in the ureters and hypotonic bladder which increases the risk of asymptomatic bacteriuria.

b) **Bacterial growth medium increased**; loss of nutrients (glucose, protein, and amino acids) provides additional substrates for bacterial growth.

c) Bladder edema and hyperemia = increased susceptibility to infection

d) Hypoactive ureters = stasis of urine facilitates ascending bacterial migration, increasing the risk of pyelonephritis.

5) Glucosuria

a) Not necessarily abnormal

b) The increase in glomerular filtration, together with impaired tubular reabsorption capacity for filtered glucose accounts for most cases of glucosuria. The increased amount of glucose filtered out is so great that the ability of the kidney to reabsorb it in the tubules is overwhelmed.

c) The possibility of diabetes cannot be ignored.

6) Proteinuria

a) Normally does not occur except in trace amounts

b) ***May be a sign of preeclampsia, UTI, or contamination by vaginal secretions***

7) Sodium intake

a) Salting food to taste will provide an plenty of sodium in the diet

b) No good evidence that Na restriction is beneficial—may be harmful to adrenals.

c) Exorbitant amounts of Na may also be harmful.

d) Filtered load of Na increases due to increased GFR but tubular reabsorption of Na also increases along with increased Na retention in last two months of pregnancy. Result is that woman remains in Na balance.

g. Reproductive system changes during pregnancy

1) Uterus

a) **Growth**

(1) Hyperplasia (increase in cells) during first 6 weeks of gestation due to estrogen

(2) Hypertrophy (growth of cells) and stretching of muscle fibers via mechanical pressure exerted by fetus after 1st trimester.

b) **Shape**

(1) **Piskacek's sign**: Slight enlargement of one part of the uterus at the implantation site

(2) Pear-shaped (piriform) to globular by 12 gestational weeks to ovoid at term

(3) Spherical in first trimester to elliptical (cylindrical)

(4) Rotation to the right as the uterus rises from pelvis, probably from pressure of rectosigmoid on the left side, is called *dextrorotation.*

c) **Contractility**

(1) Never completely quiescent

(2) Frequency of contractions increases from one contraction every 2 ½ -3 hr at 25 weeks to 2-3/hr at 40 weeks in primigravida

(3) Mild, irregular, unsynchronized; usually not felt in early pregnancy

(4) Become more intense and may assume some degree of rhythmicity as pregnancy progresses (Braxton-Hicks)

(5) Alterations in character of contractions are due to structural and functional changes in the myometrium caused by changes in the estrogen-progesterone environment. Increased estrogen activity leads to:

(a) Action potentials change in velocity and timing

(b) Myometrial cells hypertrophy and are hyperplasic with increased contractile proteins

(c) Gap junctions form (muscle bundles are in closer contact)

(d) Sarcoplasmic reticulum develops, enhancing calcium movement

(e) Energy production by the myometrial cell enhanced by increased number of mitochondria and cellular ATP

2) Cervix

a) Increases in mass, water content, and vascularization

b) 85-90% connective tissue and 10-15% smooth muscle

(1) More smooth muscle in upper part of cervix, less in lower portions

(2) Connective tissue undergoes changes in its elasticity so that by term it is soft and stretchy

c) Changes in appearance and consistency

(1) **Goodell's sign: softened consistency of cervix**

(2) **Hegar's sign :** neck of uterus is compressible

(3) **Chadwick's sign:** Cyanosis (purplish color) of cervix and vagina due to vascularity and edema

(4) **Eversion:** Endocervical cell mitosis; squamo-columnar junction becomes visible

(5) **Erosion:** Not really. Red velvety areas resulting from the proliferating endocervical glands and columnar endocervical epithelium look like erosion

(6) **Mucus increases.** Soon after conception a clot of very thick mucus obstructs the cervical canal (Mucus plug: aka...*operculum*)

3) **Ovaries and fallopian tubes**
   a) Corpus luteum of pregnancy most likely functions maximally during the first 6-7 weeks of pregnancy (4-5 weeks post-ovulation) then ceases as a source of progesterone
   b) Relaxin is a hormone secreted by the corpus luteum, myometrium, deciduas, and placenta. In late pregnancy, it plays a role in softening and effacement of the cervix
4) **Vagina**
   a) Wall
      (1) **Increased vascularity**
      (2) ***Violet color (Chadwick's sign)***
      (3) Increase in thickness of mucosa, loosening of connective tissue, and hypertrophy of the smooth muscle cells nearly to the extent of the uterus
   b) Secretions
      (1) The physiologic discharge is increased due to increased vascularity
      (2) Thick, white, acidic (lower pH) discharge due to increased production of lactobacillus

h. **Musculoskeletal**
   1) **Relaxin and progesterone** affect the cartilage and connective tissue of the sacroiliac joint and the symphysis pubis. This increases the mobility of these joints and **leads to the characteristic "waddle" gait.**
   2) **Distention of the abdomen tilts the pelvis forward**, shifting the center of gravity. The woman compensates by developing an increased curvature (**lordosis**) of the spine that may strain muscles and ligaments of the back.
   3) Stretch and decreased tone of the abdominal muscles also contribute to the lordosis.
   4) Growth of uterus causes separation of the rectus muscles in the midline of the abdominal wall called diastasis recti. In severe cases, a large portion of the anterior uterine wall is covered by only a layer of skin, attenuated fascia, and peritoneum.
   5) Bone mineralization
      a) Calcium, phosphorous, and magnesium levels decrease
      b) Parathyroid hormone (PTH), calcitonin, and Vitamin D production increase (under influence of estrogen and hPL)
      c) Rate of bone turnover increases
      d) If woman maintains calcium intake requirements for pregnancy, there is not a large change in skeletal mass or bone density (calcium homeostasis)

e) Any increase in bone reabsorption of calcium (due to hPL) is counteracted by an estrogen induced decrease in reabsorption

f) PTH increase enhances intestinal calcium reabsorption, decreases urinary calcium loss, and stabilizes bone turnover

g) Calcitonin decreases calcium release from bone while Vitamin D increases calcium release

LORDOSIS of PREGNANCY

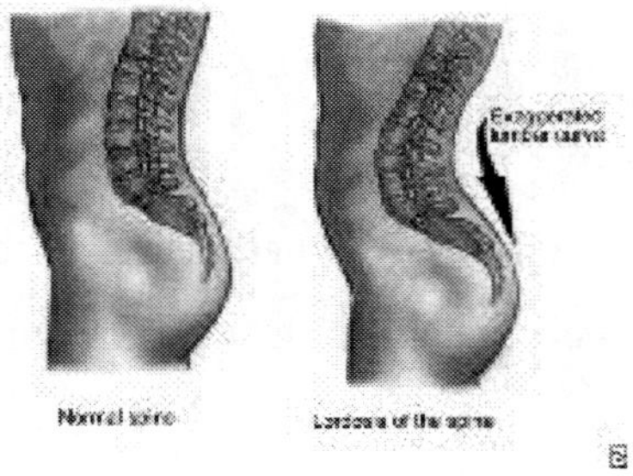

2. Genetics (also see Chapter I Primary Care), embryology, fetal development

a. ***First trimester: zygotic, embryonic, and beginning of fetal period***

1) **Zygotic period**

a) **First week of life**

b) Sex cells (GAMETES) undergo gametogenesis, producing ova and sperm

c) ***Gametogenesis:*** the pronucleus of each gamete contains only half (23 or the haploid number) of the total 46 or the diploid number) chromosomes in a human. This halving is the result of gametogenesis.

d) ***Fertilization***: the fusion of the pronuclei of a male and a female gamete, producing a ZYGOTE.

> **Remember**
>
> - ❖ Zygote becomes Morula which develops to Blastocyst
> - ❖ The Blastocyst is the form that implants in the uterine lining 6-10 days after fertilization

e) The sex of the new individual is determined at the moment of fertilization

f) The mitotic cellular division is called cleavage

g) ***As the cells divide, they become a mass of dividing cells called a morula***

h) With reorganization of the cellular mass and the entry of fluid, the ***morula develops into a blastocyst.*** This is what implants in the uterine lining 6-10 days post-fertilization.

2) **Embryonic period: post-fertilization weeks 2-7** (Gestational weeks 4-9)

a) At the time of implantation, the embryo is known as a bilaminar embryo because the embryonic disc arising from the inner cell mass consists of 2 layers of cells: ectoderm and endoderm.

b) A third layer forms in the third week: the mesoderm

Layers of cells
Ectoderm
Endoderm
Mesoderm

c) The mesoderm, ectoderm, and endoderm are 3 germ layers in the makeup of the body. All tissues, organs, and structures develop from these layers

d) ***Mullerian development starts in the mesoderm***

e) **Embryonic development by <u>conceptional weeks</u> (recall that clinical dating is by menstrual weeks, which adds 2 weeks to the conceptional age)**

Week 2 Bilaminar development of endoderm and ectoderm

Week 3 Mesoderm development (trilaminar disk)

Week 4 Heart begins to beat
Longitudinal and transverse folding occur, altering the form from a flat disk to that of a curved cylinder
The neural tube closes at separate sites, which then fuse

Week 5 Rapid brain development
Eyes begin to develop
Development is cephalic to caudal

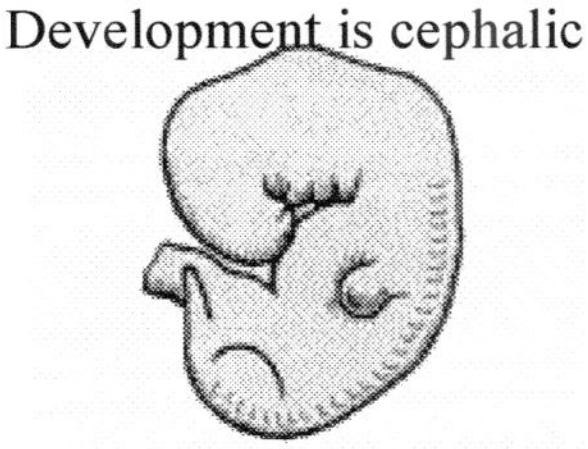

Day 29:
Crown to rump, 5.0mm

Week 6 Nose, mouth, and palate start to form
Limbs begin to differentiate
Clearly defined fingers and toes

Week 7 Neck region established
Abdomen is less protuberant but intestines are still herniated into proximal portion of umbilical cord
Distinct human characteristics

Week 8 All essential internal and external structures are present
Embryonic period is a critical time during which a teratogen may be either lethal or cause major congenital malformations

3) Beginning of fetal period

a) By end of first trimester, intestines are fully into the abdomen

b) External genitalia have male or female characteristics

c) Weight ½-1 oz; crown-rump length is ~ 2.2 inches

d) Swallows, breathes, urinates, moves limbs, squints, frowns, opens and shuts mouth.

b. Second and third trimesters

1) 13-16 weeks (4th lunar month)

a) Sex is clearly distinguishable during 14th week

b) By 16 weeks weight is 3.5 – 4 oz.; crown-rump ~ 4.5"

2) 17-20 weeks (5th lunar month)

a) Movements stronger (mother feels ~18 weeks)

b) Hiccups

c) By 20 weeks, body covered with vernix caseosa

d) Weight ~1 pound (500 grams); crown-rump ~ 6.5"

3) 21-24 weeks (6th lunar month)

a) Lanugo

b) Wrinkled, red skin without subcutaneous fat

c) Brown fat forms (source of energy and heat production and regulation)

d) Crying and sucking starts

e) Can make a fist and grip

f) By end of 24 weeks weight ~ 1.25 pounds.; crown-rump ~8"

4) 25-28 weeks (7th lunar month)

a) Some fat storage begins

b) Eyes start to open and shut

c) Fingernails

d) Substantive weight gain begins

e) By end of 28 weeks ~2.25 pounds.(1000 grams); crown-rump ~ 9"

5) 29-32 weeks (8th lunar month)

a) Lanugo on face disappears

b) Toenails

c) Eyes open

d) Fat starting to smooth out wrinkles

e) Can control body temperature and rhythmic breathing

f) By end of 32nd week ~ 3.75 pounds.; crown-rump ~ 11"

6) 33-36 weeks (9th lunar month)

a) Left testicle descends in males

b) More fat, less wrinkles, rounder body

c) By end of 36th week ~ 5.5 pounds (2500 grams).; crown-rump ~ 12.5"

7) 37-40 weeks (10th lunar month)

a) Protuberant mammary glands

b) Testes in scrotum in males

c) No lanugo

d) Nails beyond fingers and toes

e) Pulmonary, gastrointestinal, and renal systems permit extrauterine survival

f) By end of 40th week ~ 7.5 pounds; crown-rump ~ 14"

c. **Effects of teratogens on fetal development**

1) Principles

a) Genetic susceptibility of embryo

b) Timing of exposure

(1) During zygotic and first week of embryonic periods, teratogens either result in no action or a spontaneous abortion ("all or none phenomenon")

(2) Embryonic period (postconception weeks 3-8) is most critical for structural defects because this is when organogenesis occurs.

- Heart, arms, and legs susceptible in embryonic period
- Example – neural tube defects occur post conception days 22-28;
- If folic acid is to prevent the defect, it must be present in adequate amounts before and during this interval

(3) Eyes, ears, teeth, CNS, and genitalia sensitive beyond 1st trimester

(4) ***CNS sensitive throughout—has longest period of sensitivity*** (16 weeks)

(5) Teratogens have different effects depending on time of exposure

c) Dose relationship: the higher the dose of teratogen, the more likely (or more severe) defect is

d) **Weeks 8-term**: functional defects/minor anomalies

e) Many birth defects are multifactorial, i.e., they involve interaction of genetic and environmental factors

d. Mullerian development

1) Weeks 3-5

a) Mesonephric ducts emerge from mesoderm and connect with cloaca

2) Weeks 4-5
   a) Two ureteric buds develop distally from the mesonephric ducts and begin to grow cephalically toward the mesonephric duct
   b) Mullerian ducts form bilaterally between the developing gonad and the mesonephric ducts
   c) **Importance is that the close association between the Mullerian and the mesonephric ducts means that damage to either system will most often be associated with damage to both (uterus, kidneys, ureters)**

3) ~Week 10
   a) Uterus forms by union of the 2 mullerian ducts
   b) The shape of the uterus is now formed, with cellular proliferation at the upper portion of the uterus and a simultaneous dissolution of cells at the lower pole, thus establishing the uterine cavity.

4) ~Week 20
   a) The wedge of tissue (septum) at the union of the mullerian ducts is dissolved slowly until the uterine cavity is complete.
   b) Failure to fuse the Mullerian ducts or to resorb the cavity can lead to separate uterine horns or septum.

e. Placental development

1) Arises from the outer layer of cells of the blastocyst (trophoblast)
2) Trophoblast differentiates into cytotrophoblast and syncytiotrophoblast as it contacts the endometrium of the uterus.
3) **The syncytiotrophoblast penetrates the uterus.**
   a) Lacunae (blood filled lakes) form around the 8th day in the syncytiotrophoblast as it invades the endometrium.
   b) As a result, endometrial glands are eroded.
   c) Capillaries rupture to fill the lacunae with glandular secretions and maternal blood, which is nutritive to the embryo and reaches it by diffusion from the syncytiotrophoblast.

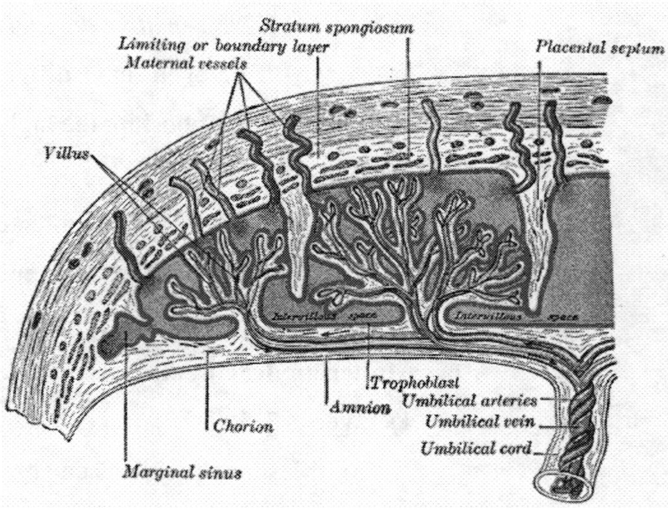

4) **Embryo is completely embedded by 12th post-fertilization day**. Lacunae now join together and form an intercommunicating network.
   a) A primitive placental circulatory system is established via the lacunar network
5) **~14th day post-fertilization, chorionic villi begin to form from the cytotrophoblast cells that reorganize into columns and extend into the core of the syncytiotrophoblast.**
   a) They invade and attach to the decidua basalis (the part of the uterine endometrium that is beneath the site of implantation of the embryo).
   b) The decidua basalis is the maternal contribution to the placenta.
   c) Thus, the placenta consists of a fetal portion of chorionic villi that interlock with the decidua basalis of the uterus, the maternal portion.
6) The capillary network of the most superficial portion of the endometrium is invaded by cytotrophoblasts.
   a) Arterioles and the spiral arteries are invaded and the walls of these vessels are destroyed.
   b) Maternal blood enters from the spiral arteries in fountain-like bursts and bathes the chorionic villi.
   c) Food substances, oxygen, and antibodies pass into fetal blood of the villi; metabolic waste products pass from the fetal blood into the mother's blood.
      (1) In general, there is no mixing of fetal and maternal blood. But as the placenta matures, the placental barrier degenerates somewhat. This provides for passage of more nutrients and immunoglobulin from the mother, and for passage of fetal blood cells to the maternal circulation.
7) **As chorionic villi invade and attach to the uterus, remnants of the decidua form the placental septa**. These septa separate incompletely into placental cotyledons.
   a) Each cotyledon consists of the main stem of a chorionic villus and all its branches.
   b) There are 15-30 cotyledons.
   c) Septa restrict the exchange of blood between the cotyledons; a problem in one cotyledon remains a localized problem.
8) **Amnion is the inner (closest to fetus) portion of the fetal membranes that surrounds the fetus.** By the end of the third month, it is in contact with the chorion, forming the amniochorionic sac.

9) **The chorion is formed from the trophoblast (outer layer of blastocyst)**
    a) Chorionic villi develop from it. It fuses with the amnion and is the outer portion of the amniochorionic sac.
10) The smooth, shiny portion of the placenta is the ***fetal side ("Shiny Schultz")***.
11) The rougher appearing portion of the placenta is the ***maternal side ("Dirty Duncan").***
12) **Hormones synthesized in the placenta**
    a) Human chorionic gonadotropin (hCG)
    b) Human placental lactogen (hPL)
    c) Estrogen
    d) Progesterone
    e) Others (there are many): corticotrophin, human chorionic thyrotropin, melanocyte stimulating hormone, β-endorphin, β-lipoprotein, corticotrophin-releasing hormones, gastrin, vasoactive intestinal peptide…
13) **Mechanisms by which the placenta transfers materials**
    a) Simple diffusion; e.g., water, electrolytes, oxygen, carbon dioxide, fatty acid, fat soluble vitamins, many medications
    b) Facilitated diffusion; e.g., glucose
    c) Active transport; e.g., amino acids, water-soluble vitamins, calcium, iron, iodine
    d) Pinocytosis (engulfing liquid molecule), endocytosis (engulfing solid molecule); e.g., globulins, phospholipids, lipoproteins, viruses
    e) Bulk flow; e.g., water, electrolytes
    f) Accidental capillary breaks: intact blood cells
    g) Independent movement: maternal leukocytes, pathogens (e.g., *T pallidum*)
14) **Placental transport increases as gestation progresses**

B. Diagnosis of pregnancy

1. Presumptive, probable and positive indicators of pregnancy

13 PRESUMPTIVE SIGNS

- Missed menses
- Fatigue
- Nausea
- Vomiting
  - ↑ urination
  - ↑ BBT
  - ↑ Salivation
- Colostrum
- Quickening
- Breast Changes
- Skin Changes
- Chadwick's Sign
- Thinks she's pregnant

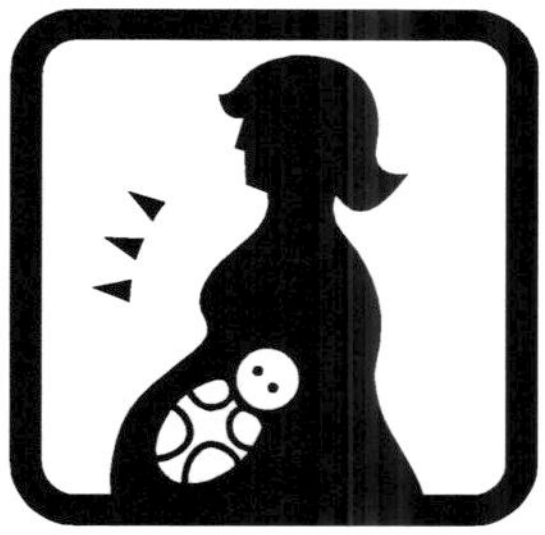

9 PROBABLE SIGNS

- Pregnancy test
- Hegar's sign
- Goddell's sign
- Piskacek's sign
- Ballotment
- Large uterus
- Enlarged abdomen
- Palpation of fetus
- Braxton-Hicks contractions

3 POSITIVE SIGNS

- ❖ Fetal heart tones
- ❖ Fetal movement felt by examiner
- ❖ Ultrasound showing intrauterine pregnancy

2. Laboratory tests

a. All pregnancy tests detect hCG (or a subunit) by an antibody to the hCG molecule or the beta subunit

1) Agglutination inhibition

a) In pregnancy, no agglutination occurs because the antibody has been complexed with the hCG in the woman's urine and is unavailable.

b) Agglutination (clumping of particles) occurs if hCG is absent (not pregnant)

c) Most tests positive 1 week after missed menses

d) Sensitivity ranges from 250 to 3000 mIU/ml of hCG

2) **ELISA (Enzyme-linked immunosorbent assay)**

a) Uses enzymes to detect hCG beta subunits

b) Commonly used for in-office or in-clinic testing. Sensitive to levels of hCG in the 25-50 mIU/mL range; performed in < 1 hr.

3) Immunochromatography with ELISA (beta specific)

a) New pregnancy test kits - convenient plastic device for urine or serum samples.

b) Antibody reaction with hCG results in color change and/or appearance of a symbol in the "window".

c) Results in < 10 minutes; can be positive any time from 1 week postconception to the time of expected menses.

d) Sensitive to levels in urine as low as 25-50 mIU/mL of hCG.

4) Radioimmunoassays

a) Used to accurately quantitate serum levels of hCG.

b) **Most sensitive test available.** Test targets beta subunit

c) Must be done in laboratories

d) ***Quantitative beta hCG can be positive several days before menses is delayed.***

e) Used to rule out early pregnancy prior to invasive procedures or x-rays.

(1) Also used to aid in dx of abnormal gestations by watching the rate hCG rises. Serum levels as low as 2 to 4 mIU/mL can be detected

3. Ultrasound

a. *Accuracy of ultrasound for dating pregnancy*

Structure measured	Gestational age (weeks)	Accuracy
Gestational sac	4-5	± 5 days
Crown-rump length	6-12	± 3-5 days
Femur length (FL)	14-26	± 7-11 days
Biparietal diameter (BPD)	14-26	± 10 days
Abdominal circumference (AC)	14-26	± 20 days
FL, BPD, AC	>26	± 14-21 days

4. Counseling regarding pregnancy options

a. Three options

1) Continue pregnancy and keep the baby

2) Continue pregnancy and give the baby up for adoption

3) Terminate the pregnancy (abortion)

b. Counseling techniques

1) Do not make assumptions, do not make judgmental statements, and do not disparage a woman as she considers the alternatives

2) Ask her what she thinks about being pregnant

3) Based on answer, provide information about prenatal care, adoption, or abortion

4) If you choose not to provide abortion counseling, relay this to the woman who desires it and refer her to someone who can provide safe, unbiased and effective counseling.

5) *Contraceptive Technology 18th ed.* (CT) recommends regarding as **urgent** any request by a woman for pregnancy confirmation, and recommends providing her with information about all options, with prompt referral if she is considering abortion.

c. Legal status of abortion

1) *Roe v. Wade* (1973) is the most commonly cited US Supreme Court decision that legalized elective termination of pregnancy in all states (CT also refers to *Doe v. Bolton*, 1973).
   - In the first trimester of pregnancy, the decision regarding abortion is between the pregnant woman and her physician
   - In the second trimester of pregnancy, each state may regulate abortion procedures with respect to the pregnant woman's health
   - In the third trimester of pregnancy, states may limit or prohibit abortion; states may not impose restrictions that interfere with the life or health of the pregnant woman

2) Abortion procedures (procedures are similar whether the abortion is elective or indicated, as for missed abortion)
   a) Surgical procedures
      - Menstrual extraction at 5-8 weeks gestation
      - Dilation and suction curettage at < 14 weeks gestation
      - Dilation and curettage (D&C) with a metal curette at <14 weeks gestation
      - Dilation and evacuation (D&E) with suction and/or surgical instruments after 16 weeks gestation
      - Hysterectomy or hysterotomy
      - Dilation is accomplished by insertion of products (e.g., laminaria) that absorb fluids, swell, and thereby soften and open the cervix, or by administration of prostaglandins that ripen the cervix (e.g., misoprostol).

   b) Medical techniques: before 8-9 weeks gestation (63 days following LMP)
      - Methotrexate is a folic acid inhibitor and causes cell death in the rapidly proliferating tissues of the embryo.
      - Misoprostol (Cytotec®) is synthetic prostaglandin E1; it causes contractions that expel uterine contents
      - Mifepristone (RU 486) is an antiprogesterone agent that is given with misoprostol

   c) Instillation procedures later in pregnancy involve injection of a hyperosmotic substance into the uterus to induce labor and stillbirth.

3) Abortions after the first trimester carry a higher maternal morbidity and mortality risk, including hemorrhage, infection, coagulopathies, and cervical or uterine damage that might affect future fertility.

d. ACNM position regarding reproductive choice:

- Every woman has the right to make reproductive choices
- Every woman has the right to factual, unbiased information about reproductive choices in order to make an informed decision;
- Women with limited means should have access to financial resources for their reproductive choices.

C. Collection of data base for pregnancy

1. Historical data

a. Menstrual history

1) Age at menarche

2) First day of last NORMAL menstrual period

3) Frequency and duration of menses

4) Does she know when she conceived?

TPAL

Term pregnancies
Premature births
Abortions (spontaneous or elective)
Live births

b. Contraceptive history

c. Obstetric history

1) Past pregnancies stories

2) TPAL system

T = number of term pregnancies

P = number of pre-term pregnancies

A = number of abortions (spontaneous, induced)

L = number of children living

The entire reproductive history cannot be reflected in the TPAL system. Multiple pregnancies count as one pregnancy, and are indicated by the number of living children. The route of birth is not evident from the TPAL system.

3) Type of delivery: Spontaneous, Cesarean Section (CS), forcep, vacuum, etc

4) Complications, e.g., gestational diabetes, hypertension, etc.

d. Medical-Surgical history

e. Sexual history

f. Abuse history (physical, emotional, sexual)

g. Family history

1) Genetic disorders

2) Medical-surgical diseases

h. Social history

i. Exercise and nutrition history

j. Immunizations

k. Medication use

l. Reaction to pregnancy – how does she feel about it?

2. Exposures and habits

a. Exercise

b. Nutritional habits, restrictions (vegetarian, cultural or religious restrictions)

c. Type of work

d. Hobbies, sports

e. Radiation exposure

f. Occupational exposure

g. Herbal or other complementary therapies used

h. Infection exposure (Toxoplasmosis, CMV, Rubella, STD, TB etc)

i. Alcohol, illicit drug, tobacco, or caffeine use

j. Use of prescription and over the counter drugs (including folic acid)

FDA Pregnancy Categories

Category A	Adequate studies in pregnant women have failed to show a risk to the fetus in the first trimester and there is no evidence of risk in later trimesters.
Category B	Animal studies have failed to show a risk to the fetus but there are no adequate studies in pregnant women: or animal studies have shown an adverse effect but human studies have not shown a risk to the fetus in the first trimester and there is no evidence of risk in later trimesters.
Category C	Animal studies have shown an adverse effect on the fetus but there are no adequate studies in humans, but the benefits may outweigh the risks; or there are no animal studies and no adequate human studies.
Category D	Positive evidence of human fetal risk but the benefits may outweigh the risks.
Category X	Animal or human studies have shown fetal abnormalities or toxicity, and the risk outweighs the benefits.

3. Genetics risks, counseling and/or referral

a. Ethnicity (Eastern European Jewish, Mediterranean, African, Caucasian)

b. Maternal and paternal age

c. Family history of genetic disorders

d. Any previous genetic screening/testing (e.g. Tay-Sachs, sickle cell, cystic fibrosis)

e. Any previous genetic counseling

4. Physical Examination

a. Height, weight, vital signs

1) Complete physical exam

b. Pelvic examination

1) To ascertain uterine size and estimate gestational age

c. Clinical pelvimetry

1) To estimate pelvic size

2) Based on the **three planes of the true pelvis**:

- The inlet, the midplane, and the outlet

3) Critical diameters of each plane:

a) Inlet: anterior-posterior, transverse

b) Midplane: anterior-posterior, transverse, posterior-sagittal

c) Outlet: anterior-posterior, transverse, posterior-sagittal

4) Measurements

- **Bituberous diameter**: Between ischial tuberosities. Gynecoid ≥8 cm.
- **Diagonal conjugate:** Only anterior-posterior diameter that can be measured directly. Gynecoid >12 cm.
- **Interspinous (Bispinous) diameter:** The distance between the ischial spines. Gynecoid 10 cm.
  - ***Smallest diameter of the pelvis***
- **Ischial spines**: Prominent, blunt, or encroaching
- **Pubic arch:** Gynecoid ≥90° (2-3 fingerbreadths)
- **Sacrosciatic notch:** Gynecoid 2-3 fingerbreadths
- **Sacrum:** Straight, concave, convex. Gynecoid: concave.
- **Coccyx:** mobile, fixed, shape. Gynecoid: mobile.
- **Sidewalls:** Straight, convergent, divergent. Gynecoid: straight.

Superior view of pelvis (not necessarily Gynecoid)

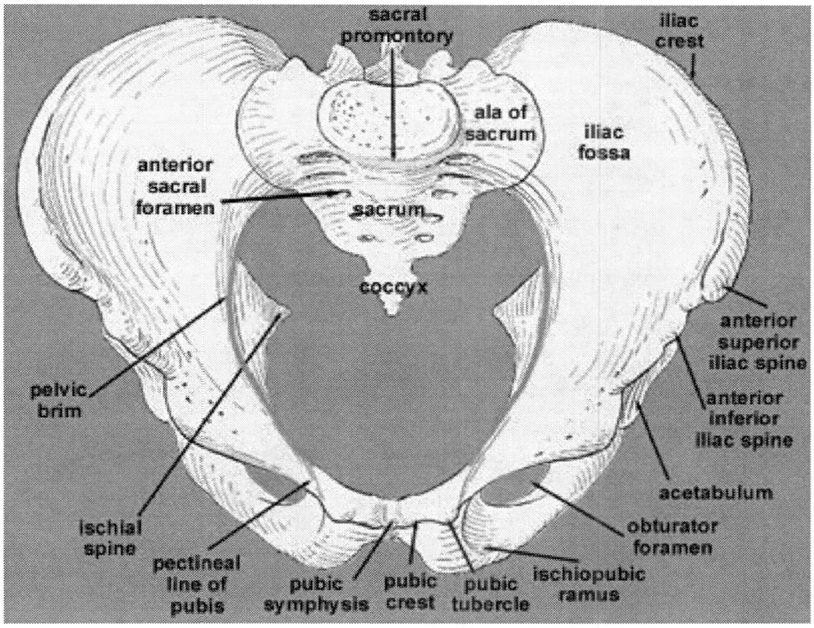

Lateral view of pelvis

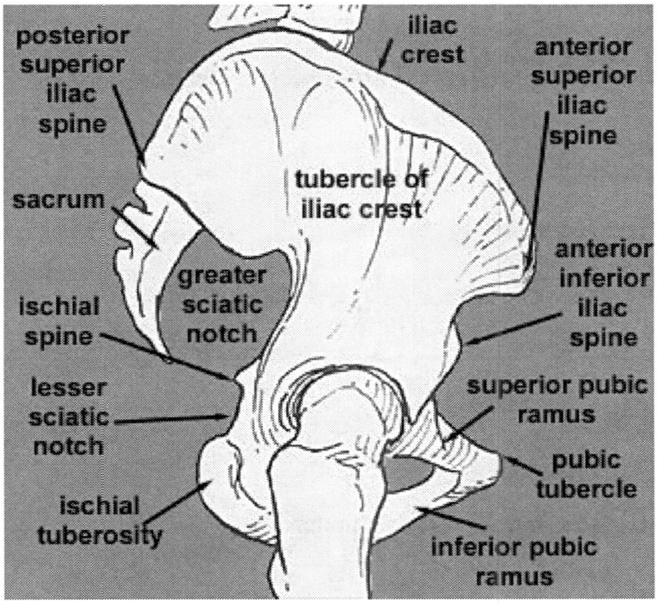

http://mywebpages.comcast.net/wnor/pelvis.htm

5) **Types of pelvis**

- Android
- Anthropoid
- Gynecoid
- Platypelloid

6) Effect of pelvic type on labor (per Oxorn-Foote)

Gynecoid: *Also called the female pelvis*

- Engages in transverse or oblique diameter
- Slight asynclitism
- Good flexion
- Early and complete internal rotation
- Spontaneous delivery
- Wide pubic arch decreases perineal tears

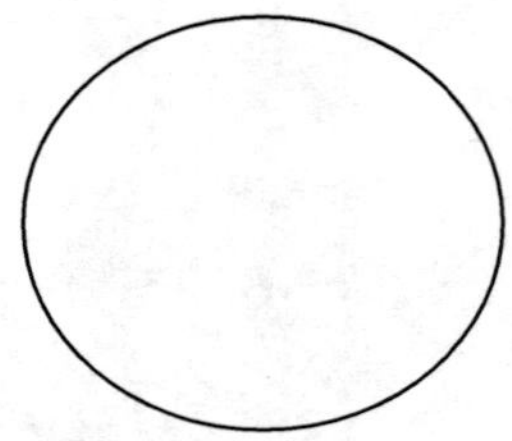

Android: Also called the male pelvis

- Engages in transverse or posterior diameter
- Asynclitism
- Extreme molding
- Deep transverse arrest common
- Arrest as OP with failure of rotation
- Frequent forceps delivery
- Narrow pubic arch increases perineal tears

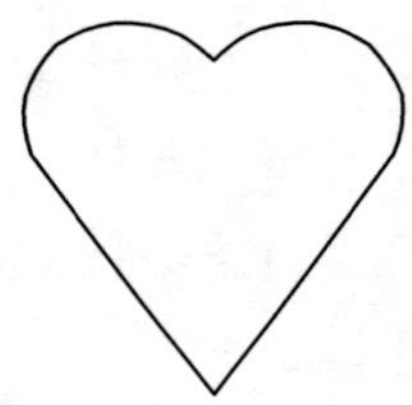

Anthropoid

- Engages in AP or oblique
- OP common
- Adequate for vaginal delivery

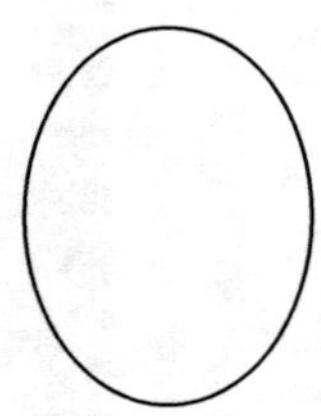

Platypelloid

- Short AP diameter
- Engages in transverse diameter
- Marked asynclitism
- Delay at inlet
- Increased chance of C/S

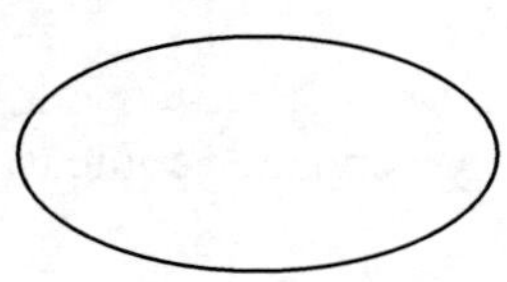

	Gynecoid	Android	Anthropoid	Platypelloid
INLET				
Shape	Round or slightly transverse oval	Heart shape	Long AP oval	Transverse oval
AP diameter	Adequate	Adequate	Long	Short
Transverse dia.	Adequate	Adequate	Short, but Adequate	Long
Post. Segment	Broad, deep	Shallow; sacral promontory indents the inlet	Deep	Shallow
Ant. Segment	Well rounded	Narrow, sharply angulated	Deep	Shallow
MIDPELVIS				
AP diameter	Adequate	Reduced	Long	Short
Transverse dia.	Adequate	Reduced	Adequate	Wide
Sacrum	Wide, deep curve; short, slopes back	Flat, long, inclined forward narrow, heavy	Narrow, long inclined backward	Wide, deep, sharply angled
Sidewalls	Parallel, straight	Convergent	Straight	Parallel
Ischial spines	Blunt	Prominent	Variable	Variable
Sacrosciatic notch	Wide; short	Narrow; long high arch	Wide	Short
Capacity	Adequate	Reduced in all diameters	Adequate	Reduced
OUTLET				
AP diameter	Long	Short	Long	Short
Bituberous dia.	Adequate	Narrow	Adequate	Wide
Pubic Arch	Wide, round	Narrow, deep	Long, relatively narrow	Very wide
Capacity	Adequate	Reduced	Adequate	Inadequate

Adapted Caldwell Classification. In Oxorn. Oxorn-Foote Human labor and birth. (5th Edition).1986, p34-38.

D. Calculation of current gestational age and estimated date of birth

1. Purpose of dating pregnancy

a. Allows for appropriate prenatal screening and management

b. Guides management of complications, including desire or indication for termination

2. Length of pregnancy

a. ***Naegele's Rule***: 1st day of LNMP, minus 3 months, plus 7 days, plus one year (280 days)

1) Caveat: based on a 28 day cycle with ovulation on day 14. Longer cycles will result in a later estimated date of delivery (EDD, also referred to as estimated date of birth EDB, or estimated date of confinement EDC); shorter cycles will result in earlier EDD.

2) Gestational wheels and electronic programs may vary in calculation of EDD. Everyone in a practice should use the same wheel and agree as to how it will be used. For example, EDD may be based on Naegele's rule and when calculating gestational age the 40 week arrow would be placed on the EDD. Go to the current date to determine gestational age.

3. Trimester definitions

General Convention		(Williams Obstetrics)
First Trimester	1-12 weeks (12 wks.)	1-14 weeks
Second Trimester	13-27 wks. (15 wks.)	15-28 weeks
Third Trimester	28-40 wks. (13 wks.)	29-42 weeks

METHODS for DATING PREGNANCY

Most accurate: 5 day to 2 week margin of error. 90% of women with due dates based on these criteria will birth within the above range.

1. **LMP which is normal, regular, and certain. **
2. Basal body temperature with coital record, showing sustained temperature elevation.
3. Ultrasound between 7 and 10 weeks of menstrual age, using crown-rump length to calculate gestational age.
4. Serum hCG levels <10,000 on two separate occasions one week apart, rising appropriately.
5. Urine pregnancy testing, which may initially be negative, but becomes positive as soon as detectable levels of hCG are present in maternal urine. Timing will vary according to the type of urine test used.
6. Two ultrasounds <26 weeks gestational age, which estimate dates of birth within 2.6 weeks of each other. Use the EDB (estimated date of birth) based upon the earlier ultrasound.

4. **Least accurate methods for dating pregnancy (≥3 week margin of error)**
    a. Ultrasound after 28 weeks
    b. First fetal heart tones (FHT) with doppler (8-12 weeks); fetoscope (16-21 weeks)
    c. Quickening
    d. Signs and symptoms of pregnancy
    e. Lightening occurs approximately 2 weeks before the onset of labor (nullipara)
5. **Pregnancy test**
    a. Reliable test can be positive 7-10 days after conception. If there were a negative test followed by a positive test, a range of minimum to maximum gestational age can be determined.
6. **Clinical landmarks**
    a. **Fetal heart tones by doppler** are present by 10-12 weeks gestational age
    b. **FHT by fetoscope** are present by 18-21 weeks EGA
    c. **Fundal height** should be approx. the same number in centimeters (+/-_2-3) as number of weeks gestation .(Between 18 and 32 weeks depending on the study)
    d. **Other fundal landmarks**
        1) Uterus palpable at pubis about 12 weeks.
        2) Uterus halfway between pubis and umbilicus at about 16 weeks
        3) Uterus 1 fingerbreadth below or at umbilicus at about 20 weeks

> **4** is the normal pH of the vagina.
> **40** weeks is the normal gestation period.
> **400** oocytes released between menarche and menopause.
> **400,000** oocytes present at puberty.
> **28** days in a normal menstrual cycle.
> **280** days (from last normal menstrual period) in a normal gestation period.

E. Baseline laboratory tests (order/obtain/interpret)

1. **Serum tests**
    a. Initial screening serum laboratory tests for all women
        1) **Hemoglobin (Hb) or hematocrit (Hct)**
            a) Normal ranges
            First and third trimester: Hb ≥11.0 g/dL; Hct ≥33%
            Second trimester: Hb >10.5 g/dL; Hct >32%
            b) Hb or Hct is repeated in the 3rd trimester to assess need for iron therapy

2) **Blood type and Rh status**
   a) Normal: A positive or negative, B positive or negative, O positive or negative, AB positive or negative
3) **RBC antibody screen (ABS)**
   a) Identifies antibodies dangerous to fetus, e.g., Kell, Duffy, anti-D.
   b) 2% of hemolytic disease in newborns results from rare red blood cell antigens
   c) Rh-negative woman with a positive antibody screen (anti-D or other antibody causing severe hemolytic disease of the newborn) should be referred
   d) ***A repeat antibody screen should be done for Rh negative women at 26-28 weeks.***
   e) Some antibodies do not usually cause hemolytic disease but may be of concern if the woman needs a transfusion, e.g., Lewis
4) **Syphilis test**
   a) **VDRL or RPR:** Normal is non-reactive.
   b) If reactive, a titer will be reported. Treponema -specific testing is necessary to rule out false positives: FTA-ABS or MHA-TP
   c) RPR is repeated in 3rd trimester if at risk
5) **HIV**
   a) ELISA
   b) Perinatal acquisition of HIV associated with morbidity and mortality
   c) CDC recommends all women be counseled for HIV testing and antiviral therapy during pregnancy
   d) If HIV +, Cesarean delivery should be anticipated in most settings
6) **Rubella immunity**
   a) ***Most devastating effects occur when rubella infection in first trimester***
   b) After 16 weeks gestation, teratogenic effects are small
   c) Do not immunize during pregnancy or within 1 month of conception
   d) Non-immune women should be vaccinated after delivery; breast feeding is not a contraindication
7) **Hepatitis B surface antigen (HBsAg)**
   a) CDC recommends hepatitis B vaccine for individuals at risk
   b) **Can initiate vaccinations antepartum**
8) **Screening of serum for women at risk**
   a) Toxoplasmosis
   b) Hemoglobinopathies
   c) Tay-Sachs, cystic fibrosis, coagulopathies, or other genetic defects

d) Varicella

e) Illicit drug screen

f) Thyroid stimulating hormone

9) Interval pregnancy serum assessments

a) Glucose screening tests

(1) **Random glucose: If ≥ 130mg/dl, order 1 hour glucose tolerance test (GTT)**

(2) 1 Hour glucose challenge test (GCT): administer 50 g glucose oral load between 24-28 weeks or earlier for high risk women

(a) Last meal and time of day irrelevant

(b) Serum test 1 hour after administration

(c) ≥140 mg/dL requires diagnostic testing (i.e., 3 hour glucose tolerance test)

(d) Carpenter & Coustan suggested using 130 mg/dL as cut off for GCT

(e) ACOG suggests if 1 hour screen is ≥ 200 mg/dL, treat as gestational diabetic

(f) Glucose testing with jelly beans and other sources of glucose is not standardized and not recommended by most authors and panels

(g) Women at risk should be tested at the first prenatal visit and again at 32 weeks gestation. Risk factors are obesity, history of gestational diabetes or macrosomic infant, stillbirth, strong family history of diabetes, etc

(3) **3 Hour GTT:** administer 100-g oral glucose load

Two or more of the following values must be exceeded for diagnosis of gestational diabetes (Plasma levels)—

National Diabetes Data Group values (listed here) are most often used:

Fasting ≥ 105mg/dL
1 hour ≥ 190mg/dL
2 hour ≥ 165mg/dL
3 hour ≥ 145mg/dL

(4) **Carpenter & Coustan levels are acceptable**, but not used as widely

Fasting ≥ 95mg/dL
1 hour ≥ 180mg/dL
2 hour ≥ 155mg/dL
3 hour ≥ 140mg/dL

(5) WHO recommends the 75 g 2 hour GTT; used more in Europe than U.S.
   (a) Most, including ACOG, do not recommend universal diabetes serum screening. HOWEVER, they acknowledge that it may be difficult in a busy practice to determine who does not need to be screened since the criteria are so broad
   (b) Criteria for diabetic screening in pregnancy: age >25 years, obesity, history of gestational diabetes, history of macrosomic infant or stillbirth, high risk populations (African American, Hispanic, Native Americans, Pacific Islanders)

b) Screening for neural tube defects: Maternal Serum Alpha Fetoprotein (MSAFP)

(1) AFP is produced by fetal liver and excreted in urine. It passes into the maternal circulation.
(2) In some fetal deviations, abnormal amounts of AFP are produced; e.g., **neural tube defects, Down Syndrome, Trisomy 18,**
(3) Usually tested 15-19 weeks (labs vary in reference ranges – may be able to test as early as 13weeks and as late as 22 weeks; know your lab's parameters). Earlier testing is better to give parents time for decision making if result is abnormal.
(4) Note: AFP is not elevated in skin-covered lesions or closed neural tube defects. Encephalocele, for example, may be missed. Many other conditions are associated with abnormally elevated MSAFP levels; most of them will be detected with follow-up ultrasound (e.g., gastroschisis, fetal demise). DeCherney recommends amniotic fluid AFP and acetylcholinesterase testing if the level remains elevated and no cause is found.
(5) **Interpretation:**
   (a) Value > 2.5 multiples of the median (MoM) elevated and high-resolution ultrasound is recommended.
   (b) Value <.5 MoM indicates need for further testing (confirm gestational age, rule out Down syndrome)
   (c) Many labs will not report MoM, but report risk of defect, e.g., risk of Down is 1:1,000, so tests are never absolutely positive or negative. When the risk of Down is 1:250 or higher, follow-up is recommended.

- ➢ 1:250 is the cutoff because it approximates the risk of pregnancy loss with amniocentesis, which is the followup diagnostic test

(6) Factors that influence test results

(a) Discrepancy of gestation age (GA): if GA is longer than estimated, MSAFP is higher than expected; if GA is lower than estimated, MSAFP is lower than expected. *Most common reason for discrepancies.*

(b) Obesity – decreased

(c) Low maternal weight – increased

(d) Black race – slight increase

(e) Insulin dependent diabetic – decreased

(f) Multiple gestation – increased

(g) Down syndrome – decreased

c) **Multiple Markers Screens**

(1) ***Triple: MSAFP, β hCG, unconjugated Estriol (uE_3)***

(a) MSAFP is low in Down syndrome, high in open neural tube defects and abdominal wall defects.

(b) β hCG is high in Down syndrome

(c) Estriol is low in Down syndrome

(2) ***Quadruple ("Quad"): MSAFP, hCG, uE_3, inhibin A***

(a) Inhibin A is elevated in Down syndrome

(b) Most accurate <u>second</u> trimester screen for Down

(3) Other screening tests for Down

(a) First trimester screening: ultrasound measurement of nuchal translucency thickness at 10 weeks combined with Pregnancy Associated Plasma Protein A (PAPP-A). PAPP-A is low in Down syndrome

(b) Combining first and second trimester screening tests provides best overall non invasive screening for Down syndrome.

(c) Earlier testing gives mother more choices and safer alternatives for pregnancy termination if desired.

(d) Ultrasonographer must be qualified.

d) CBC

(1)**Anemia in pregnancy is usually iron deficiency:** ***RBCs*** are

(a) Microcytic (low MCV) and

(b) Hypochromic (low MCH)

(2)**Categories of anemia based on RBC indices**

(a) ***Microcytic anemia (MCV < 80 fL): Suspect iron deficiency***

(b) ***Macrocytic anemia (MCV > 95 fL): Suspect B_{12} or folate deficiency***

(c) ***Normocytic anemia (MCV 81-94 fL): Underproduction - suspect chronic disease, bone marrow failure***

(3) White blood count (WBC) is normally 4K to 11K/μL.

(4) ***Platelet count should be above 150,000 per ml***

2. Pap smear and cultures

a. Initial non-serum screening laboratory tests for all women

1) Urine dipstick for protein, glucose, nitrites; urine culture

2) Gonorrhea culture or DNA probe

3) Chlamydia screen for women at risk, includes all women <25 years age

4) Pap smear

b. Screening for women at risk or part of at risk population

1) Tuberculin skin test- PPD

a) Screen women from countries with high TB prevalence rate, as well as women associated with high-risk groups

2) Herpes simplex - culture if history of lesions or suspicious lesion

3) Asymptomatic bacteriuria (ASB), urinary tract infection (UTI)

a) Nitrites by dipstick

(1) Measures conversion of nitrate to nitrite

(2) Valid for gram negative bacteria only

(3) **+nitrite correlates with infected urine 90% of the time**

(4) False negative rate of 50%

(5) **+nitrites can be treated for UTI**

b) Urine culture

(1) Urine culture often performed routinely at initial prenatal visit

(2) Colony count of 100,000 is often used as criteria for diagnosis

(3) Urine culture that reports "mixed gram positive" growth: specimen probably contaminated with vaginal secretions and should be repeated, confirming instructions for clean catch

(4) Any colony count group B streptococcus should be treated and the woman is considered GBS positive; she is a candidate for Intrapartum antibiotic prophylaxis.

4) **Group B Streptococcus (GBS): CDC recommendations**
   a) ***GBS culture on all pregnant women at 35-37 weeks gestation***
      (1) Unless previous pregnancy resulted in affected child (woman will be treated intrapartum regardless of culture results)
      (2) Unless previous urine culture positive for GBS any time in pregnancy (woman will be treated intrapartum)
   b) ***Specimen obtained from lower (distal) vagina and anorectum***
   c) Woman may collect specimen herself
   d) Women planning elective cesarean should be tested but will not have IP prophylaxis
   e) See Chapter III Intrapartum for complete discussion of intrapartum prophylaxis criteria

   Source: http://www.cdc.gov/mmwr/PDF/RR/RR5111.pdf

c. **Pap smears/cervical cytology**
   1) Invasive cervical cancer is rare in pregnancy
   2) Approximately 5% of pregnant women will have abnormal Pap test
   3) Challenges of sampling in pregnancy
      a) Due to increase in cervical volume from hypertrophy of stroma, there is a larger area to sample
      b) Endocervical mucus becomes thick and tenacious; may diminish visibility and lead to scant cellularity
      c) Treat cervicovaginal infections before obtaining Pap smear
   4) Sampling devices
      a) **Spatula:** ectocervix: 360 degree rotation of entire cervix
         plus
      b) **Endocervical brush**: 180 degree rotation in endocervix
         or
      c) **Combined endocervical/ectocervical** "broom" device: 5 360 degree rotations around cervix
      d) Traditional slide or liquid-based technique may be used.
   5) ***Results and recommendations in pregnancy using Bethesda System (2001)***
      a) **ASC-US (atypical squamous cells of undetermined significance)**
         (1) Human papillomavirus (HPV) negative: Repeat postpartum/annual visit
         (2) HPV positive: Colposcopy

b) ASC-H (atypical squamous cells, cannot exclude HSIL)

(1) Colposcopy

c) LSIL (LGSIL; low grade squamous intraepithelial lesion)

(1) Previously designated mild dysplasia, CIN 1

(2) May repeat Pap in 6 & 12 months, get HPV type, or colposcopy in adolescent

d) HSIL (HGSIL; high grade squamous intraepithelial lesion)

(1) Previously called moderate or severe dysplasia, CIN 2 or CIN 3 (Carcinoma in situ, CIS)

(2) Refer for colposcopy

e) AGC (Atypical glandular cells)

(1) Abnormal endocervical or endometrial cells

(2) Refer for colposcopy

F. Management of pregnancy

1. Interval assessments to evaluate status of pregnancy

According to *Caring for Our Future: The Content of Prenatal Care*

Visit Schedule

Nullipara Prenatal Visit	Timing	Multipara Prenatal Visit	Timing
First	6-8 Weeks	First	6-8 weeks
Second	Within 4 weeks of 1st	Second	14-16 weeks
Third	14-16 weeks	Third	24-28 weeks
Fourth	24-28 weeks	Fourth	32 weeks
Fifth	32 weeks	Fifth	35 weeks
Sixth	36 weeks	Sixth	39 weeks
Seventh	38 weeks	Seventh	41 weeks
Eight	40 weeks		
Ninth	41 weeks		

From Public Health Service Expert Panel on the Content of Prenatal Care. (1989). Caring for our Future: The content of prenatal care. Washington, D.C. Department of Health and Human Services (NIH Publication No. 90-3182).

✓ **First pregnancy visit**

> **Midwifery Message**
> Remember the best first prenatal visit is the one that is conducted preconceptionally—(12 months or less before conception) when changes in health habits, diagnosis and treatment of conditions etc. can be made—and folic acid started.

1) History
    - Menstrual
    - Obstetric
    - Contraceptive
    - Sexual
    - Infection
    - Family and genetic
    - Medical/surgical
    - Nutrition
    - Smoking
    - Alcohol use
    - Mental illness/status
    - Drug use (including folic acid)
    - Physical activity
    - Social support
    - Stress levels
    - Physical abuse
    - Exposure to teratogens

2) Physical examination

a) Complete physical exam, with special attention to:
    - Blood pressure/pulse
    - Height/weight
    - Body mass index (BMI)
    - Pelvic examination/clinical pelvimetry/uterine size, dating, pathology
    - Breast examination

b) Laboratory tests (see Section E, baseline laboratory tests)

c) Health promotion activities
    - Nutrition counseling
    - Avoidance of teratogens
    - Safer sex
    - Physiologic and emotional changes in pregnancy
    - Sexuality
    - Fetal growth and development
    - Self-help strategies for discomforts
    - Early pregnancy classes
    - Preparation for screening and diagnostic tests
    - Content and timing of prenatal visits
    - Need to report danger signs

- ✓ **Second pregnancy visit (within 4 weeks of first visit)**
  1) In person contact with nulliparous women
  2) May contact parous women by phone

     Interval history
     - Nausea, vomiting
     - Vaginal bleeding, etc
     - Other discomforts of pregnancy
     - Psychosocial adaptation
  3) Review of laboratory results
  4) Counseling to promote and support healthful behaviors
  5) General knowledge of pregnancy and parenting
  6) Information on proposed care
- ✓ **Third pregnancy visit (14-16 weeks): 2nd visit for parous women**
  1) Interval history
     - Nausea, vomiting, other discomforts of pregnancy
     - Vaginal bleeding
  2) Psychosocial factors
  3) Partial physical exam
     - Auscultation of FHR (doppler)
     - Fundal height
     - Weight
     - Blood pressure
  4) Laboratory tests
     - Offer MSAFP or triple screen
  5) Counseling to promote and support healthful behaviors
  6) General knowledge of pregnancy and parenting
  7) Information on proposed care
- ✓ **Fourth pregnancy visit (24-28 weeks): 3rd visit for parous women**
  1) Interval history
     - Fetal movement
     - General health
     - Nutrition
     - Discomforts of pregnancy
     - Psychosocial adaptation

2) Partial physical exam
    - Auscultation of FHR (Doppler or fetoscope)
    - Fundal height
    - Weight
    - Blood pressure
3) Laboratory tests
    - Hemoglobin or Hematocrit
    - Glucose screen for diabetes
    - Antibody screen for Rh negative women with negative ABS
        - RhIG at 28-30 weeks if negative ABS
4) Counseling to promote and support healthful behaviors
5) General knowledge of pregnancy and parenting
    - Promotion of breastfeeding and other newborn care issues e.g., pediatrician, circumcision
    - Encourage prepared childbirth classes
    - Preterm labor information
6) Information on proposed care

✓ **Fifth pregnancy visit (32 weeks): 4th visit for parous women**

1) Interval history - same as 24-28 weeks
2) Partial physical exam – same as 24-28 weeks
3) Counseling to promote and support healthful behaviors
4) General knowledge of pregnancy and parenting
    - Including infant car seat use
5) Information on proposed care

✓ **Sixth pregnancy visit (36 weeks): 5th visit for parous women**

1) Interval history – same as 24-28 weeks
2) Partial physical exam – same as 32 weeks
    - Add: Fetal lie, presentation, descent
3) GBS culture
4) Counseling to promote and support healthful behaviors
5) General knowledge of pregnancy and parenting
    - Include signs and symptoms of labor
6) Information on proposed care
    - Include preparation for labor and birth
    - Birth plan
    - When to call, where to go in labor

✓ **Seventh pregnancy visit: 6th visit for parous women**

- Nullipara – 38 weeks
- Multipara – 39 weeks

1) Interval history - same as 24-28 gestational weeks
2) Partial physical exam – same as 36 weeks
    - Including fetal lie, presentation, descent
3) Counseling to promote and support healthful behaviors
4) General knowledge of pregnancy and parenting
    - Including postpartum activity, family planning
    - Newborn care
    - Family roles and adjustments
5) Information on proposed care

✓ **Eighth pregnancy visit (40 weeks) for nulliparous women**

1) Interval history, same as before, but add
    - Fetal movement counts
    - Signs and symptoms of labor
2) Partial physical –same as 38 weeks
3) Counseling to promote and support healthful behaviors
4) General knowledge of pregnancy and parenting
5) Information on proposed care
    - Including preparation for postterm tests

✓ **Ninth pregnancy visit (41 weeks): 7th visit for parous women**

1) Interval history
2) Partial physical – same as 40 weeks, but add:
    - Cervical examination
3) Counseling to promote and support healthful behaviors
4) General knowledge of pregnancy and parenting
5) Information on proposed care
    - Including antenatal testing
    - Preparation for possible induction

a. Vital signs/urine

1) Vital signs

a) Height (short stature may be an indicator of a genetic disorder)

b) Weight: recommend weight gain for pregnancy based on BMI

c) Blood pressure normally declines slightly after 8th gestational week and stays down through 2nd trimester; rises toward prepregnant levels in third trimester

(1) Use appropriate cuff

(2) Arm greater than 35 cm around - use large cuff

(3) Sitting position, same arm each time

d) ***Pulse (If > 100 suspect hyperthyroidism)***

> **Remember**
> Baseline BP refers to preconception or first trimester -- After first trimester, no baseline BP is available

2) Urine testing

a) Routine dipstick testing for protein, glucose and nitrites is commonly performed during well prenatal visits, but is not universally recommended.

b) Routine urine culture and urinalysis for protein are recommended ***only at the initial visit*** by Williams Obstetrics 22nd ed. and Gabbe 4th ed., AHRQ (http://www.guideline.gov/summary/summary.aspx?doc_id=5702), and others.

b. Weight gain patterns

1) **Weight gain recommendations in pregnancy**

1990 Institute of Medicine recommendations were designed to decrease low birth weight (LBW):

BMI < 19.8	**28-40 pounds**
BMI 19.8 to 26.0	**25-35 pounds**
BMI 26 to 29	**15-25 pounds**
BMI >29	**15 pounds minimum**

2) In 2001 almost 1 in 3 women had weight gains outside recommended guidelines.

3) Wide range is compatible with good outcome in individual women

4) Short women should strive for gain in lower end of range

5) Pattern of weight gain is significant

a) Weight gain of early pregnancy is attributable to growth of maternal tissue and expanded blood volume

b) Weight gain of <10 pounds by 20 weeks: nutrition counseling

c) Weight gain <2 pounds/month or >6.5 pounds/month: diet counseling

6) Differential diagnoses associated with inadequate weight gain

a) Hyperemesis

b) Anorexia nervosa or bulimia

c) Hypermetabolic conditions

d) Malabsorption syndrome

7) Outcomes of pregnancies in obese women related to weight gain
   a) Williams Obstetrics 22nd ed. recommends no more than 15 pound weight gain for obese women
   b) Antepartum and intrapartum complications are highest for women who gain >44 pounds (e.g., fetal macrosomia)

8) Risks of being moderately overweight to obese
   a) Hypertension
   b) Preeclampsia
   c) Gestational diabetes
   d) Insulin treatment
   e) Urinary tract
   f) Macrosomia
   g) Cesarean section
   h) Shoulder dystocia
   i) Two-fold increased risk of neural tube defect, mostly spina bifida
   j) Late intrauterine fetal death

9) Complications associated with weight greater than 300 pounds
   a) Chronic hypertension
   b) Diabetes
   c) Cesarean for cephalopelvic disproportion
   d) Postpartum infection

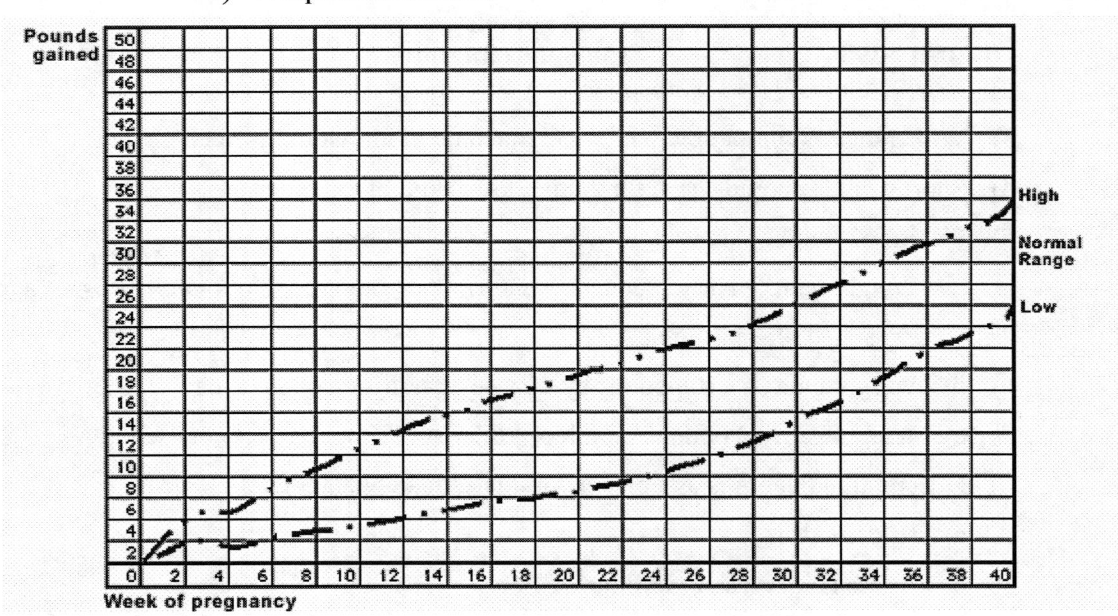

Approximate Average Weight Gain By BMI in Pounds

	BMI <19.8	BMI 19.8-26.0	BMI > 26.0
12 weeks	5	7-8	2-3
16 weeks	7.8	6-7	4-5
20 weeks	14	10	7
24 weeks	17	15	9-10
28 weeks	22	18-19	11-12
32 weeks	26	22	15
36 weeks	30	26	17-18
40 weeks	35	30	20

c. **Auscultation of the fetal heart (FHT)**

1) FHT can be heard with a Doppler at 10-12 week, occasionally earlier
2) If no FHTs by 13 weeks, confirm viability and gestational age with sonogram
3) **Check FHT each prenatal visit after 10 weeks**
4) **Auscultate with fetoscope between 18-21 weeks**
   a) Supports an EDD determined by LMP
   b) Document for dating validation
5) ***Baseline FHT rate should be 120-160 bpm***
6) Short periods of increased heart rate associated with fetal activity
7) **FHT best heard in upper abdominal quadrants may indicate breech position**

d. **Assessment of fetal movement (includes fetal movement counts): Fetal Kick Counts**

1) **Fetal movement**
   a) Fetal movements begin in 3rd month of pregnancy
   b) **Quickening** (mother's perception of fetal movement) approximately at 19 weeks in primigravida, 17 weeks in multipara
   c) Most fetuses move frequently
   d) A decrease in fetal movement can indicate fetal jeopardy
2) **Indications for fetal movement counting**
   a) Maternal medical conditions, including pregnancy complications
   b) Intrauterine growth restriction, oligohydramnios, polyhydramnios
   c) Multiple gestation
   d) Post term gestation
   e) Previous fetal demise
3) **Wide variety in methods**
   a) One example of fetal movement assessment: Instructions to mother
      (1) Begin counts at 38 weeks
      (2) Begin count one hour after a meal and count for one hour
      (3) If <4 movements, continue to count for additional hour
      (4) If fetal movement continues to be diminished, contact CNM

b) Some practices instruct all pregnant women in 3rd trimester to periodically observe fetal activity

c) Instruct mothers to count movements if/when she perceives a decrease in usual pattern

4) **Cardiff count-to-ten method:**

a) Woman counts fetal movement as she goes about the day, noting how long it takes to arrive at 10 movements

b) If unable to perceive 10 movements in 12 hours, report

5) Take seriously reports of absent or decreased fetal movements

6) Fetuses continue to move in labor

e. Assessment of fundal height

1) **First trimester:** Subjective assessment of uterine size per bimanual examination

- 8 gestational weeks – size of tennis ball
- 10 gestational weeks – size of orange
- 12 gestational weeks – size of grapefruit, fundus usually palpable above symphysis pubis if not retroflexed

2) **Second trimester**

- **13-18 weeks -- fundus in relation to umbilicus** (or measure with centimeter tape to document growth; not necessarily consistent with gestational age)
  - 16 weeks -- 3-4 fingerbreadths below umbilicus, or half way between pubis and umbilicus
  - 18 weeks -- 1-2 fingerbreadths below umbilicus
- **18-27 weeks – measure with centimeter tape**
  - Measurement in cm equals gestational age +/– 2-3 cm

3) **Third trimester**

- 28-32 weeks – measurement in centimeters equals gestational age +/– 2-3 cm
- 32 weeks to term – estimate fetal weight, measure for growth of approximately 1 cm per week
  - ➢ S>D consider multiple gestation, macrosomia, hydramnios
  - ➢ S<D consider intrauterine growth restriction, oligohydramnios
  - ➢ For significant deviations (>2-3 cm by same examiner), follow up with ultrasonography

4) Confounding factors of fundal height

a) Fetal descent into pelvis

b) Obesity

c) Malpresentation

d) Breech or transverse

e) Uterine fibroids

f) Amniotic fluid volume

g) Multiple providers with various techniques

Expected location of uterine fundus using maternal anatomical landmarks

Weeks Gestation	Approximate Expected Fundal Height
12	Level of symphysis pubis
16	Halfway between symphysis pubis and umbilicus
20	1-2 finger breadths below umbilicus
24	1-2 finger breadths above umbilicus
28-30	1/3 of the way between umbilicus and xiphoid process
32	2/3 of the way between umbilicus and xiphoid process
36-38	1 finger breadth below xiphoid process
40	2-3 finger breadths below xiphoid process if lightening occurs

Adapted from Varney et al, 2004

f. Leopold (or Leopold's) maneuvers

1) Systematic method of assessing the gravid abdomen

2) Maternal obesity, excessive amniotic fluid, anterior placenta may obscure fetal outline

3) Woman should be comfortable, with empty bladder and reclining on back with one pillow; may elevate knees slightly

4) **NOTE:** *There are discrepancies in obstetric & midwifery texts regarding the technique. Williams 22nd ed, Gabbe 4th ed, Oxorn 5th ed, all describe slightly different techniques. Myles 14th does not refer to Leopold maneuvers, but presents a method of palpating the abdomen. Varney 4th, Walsh, & Sinclair describe the same technique as Williams:*

❖ **First Maneuver: Lie and presentation**

- Examiner faces woman's head
- Palpate uterine fundus with pads of finger of both hands

❖ **Second Maneuver: Position**

- Examiner still facing woman's head
- Palpate with one hand on each side of uterus
- Palpate fetus between two hands
- Assess which side is spine and which extremities

❖ **Third maneuver: Confirms lie and presentation, determines engagement**

- Pawlik's grip, or combined Pawlik's grip
- Examiner still facing woman's head
- Grasp abdomen just above pubic symphysis with outstretched thumb and third finger; may combine with grasping fundus similarly with other hand.
- The suprapubic grip is uncomfortable for the woman.
- Assess character and mobility of presenting part, confirming first maneuver

❖ **Fourth maneuver: Attitude and descent of presenting part**

- Face the woman's feet.
- With finger pads of both hands, press inward and down, moving toward axis of pelvic inlet.
- Evaluate for degree of descent and cephalic prominence, which will be on the opposite side of the spine if the head is flexed.

Significance of prenatal abdominal examination findings

Abdominal Assessment	Findings	Significance
Palpation of fundus	Fetal parts round & hard. Readily movable. Ballotable.	Fetal head moves independently of the trunk. Cephalic presentation.
	Fetal part is irregular. Larger, bulkier and less firm than a head. Cannot be well delineated or readily moved or balloted.	Fetal breech does not move independently of fetal trunk. Breech presentation
Palpation of sides of uterus	No smooth, firm surface on one side. Small parts all over abdomen	Possible posterior position or multiple gestation
Palpation of lower uterus	One hand detects a hard, round mass while the other hand continues in the direction of the pelvis	The hard, round mass is the cephalic prominence. If it is on the same side as the fetal back, the cephalic prominence is the occiput and indicates a face presentation because the head is extended. If cephalic prominence is on the same side as fetal small parts, it is the forehead and indicates a vertex presentation with a well-flexed head.
	Both hands encounter simultaneously a hard, round mass, which is equally prominent on both sides	This indicates a sincipital (military) presentation, i.e., no flexion of the fetal head.
Inspection	A saucer-like depression appears just below the umbilicus and a bulge like a full bladder appears above the symphysis pubis	Indicates a posterior presentation
	Movement of fetal small parts can be seen all over the abdomen.	Indicates a posterior position.
Fundal height measurement	Larger than expected	Inaccurate dates, multiple gestation, uterine fibroids, full bladder or other maternal factors, fetal anomaly, polyhydramnios etc
	Smaller than expected	Inaccurate dates, fetal growth restriction, oligohydramnios, fetal engagement, abnormal presentation such as transverse lie, breech etc
Auscultation of fetal heart tones	Below the umbilicus, close to midline	Cephalic presentation
	Below the umbilicus, either directly midline or far lateral	Posterior presentation
	Above the umbilicus	Breech presentation, transverse lie
	Not able to find	Gestation is earlier than expected Fetal demise

Adapted from Varney et al, 2004

2. Laboratory tests (order/obtain/interpret) See Sections B 2 and E 1 also

Laboratory tests frequently performed in pregnancy

Test	Normal	Comments
ABO type	A, B, AB, O	Type O potential for ABO incompatibility
Antibody screen	Negative	Tests for irregular & Rh antibodies. ("Kell kills, Lewis lives, Duffy dies")
Chlamydia	Negative	<25 years at risk
Cystic fibrosis (CF) screen	Negative	Identifies CF carrier for genetic counseling.
Cytomegalovirus (CMV)	Negative	IgG indicates past infection; IgM indicates active or recent infection.
Ferritin	10-300 ng/mL	<20 - iron deficiency anemia; >100 - anemia other than iron deficiency
Glucose Tolerance Test (GTT)		
Screen: 1 hour 50 g oral load	<140 mg/dL	For diagnosis, follow with 3 hour 100 g test. Carpenter/Coustan: <130 mg/dL is normal. Some consider >200 mg/dL contraindication to 3 hour GTT and proceed with diabetic management
Diagnosis: 3 hour 100 g oral load	Fasting: <105mg/dL 1 hr: <190 mg/dL 2 hr: <165 mg/dL 3 hr: <145 mg/dL	Two abnormal values diagnostic of gestational diabetes mellitus. C/C normal: Fasting: <95, 1 hr: <180, 2 hr: <155, 3 hr: <140
Gonorrhea	Negative	Repeat at term if at risk
GBS (*S. agalactiae*)	Negative	Positive recto/vaginal or urine culture requires antibiotic prophylaxis in labor
Hematocrit	1st trimester:>33% 2nd trimester: >32% 3rd trimester: >33%	Drop in 2nd trimester confirms plasma volume expansion
Hemoglobin (Hb) electrophoresis	Hb A: 95-98% Hb A_2: 1.5-3.5% Hb F: <2%	For diagnosis of sickle cell or thalassemia carrier or disease status, other hemoglobinopathies
Hepatitis B surface antigen (HBsAg)	Negative	+HBsAg indicates HBV infection. Presence for more than 6 months indicates chronic status
	+HBsAg order HBeAg	+HBeAg associated with high viral load; more highly infectious
	+HBsAb (Anti HBs)	Indicates immunity to HBV
Herpes simplex (HSV) culture	Negative	
HSV-1, HSV-2 titers	Negative	May be useful in counseling woman with no history of HSV if her partner has history of HSV infection
HIV	Negative	
Human parvovirus	Negative or positive	IgG indicates past infection; IgM indicates active or recent infection.
Karyotype	46, XX if maternal, 46, XY if paternal, either if fetal	Identifies specific chromosomal defects, e.g., aneuploidies, structural abnormalities, etc.
Platelet count	150,000-400,000/mm^3	Low, >70K: Gestational thrombocytic purpura; <70K probably idiopathic thrombocytic purpura (ITP). Treatment started if <50K. <100K associated with preeclampsia, HELLP syndrome.

Test	Normal	Comments
PPD (TB skin test)	Read in 48-72 hr; positive reaction may be measurable up to 1 week. Induration is significant, not redness.	Criteria: 1. Induration $\geq$5 mm and recent contact; x-ray suggesting old lesion; suspected HIV; IV drug user. 2. Induration $\geq$10 mm and TB risk factors; birth in Asia, Africa, Latin America; Low SES; IV drug user; member of local high prevalence group.
Preeclampsia "PIH labs"	Creatinine: <0.9 mg/dL Uric acid: <5.4 mg/dL AST: <40 U/L Hct: <38% Platelets: >150K/ mm^3 urine protein: <300 mg/24 h	NIH guidelines suggest 2 g protein in 24 hour urine raises probability of preeclampsia; 5 g/24 hr indicates severe preeclampsia.
RBC indices	MCV: 80-100 fL MCH: >27% MCHC: 31-36 g/dL	MCV<80 = microcytic anemia; MCV>80 = Macrocytic anemia; MCV in 60s, consider hemoglobinopathy; Low MCH = hypochromic anemia
Quad screen	MSAFP, hCG, uE_3, Inhibin A	Improves screening for Down syndrome (DS). Neural tube defect (NTD) : high MSAFP; DS: low MSAFP, high hCG, low uE_3, low Inhibin A.
Rh factor	Positive or negative	Either is normal; no risk of Rh sensitization if positive.
Rubella titer	>1:10 = immunity	If negative, counsel to avoid infection and get PP immunization
Sickle cell screen	`Negative	Identifies Hb S, not Hb C or thalassemia
Syphilis (RPR or VDRL)	Negative	Nontreponemal tests for screening. If positive, follow with treponemal specific test, e.g., FTA-ABS. False negative, consider lupus.
Thrombophilia screen	Negative	Identifies women at risk for deep vein thrombosis, e.g., Factor V Leiden, Protein C, Protein S, Hyperhomocysteinemia.
Thyroid screen: TSH	0.2-4.0 μIU/mL	Depressed in hyperthyroidism and elevated in hypothyroidism; follow abnormal with free T_4.
Toxoplasmosis titer	Positive or negative	IgG: convalescent IgM: active or recent infection
Triple screen	MSAFP, hCG, uE_3	NTD: high MSAFP; DS: low MSAFP, high hCG, low uE_3.
Urine culture	Negative	If colony count >100,000, treat; if Proteus, Klebsiella, GBS, treat with colony count <100,000. Contaminants are diptheroids, lactobacilli, alpha-hemolytic streptococci; mixed flora, even if >100K colonies usually indicates contamination
Urine drug screen	Negative	Most drugs clear in 28 hr; marijuana is fat soluble and may be detected in urine for up to 3 weeks.
Urine protein	<300 mg in 24 hr	300 mg –5 g = mild preeclampsia 2-5 g/24 hr = preeclampsia
Varicella titer	Positive; immune	If negative, counsel woman to avoid infection; vaccinate post partum

Adapted from Wheeler L, 2002

3. Diagnostic tests and procedures

   a. **Nonstress testing** (NST)

      1) Antepartal fetal surveillance method that observes the fetal heart rate response to fetal movement or other stimulus (e.g., vibroacoustic stimulation) using continuous electronic fetal monitoring.
      2) Based on concept that fetal hypoxia depresses the medullary center of the brain (which controls fetal heart rate response). Thus, hypoxia causes a decrease in the frequency of accelerations or less amplitude of the fetal heart rate accelerations.
      3) **Indications for NST**
         a) Decreased fetal movement
         b) Postdates
         c) Insulin dependent diabetes
         d) Hypertension
         e) Fetal growth restriction, intrauterine growth restriction (FGR, IUGR)
         f) Other chronic maternal diseases, e.g., lupus, anemia
         g) History of stillbirth, etc
      4) **Evaluation of fetal monitor strip**
         a) Consider gestational age. <30-32 weeks EGA are less likely to meet criteria
         b) **Reactive**: 2 or more accelerations of the fetal heart rate of ≥15 beats per minute, lasting at least 15 seconds within 20 minutes
         c) **Non-reactive**: Criteria not met within 40 minutes
         d) **Inconclusive**: Fetal heart rate tracing uninterpretable
         e) **Note:** Variable decelerations may be indicative of oligohydramnios.

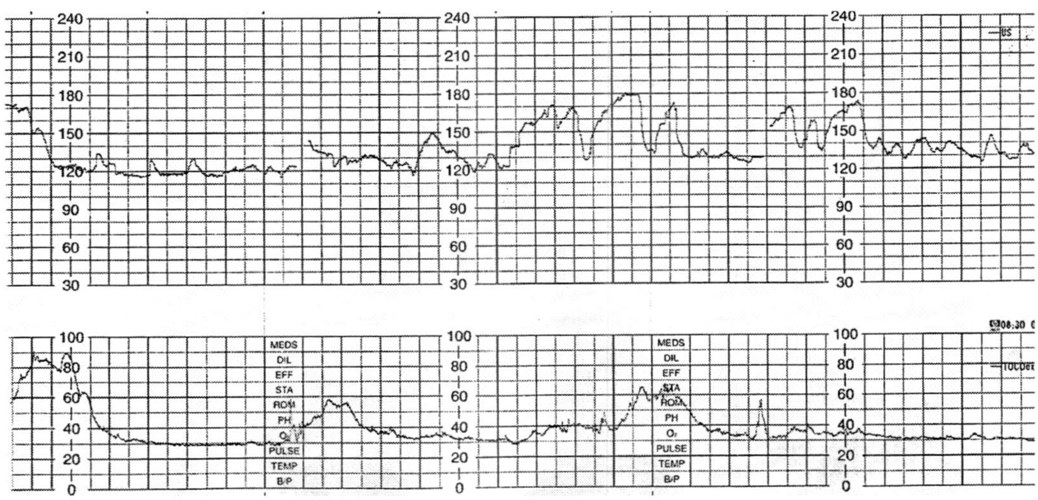

Reactive NST (and negative spontaneous contraction stress test)

5) **Factors that affect NST**
    a) Sleeping fetus
    b) Medications
    c) Fetal CNS abnormalities
    d) Smoking prior to testing
    e) Fetal hypoxia

> **Note:**
> There is no evidence that feeding a mother will increase success of obtaining reactive NST

6) **Nonreactive NST is usually followed by a biophysical profile**
7) If inconclusive, repeat.
8) If reactive, may repeat weekly or twice weekly

b. **Contraction stress testing** (CST) -- includes nipple stimulation
1) Antepartal fetal surveillance method that observes fetal heart rate response to uterine contractions while using continuous electronic fetal monitoring.
2) ***Based on the physiology that placental blood flow is decreased from compression during a contraction. A compromised fetus does not have the reserves to accommodate this decreased blood flow.***
3) Indications: Nonreactive NST; abnormal biophysical profile (BPP)
4) Method
    a) Done in the hospital with electronic fetal monitor.
    b) Contractions may be spontaneous or induced with oxytocin or nipple stimulation
    c) **An acceptable test is one with 3 contractions lasting 40-60 seconds within a 10 minute period.**
    d) **Evaluation of fetal monitor strip**
        (1) **Negative:** No late or variable decelerations
        (2) **Equivocal/Suspicious:** No long term variability or non-repetitive decelerations
        (3) **Positive:** Persistent late decelerations (>50% of contractions)
        (4) **Note:** If a late deceleration is noted during or after hyperstimulation (i.e. contractions closer than every 2 minutes or lasting >90 seconds), the test is not interpretable.
    e) Contraindications to CST include contraindications to labor, e.g., placenta previa

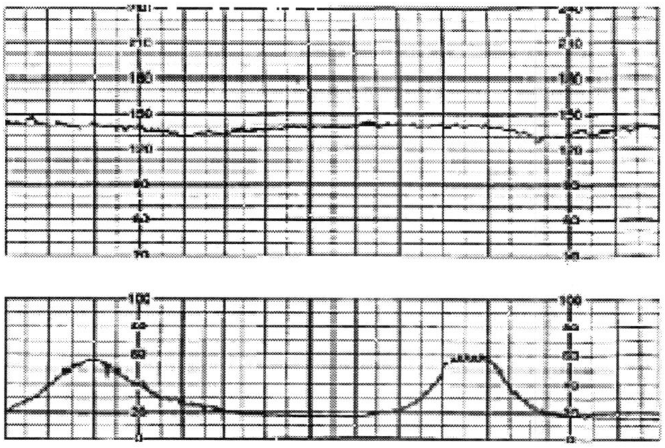

Positive contraction stress test

c. **Ultrasound**

1) Use of intermittent, high frequency sound waves for antepartal fetal surveillance. Sound waves are transmitted through the tissues via a transducer on the abdomen or in the vagina. The waves are then reflected by the underlying structures. Fetal tissues, bones, fluid, heart and lung activity, and vessel pulsations can be detected.
2) Real-time ultrasound is most common for diagnostic purposes. (Doppler fetoscopes and external fetal heart monitors utilize same principle)

A hallmark of midwifery is the appropriate use of technology in providing care to women.

Indications for Ultrasonography during Pregnancy

- Estimation of gestational age
- Size/date discrepancy
- Suspected multiple gestation
- Abnormal maternal serum marker screen, e.g., triple screen, quad screen
- Adjunct to special procedures (e.g. amnio, CVS)
- Identification or follow-up of fetal anomaly
- Intrauterine contraceptive device localization
- Pelvic, abdominal mass
- Suspected uterine abnormality, including cervical length
- Suspected hydatidiform mole
- Suspected ectopic pregnancy
- Suspected fetal death
- Suspected polyhydramnios or oligohydramnios
- Vaginal bleeding
- Follow-up evaluation of placental location for placenta previa
- Evaluation of fetal growth
- Serial evaluation of fetal growth in multiple gestation
- Fetal presentation
- Adjunct to external breech version
- Estimation of fetal weight and presentation in premature rupture of membranes, premature labor
- Biophysical evaluation for fetal well-being
- History of previous congenital anomaly

Adapted from Williams Obstetrics 22nd ed, which cited U.S. Department of Health and Human Services. Diagnostic ultrasound in pregnancy. Bethesda, Maryland: National Institutes of Health, 1984; NIH publication no. 84-667

d. Amniotic fluid index (AFI)/ Biophysical Profile (BPP)

1) Amniotic Fluid Index (AFI)/Volume

a) Calculated ultrasonically by adding the vertical depths of the largest pocket in each of four equal uterine quadrants.

b) Polyhydramnios (also called hydramnios) is more frequently present with chromosomal disorders, structural anomalies, and diabetes. Frequently, the cause of polyhydramnios is not known.

Polyhydramnios: AFI > 24-25 cm

c) Oligohydramnios is associated with uteroplacental insufficiency, fetal hypoxia, and genitourinary anomalies. A woman with oligohydramnios is more likely to encounter fetal distress in labor with meconium-stained amniotic fluid, fetal meconium aspiration, and fetal postmaturity syndrome.

Oligohydramnios: AFI ≤5 cm

2) **Biophysical Profile (BPP)**

a) Antepartal fetal surveillance that evaluates five parameters of fetal well being. It is based on the concept that evaluation of multiple components increases the accuracy of identification of a compromised fetus. Real time ultrasound coupled with a nonstress test.

b) 5 components; each receives score of 0 or 2; added together for final score

(1) **Fetal heart rate acceleration (NST)**

(2) **Fetal breathing movements**

(3) **Fetal body movements**

(4) **Fetal tone**

(5) **Amniotic fluid index**

c) Scoring

(1) **Score of 8 or 10 is normal** (unless AFI is score is 0).

(2) **Score of 6 is equivocal** and requires a **repeat test in 24 hr**.

(3) **<6 indicates fetal compromise and need for immediate delivery.**

(4) **AFI of 0 indicates oligohydramnios. Delivery usually initiated**

d) Modified biophysical profile (per Williams Obstetrics 22nd ed, 2005)

(1) Vibroacoustic NST and AFI are performed twice weekly.

(2) This method requires approximately 10 minutes for the ultrasonic evaluation.

(3) If NST is reactive and AFI is normal, it is considered a reassuring test and equivalent to the complete BPP.

Scoring the Biophysical Profile

Component	Score 2	Score 0
Nonstress Test (may be omitted if all four sono components are normal)	2 or more accelerations of 15 or more beats per minute for 15 seconds or more in 20-40 minute interval	0 or 1 acceleration in 20-40 minute interval
Fetal Breathing	1 or more episodes of rhythmic breathing lasting 30 seconds or more within 30 minutes	Less than 30 seconds of breathing in 30 minutes
Fetal Movement	3 or more discrete body or limb movements within 30 minutes	2 or more movements in 30 minutes
Fetal Tone	1 or more episodes of extension of a fetal extremity with return to flexion, or opening or closing of hand	No movements or no extension/flexion
Amniotic fluid volume (further evaluation is warranted, regardless of total score if largest fluid pocket is ≤ 2 cm deep)	Single vertical pocket > 2 cm	Largest single vertical pocket ≤ 2 cm
From ACOG, 1999; in Cunningham et al. (2005). Williams Obstetrics, p 381		

4. Counseling regarding normal pregnancy

a. Common discomforts, including use of alternative and complementary therapies

Condition	Etiology	Remedies	Avoid	Differential Diagnosis
Backache	Mechanical issue of increase in uterine size. Exacerbated by poor posture	Awareness and correction of posture Pelvic Tilt exercise Pelvic Rock exercise Supportive bra Heat, ice Girdle Chiropractic, acupuncture, osteopathy, physical therapy, yoga, massage	High heel shoes	Labor (preterm or term) Pyelonephritis Cholecystitis Heart disease
Bell's Palsy	Unknown why it is more common during pregnancy	Acyclovir and corticosteroids or supportive treatment only	--	Stroke, CNS disease
Bleeding of gums and/or nose	Hyperemia induced by hormonal changes	Gums—good oral hygiene Frequent flossing and brushing Dental visit during pregnancy Nose—normal saline drops for palliative relief	Decongestants and Antihistamines are ineffective and may cause rebound hyperemia	Gingivitis Coagulopathy URI, allergies
Carpal Tunnel Syndrome	Due to fluid retention placing pressure on nerves, especially wrists	Elevation of hands on pillows during sleep, increased intake of fluids. Splint; chiropractic, acupuncture, acupressure, vitamin B6, magnesium	Surgical treatment since probably will resolve after birth Repetitive motions	____________________

Condition	Etiology	Remedies	Avoid	Differential Diagnosis
Constipation	Related to slowed GI system due to progesterone and lack of fiber in normal American diet	Dietary manipulation Increase fiber, water Exercise Glycerin suppository, bulk forming laxative, stool softener Change iron preparation Regular bowel habit Acupuncture, homeopathy, reflexology, psyllium seeds.	Laxatives Avoid foods that are constipating to the individual woman	Obstruction
Dyspnea (shortness of breath)	Pressure on diaphragm, influence of progesterone Exacerbated by anemia and/or smoking	Posture Extra pillows during sleep Shiatsu	Smoking Allergens, asthma triggers	Pneumonia Asthma Pulmonary embolism Cardiac disease
Fatigue	Probably related to increase in progesterone in first trimester; rarely related to anemia	Anticipatory guidance; reassurance, Adequate sleep, rest Adequate diet – B vitamins, protein Shiatsu	Avoid dependency on pharmaceuticals including caffeine	Depression, anxiety Anemia Thyroid disease
Gestational Nausea and Vomiting	Uncertain Theorized to be associated with hormone levels Associated with positive pregnancy outcomes	Dietary manipulation, guided imagery, reassurance Anecdotal remedies include complex carbohydrates, small frequent meals, separation of foods and fluids, crackers upon arising Sea bands (for Accupressure) Vitamin B 6, Ginger, hypnosis	Anecdotally it is said to avoid spicy foods and fatty foods	Hyperemesis gravidarum, hydatidiform mole, pancreatitis, hepatitis, appendicitis, Pyelonephritis, Cholecystitis, peptic ulcer, HELLP (late pregnancy
Headache	Relatively common and thought to be related to hormones Benign headaches more likely in first trimester	Rest, darkened room, adequate fluid intake, ice pack to eyes/neck, relaxation techniques, acetaminophen Adequate rest, diet, massage Biofeedback, magnet therapy, homeopathy, shiatsu	NSAIDs, including ASA	Sinusitis, allergy, migraine, tension, intracranial mass, stroke etc. Preeclampsia
Hemorrhoids	Relaxation of vessels by progesterone and aggravation by dependent edema and constipation	Increase fiber in diet If painful, ice If enlarged, astringent like witch hazel or kerolytic or hydrocortisone cream If irritated, protectant like petroleum jelly Garlic clove, grated potato in rectum	Avoid constipation Avoid laxatives	Thrombosis of hemorrhoid if painful and no relief

II. Antepartum Care (25-30%)

Condition	Etiology	Remedies	Avoid	Differential Diagnosis
Insomnia	Potentially due to other minor discomforts like backaches, urinary frequency etc. Anxiety	Anecdotal reports: exercise (early in day), warm bath, chamomile tea, If necessary consider Diphenhydramine HCl (Benadryl) Acupuncture, acupressure, homeopathy, shiatsu., massage. Valerian root, catnip tea	Avoid sedatives and hypnotics, bedtime fluids or large meals, exercise within 2 hours of sleep	Underlying psychological issues, stresses etc.
Leg Cramps	May be caused by circulatory derangements or unknown reasons Commonly called "Charlie Horses" by many women	Dorsiflex the foot, especially after it is placed flat on firm surface Possibly use support hose Water immersion, calcium, magnesium supplements	Avoid standing for long times. No evidence for dietary manipulation of calcium/phosphorus or increase of calcium rich foods	Deep vein thrombosis
Leukorrhea	Increase in vaginal secretions due to hormonal changes	General body hygiene, cotton underwear	Douches and other feminine hygiene products	Vaginitis, STD, ROM
Ptyalism (increased saliva)	Unknown, but probably hormonally related	No easy solution, consider hard candies, gums etc.	Pharmaceutical agents rarely very effective; Starchy or dairy foods	---
Pyrosis (Heart burn)	Hormonally influenced relaxation of gastric sphincters, allowing reflux to occur	Dietary manipulation to reduce fats and spices Maintain upright position for at least an hour after eating Hazelnuts, Papaya, Garlic, marshmallow root, catnip, ginger. If pharmaceutical agents are needed, use antacids and antisecretory antihistamines	Bismuth (e.g. Pepto Bismol); probably not effective and metabolizes to a salicylate (contraindicated in pregnancy)	Gastrointestinal diseases, e.g., GERD, peptic ulcer
Round ligament pain	Mechanical stretching of ligaments; usually occurs in early second trimester when uterus becomes an abdominal organ. Usually onset around 14-20 weeks; Location is around symphysis pubis	Rest on side Warm or cold packs for symptomatic relief Consider clothing to provide some support Acetaminophen if necessary	NSAIDs including ASA	labor (preterm or term) UTI GI disease e.g., appendicitis, abdominal mass (e.g., adnexal tumor)

Condition	Etiology	Remedies	Avoid	Differential Diagnosis
Striae Gravidarum (Stretch Marks)	Hormonally based, and genetically influenced	No evidence that any creams or ointments influence development of striae. Postpartum Retin A	Expensive creams and ointments since they are not efficacious	Dermatologic conditions
Swollen feet and ankles	Usually dependent edema, most pronounced in late pregnancy Exacerbated by different situations (e.g. working, hot weather)	Elevation of feet at frequent intervals Loose clothing Rest, especially on side to mobilize fluid Drink additional fluids High protein diet Water immersion	Avoid standing for long intervals, knee-high socks and diuretics	Renal failure, cardiac disease
Varicose Veins	Relaxation of vessels by progesterone and aggravation by dependent edema	Support Hose Frequent rest with feet elevated Vulvar: 2 peripads held tight against labia, ice	Constricting clothing and especially knee highs	Thrombophlebitis

Reference: Sinclair C. (2004). A Midwife's Handbook. St Louis: Saunders.

b. Health promotion and disease prevention (includes exercise, hygiene, and prenatal Rh immune globulin

1) Exercise in Pregnancy

a) Moderate exercise in pregnancy does not have adverse effect on pregnancy outcome

b) Stretching and strengthening decrease incidence of minor discomforts in pregnancy (e.g. backache, constipation)

c) Safety Guidelines: established by ACOG and the American College of Sports Medicine (ACSM)

(1) Teach pregnancy women how to monitor their intensity level (e.g. can they talk and engage in a conversation while exercising)

d) Research related to exercise in pregnancy

(1) No increase in pregnancy loss

(2) Lower incidence of obstetrical intervention, labor stimulation, episiotomy, epidural and cesarean deliveries

(3) Compared to sedentary women, no difference in birth weights, maternal weight gain, length of gestation, length of labor or Apgar scores.

(4) Exercise is good primary prevention of gestational diabetes, especially in morbidly obese women (BMI >33)

> ***Midwifery Message***: The type and amount of exercise during pregnancy depends on the woman's past conditioning and the status of her pregnancy

Exercise Guidelines (ACOG 2002 and others)
• Pregnancy is a good time to begin healthy lifestyle, including participation in a wide range of recreational activities • Evaluate previously inactive women before recommending physical activity • Second trimester is best time to initiate or increase an exercise program, avoiding discomforts of first trimester, high rate of miscarriages, and possible deleterious effect of elevated body temperature on closure of neural tube (though ACOG denies Teratogenicity of exercise-induced hyperthermia) • Because of high fetal needs for oxygenated blood, glucose, and heat dissipation in late gestation, the third trimester is a poor time to increase the quantity and quality of physical activity. • Exercise (moderate) at least 30 minutes per day on most, if not all, days • Avoid the supine position and motionless standing • Modify intensity according to maternal symptoms and fatigue levels • Avoid exercises that may cause loss of balance, contact sports, high risk for trauma, scuba diving • Extra care when exercising at high altitudes • Retraining postpartum should be gradual

e) **Absolute contraindications** to aerobic exercise in pregnancy (ACOG 2002)

(1) Significant heart, lung disease

(2) Incompetent cervix, cervical cerclage

(3) Multiple gestation

(4) Second or third trimester bleeding, placenta previa in third trimester

(5) Premature labor (current gestation)

(6) Ruptured membranes

(7) Preeclampsia

f) **Relative contraindications** to aerobic exercise in pregnancy (ACOG 2002)

(1) Severe anemia

(2) Undiagnosed maternal cardiac arrhythmia

(3) Extreme underweight (BMI <12) or extreme morbid obesity

(4) IUGR in current pregnancy

(5) Poorly controlled chronic diseases, e.g., hypertension, bronchitis, seizure disorder, hyperthyroidism, Type 1 Diabetes

(6) Orthopedic limitations

(7) Heavy smoker

g) **Warning signs to stop exercising (ACOG 2002)**

(1) Any pain including back, pubic, headache, chest, calf etc

(2) Bleeding

(3) Dizziness, shortness of breath, faintness, and/or heart palpitations

(4) Preterm labor

(5) Decreased fetal movement

(6) Rupture of membranes

(7) Muscle weakness

h) Specific exercises to recommend in pregnancy
   (1) Pelvic tilt strengthens abdominal muscles, relieves low back pain
   (2) Squatting improves leg strength and reduces leg cramping
   (3) Kegel's (contraction and release of pubococcygeal muscle) improves vaginal tone and elasticity for birth, and prevents stress incontinence. May be taught as stopping the flow of urine but do not use buttocks or abdominal muscles

2) Rh Factor

a) The Rh (D) factor) is a red blood cell antigen expressed in the majority of humans
   (1) When the factor is found on the surface of the RBC, the individual is Rh (D) positive
   (2) If the individual lacks the Rh factor, she is Rh negative

b) A woman who is Rh negative and sensitized has a high risk of carrying a fetus affected by erythroblastosis fetalis or a neonate affected by hemolytic disease if the fetus is Rh positive

c) Normal maternal fetal blood communication
   (1) Maternal and fetal red blood cells usually do not communicate early in pregnancy
   (2) However, antibodies, antigens, nutrients etc. are small and readily cross the placenta
   (3) **If the woman is Rh negative and the fetus Rh positive, the fetal blood cells carrying the Rh antigen escape into the maternal blood stream during placental separation**. In most cases, the woman will mount the normal immunological reaction: namely development of antibodies against those antigens (Williams uses the term isoimmunization; Gabbe uses alloimmunization).
   (4) Other conditions in which fetal blood may enter the maternal circulation:
      (a) Spontaneous or planned abortion
      (b) Third trimester bleeding (e.g. previa)
      (c) Obstetrical interventions such as amniocentesis, external version
   (5) Maternal trauma such as domestic violence, motor vehicle accident
   (6) In future pregnancies those antibodies can pass through the placenta into the circulation of the new fetus, causing erythroblastosis fetalis (hemolysis) and hydrops (generalized edema).

(7) If the mother is Rh positive and the fetus is Rh negative, there is no problem as the fetus has no antigen to provoke an antibody/antigen reaction.

(8) If the mother is Rh negative and fetus also is Rh negative there is also no problem.

d) **Prevention of isoimmunization**

(1) ***Rh Immune Globulin** (Rh IG, **RhoGAM), if administered within 72 hours of feto maternal bleed prevents development of antibodies in more than 98% of Rh negative women.***

(2) Rh IG may provide benefits even if given after 72 hours, so it should not be withheld if the 72 hour window was missed

(3) ***Administration of Rh IG in the third trimester prevents the majority (albeit a small number) of isoimmunization caused by occult third trimester bleeding episodes.***

(a) Since protection theoretically lasts 12 weeks, it is administered at 28-30 weeks gestation.

(4) No harm seems to be linked to Anti D serum administration. Because it is a blood product, it is screened for bacteria and HIV. (For some women, usage of blood products is an important issue for their religion i.e., *Jehovah's Witnesses*),

(5) Anti D serum comes in two doses

(a) 50 micrograms Rh IG is given IM after first trimester loss or early amniocentesis; it neutralizes 5 mL of fetal blood

(b) 300 micrograms Rh IG is given IM after a birth, amniocentesis beyond 12 weeks, abruption etc to neutralize up to 30 mL of fetal blood

> **Midwifery Reminder**
> A woman who has received antenatal AntiD serum has essentially had a passive immunization and her antibody screen will be positive due to the injection for several weeks thereafter.

(6) In the case of multiple gestation, profound abruption, hemorrhage etc., more than expected fetal blood may have escaped into the maternal circulation. A Rosette test or Kleihauer Betke can determine the amount of fetal blood and additional doses of Anti D serum (Rh IG, *RhoGAM*) can be administered. (10 micrograms Rh IG for every 1 mL fetal blood). The Kleihauer Betke is also used to determine if there has been a feto-maternal bleed from abdominal trauma.

e) Testing for Rh isoimmunization

(1) Blood type, Rh and antibody screen with her initial laboratory testing

(2) If antibody screen is positive for anti D antibodies (or another RBC antibody associated with hemolytic disease), she should be referred to a perinatologist.

(3) Treatments will include close fetal surveillance, potentially percutaneous cord sampling and even fetal blood transfusions

c. Nutritional assessment and counseling

1) Calories

a) Basic components of energy expenditure (basal metabolism increases ~25%)

b) Institute of Medicine states total energy cost of pregnancy is ~55,000-85,000kcal.

c) RDA of calories for pregnancy is 300/day extra (ACOG 2002: 100-300 calorie increase)

d) Needs tied in to protein.

e) If insufficient calories, will burn protein

f) ***Note that the woman does not necessarily have to ingest the additional calories; additional energy needs might be met by a reduction in activity during pregnancy. Nutritional needs increase with multiple gestations.***

2) Protein

a) Needed for expansion of blood volume, growth of maternal tissues, growth of the fetus, and the development/activity of the placenta.

b) ***RDA of protein for pregnancy is 60 grams per day*** (~ 10 g extra)

c) Major food sources: Meat, fish, grains, legumes, nuts, eggs, dairy

3) **Trace elements**

a) Potential for interactions of more concern than overt toxicity (e.g. large doses of iron may interfere with absorption of zinc in pregnancy. Zinc supplementation in turn may affect copper metabolism.)

b) Zinc involved in nucleic acid and protein metabolism

(1) Conflicting reports of zinc preventing hypertension in pregnancy

(2) Zinc associated with lower incidence of premature birth in one study

(3) Zinc RDA: 15-45 mg/day

(4) If woman is on > 30 mg./day of iron, zinc supplementation is recommended

c) Copper plays a role in the production of energy for metabolism

(1) Copper supplementation = 2 mg/day

d) Iodine is an essential component of thyroid hormones

(1) Iodine RDA in pregnancy: 175 mcg. /day

4) **Essential fatty acids** *according to WHO and UN:*
   a) Essential for perinatal brain and retinal development and maintenance of neurologic function throughout life
   b) If deficient in diet, will be deficient in breast milk
   c) European studies have found no pregnancy induced hypertension in women on diets high in omega 3 and 6.
   d) Major food sources: cold water fish (salmon, tuna, mackerel), organ meats, eggs. Note that pregnant women should eat no more than 6 ounces twice a week of salmon or light tuna, and no more than 6ounces per week of white (albacore) tuna. Mackerel should not be eaten by women of childbearing age.
5) **Food pyramid: See Chapter I Primary Care.**
6) **Counseling**
   - 24-hour diet recall
   - Calculate BMI
   - Set weight gain goal
   - Use same scale for weight each visit
   - Complete vegetarians need supplementation of Vitamin D and Vitamin B_{12}
   - Average rate of weight gain may be slightly higher in 2nd trimester than in 3rd
   - Routine vitamin supplementation for normal pregnancy is not recommended
   - Same debate today regarding issues such as cultural appropriateness of one pyramid (others available)
   - Use of a glycemic index
   - Fun foods
7) **Common problems affecting nutrition (see table on common discomforts)**
   a) Nausea and vomiting
   b) Cravings
   c) Pica
   d) Pyrosis (aka heartburn)
   e) Lactose intolerance/milk allergies
8) **Vitamins**
   a) Routine supplementation with a prenatal vitamin is not recommended by the Food and Nutrition Board (FNB) except for iron, folic acid and calcium if the diet is inadequate.

b) FNB recommends that special attention to diet and administration of supplements be given to
   (1) Adolescents
   (2) Women with multiple gestations
   (3) Cigarette smokers and drug users
   (4) Alcohol abusers
   (5) Financially challenged women
   (6) Women with a knowledge deficit

c) Note that IOM recognizes no adverse effects of excess vitamin intake by ingestion of foods. There are adverse effects of excess vitamin/mineral intake when supplements are used, especially iron, zinc, selenium, and Vitamins A, B_6, C, and D

d) ***Vitamin and mineral intake during pregnancy should be no more than twice the RDA.***

e) The following recommended daily allowances (RDA) are based on the 2001 IOM report. (Institute of Medicine, National Academy of Sciences, 2001, accessed at http://www.iom.edu/Object.File/Master/7/296/0.pdf).

f) **Folate**
   (1) Up to 50% of neural tube defects can be prevented with folic acid supplementation.
   (2) RDA: 600 μg (Non-pregnant 400 μg/day)
   (3) A water soluble B vitamin (also known as folic acid, folacin)
   (4) Action: Folic acid needed for protein metabolism and production of RBCs. Involved in almost all aspects of DNA and RNA synthesis
   (5) If lacking cell division can not proceed normally.
   (6) Sources of folate:
      (a) Leafy green vegetables; Spinach, cooked beans, orange juice, liver, asparagus, broccoli, and most grains, and food fortification.
      (b) 80% of vitamin can be lost during food storage and preparation
      (c) Folic acid is the vitamin form, Folate is the food form.
   (7) In 1996, the FDA instituted a program to fortify food with folic acid (140 micrograms per 100g.)

> **Remember**
> All women - 400 mcg or 0.4 mg daily.
>
> If had baby with NTD before 4 mg or 4000 mcg a month before conception and first weeks of pregnancy, then 400 mcg throughout pregnancy

(8) Indications for folate/folic acid supplementation:

(a) ***Secondary prevention*** of neural tube defects (i.e. has had a baby with an open neural tube defect before or is currently taking antiseizure medication such as phenytoin): ***4 mg per day*** given 4 weeks before conception and during first six weeks of pregnancy

(b) ***Primary prevention*** of neural tube defects (e.g. primigravidas): ***0.4 mg (400 μg) a day***

(c) All childbearing age women should take in 400 mcg folic acid per day

(d) In women affected with HPV-16 to decrease incidence of pre-cancerous lesions

(e) Prevention of Alzheimer's as evidenced in longitudinal nun study

(f) Prevention of heart disease: regulates the level of the amino acid homocysteine; high levels of homocysteine are associated with increased risk of atherosclerosis

(9) Adverse effects

(a) May mask pernicious anemia with daily supplementation greater than 1mg/day

g) Calcium

(1) Necessary for muscle contraction, cardiac function, coagulation of blood

(2) Requirements

(a) RDA: 1000mg/day for pregnant women 19 and older; 1300mg/day for pregnant women 14-18 years of age

(3) Sources: Milk, yogurt, cheese, egg yolk, leafy vegetables, whole grains

(4) Research is conflicting regarding whether calcium supplementation has a role in prevention of preeclampsia

(5) Supplements

(a) Not absorbed as well as food which contains lactose, vitamin D, protein, and magnesium

(b) All supplements absorbed equally; calcium carbonate is the most concentrated form

(c) Supplement absorption improved when taken with food and spaced throughout the day.

h) Iron

(1) Needed for the production of heme (the basic protein of hemoglobin)

(2) Total body iron about 2-3g in women; two-thirds in the form of hemoglobin

(3) Serum ferritin reflects iron stores in the liver, spleen and bone marrow (~1g)

(4) RDA: 27 mg per day starting 12th week; continue for 6 to 8 months after birth to replace iron stores

(5) ACOG (2002) recommends supplementation of 27 mg per day, the amount included in most prenatal vitamins

Iron Needs of Pregnancy

Increased RBCs and blood volume	500 mg
Fetus	300 mg
Daily excretion	200 mg
Total iron needs in pregnancy	1000-1200mg

Williams Obstetrics 2005

(6) Sources

(a) Heme iron: Meat, poultry and fish (absorbed 20-40%)

(b) Nonheme iron: plant foods; pinto beans, fortified cereals, whole grains (absorbed 5%, influenced by inhibitors and enhancers).

(c) Meat enhances absorption of nonheme iron as does ascorbic acid (baked potatoes and apples with skin, citrus fruit, tomatoes, broccoli).

(d) Inhibitors: tannins, coffee, antacids, dairy products, and phytates in whole grains

(e) Approximately 6 mg of iron is obtained from each 1000Kcal of food

(7) Absorption of iron:

(a) In deficient states, absorption increases to about 25%

(b) In pregnancy, absorption increases from 7% in first trimester to 36% in second and up to 66% in the third trimester.

(c) Slow release formulations have variable absorption rates but less GI side effects

(d) ***Absorption better if given between meals***

(e) Absorption better with pure iron salts compared to iron in multiple vitamin/mineral supplements.

(f) ***Calcium carbonate and Magnesium-oxide inhibit iron absorption***

(g) Ascorbic acid does not increase iron absorption unless 250 milligrams or more (1 glass of orange juice contains 80 milligrams)

(h) Side effects are increased with vitamin C supplements of 200 mg or more

(i) High doses of iron may inhibit zinc and iron absorption

d. Psychologic/emotional response to pregnancy (includes family relationships)

1) Pregnancy is a crisis, a developmental stage, and a biological event
2) Profound metabolic changes
   a) Altered hormonal/systemic functions
   b) Altered body image
3) Pregnancy is a psychological event
   a) Major changes in
      (1) Ego functions
      (2) Reality testing
      (3) Defensive mechanisms
      (4) Mood swings
      (5) Dreams
      (6) Object relations
4) Pregnancy is a social event
   a) Realignment of roles
   b) Learning new expectations
   c) Developing new expectations
5) **Pregnancy is a transitional event**
   a) Bridges youth and adulthood
   b) Change in mother-daughter relationships
   c) Transitions of new generations
6) Psychological stages of pregnancy
   a) **First trimester**
      (1) Growing awareness of fertilized ovum
      (2) Fetus first seen as outsider
      (3) Then fetus merged with self
      (4) Major developmental tasks of first trimester
         (a) Incorporation of intruding fetus
         (b) Gradual alteration of body image and ego identification
         (c) Acceptance of fetus/infant by significant other
      (5) First trimester cognitive/affective/ behavioral processes
         (a) Increase in introversion, somatization, narcissism and dependency
         (b) Initial ambivalence and rejection of pregnancy is normal
         (c) Major cognitive focus is self and changing body

b) Second trimester

(1) Beginning separation of fetus as object rather than self

(2) Shift of major object relations from mother to mate

(3) Secondary objects are peers

(4) Second trimester major developmental tasks

(a) Acceptance of growing fetus by self and others

(b) Willingness to "house" fetus with resulting major body/role/ego changes

(5) Second trimester cognitive/affective/behavioral processes

(a) Slight decrease in introversion, dependency and anxiety

(b) Rising attachment to fetus

(c) Acute openness to environment

(d) Increase in susceptibility to suggestions

(e) Increase in emotional liability

(f) Increase in transient compulsions and ruminations

(g) Acquisition of maternal role

Mimicry

Role play

Introjection

Identification

c) Third trimester

(1) Fetus seen as separate object with own identify

(2) Sometimes increase in confusion between self and mother

(3) Major significant object mate

(4) Third trimester cognitive/affective/ behavioral processes

(a) Increase in introversion

(b) Increase in dependency and ego rigidity

(c) Increased preoccupation with impending birth

(5) Third trimester major developmental tasks

(a) Separation of fetus and self

(b) Mastery and integration of primitive anxieties and fantasies regarding birth

d) Labor and birth major developmental tasks

(1) Safe passage for self and baby

(2 Identification of infant as own

(3) Association and differentiation of infant

e) Labor and birth object relations
   (1) Major significant object: fetus/baby
f) Labor and birth cognitive/affective/ behavioral processes
   (1) Extreme ego constriction during labor
   (2) Sense of void immediately after birth
   (3) Recognition and attachment to infant

e. Referral to community resources

1) It is the responsibility of the midwife to know personal limitations and refer women and families not only to physicians in the case of high-risk complications, but to community resources for various situations.
2) Among the examples of community resources are those that deal with
   a) Finances
   b) Housing/utilities
   c) Social issues such as education
   d) Women's shelter, domestic violence hot line
   e) Clothing, food
   f) Child care
   g) Transportation
3) Professionals
   a) Dieticians
   b) Social workers
   c) Physical therapists
   e) Childbirth educators
   f) Alternative healing therapists, e.g., chiropractors, massage therapists, acupuncturists, herbalists, homeopathy, etc
   g) Pastors for spiritual guidance, churches, synagogues
4) Peer groups
   a) Mothers of Multiples groups
   b) Compassionate Friends (for miscarriage, stillbirth or neonatal loss)
   c) Resolve to Share (the same group as compassionate friends)
   d) Other support and therapy groups, e.g., Alcoholics Anonymous
5) Information
   a) Classes for credit and non credit
   b) Libraries, reading rooms
   c) On-line computers

d) Resources should be evaluated by the CNM/CM and not capriciously recommended. Evaluation should include such issues as usability, user friendliness, attractiveness, accuracy of information, authority (are credible sources used?), sponsorship (if a pharmaceutical agency or trade organization, is the information unbiased?), currency, links to other resources and quality of the writing. Does it appear appropriate for all pregnant women and couples, or specific groups, such as those with a reading level at or greater than college?

G. Patient and family education to prepare for childbirth and parenthood

1. Informed childbirth methods/pain management options/birth plan/assisted delivery techniques

a. Informed childbirth methods

1) Goal is to assist women and their families to make informed decisions about pregnancy and birth by providing information about healthy pregnancy, labor and birth; alternatives for coping with discomforts of pregnancy, self help during labor, and the role of partners during pregnancy and birth are provided.

2) Enkin et al (2000) noted that positive effects of childbirth education have been identified, i.e. decreased analgesic use and increased satisfaction with some aspects of birth, and no significant adverse effects. Potential adverse effects include fear instigated by classes; submission to peer or educator pressures to conform; feelings of anger, guilt or inadequacy if the woman does not meet up to partner's expectations; acquiescence to conventional obstetric routines without adequate information. Much depends on the educator's knowledge, attitudes, and competence, and the objectives of the particular course.

3) History

a) **Natural Childbirth** and childbirth preparation classes: **Grantly Dick- Read** (*Natural Childbirth,* 1933; *Childbirth Without Fear,* 1944); rejected the need for pain relieving drugs during childbirth on the grounds that pain was principally a product of the 'fear-tension-pain' syndrome. He eventually acknowledged that there might be some pain during the later contractions of labor.

b) **Lamaze: Fernand Lamaze** (*Painless Childbirth: The Lamaze Method*); French obstetrician; modified Grantly Dick Read's approach and developed psychoprophylaxis, based on Pavlovian principles of conditioned reflexes. Promoted specific breathing techniques for different stages of labor, effleurage (gentle massage), and controlled relaxation. Currently, the Lamaze web site cites the following objectives for childbirth education (http://www.lamaze.org)

- Avoidance of induction without a clear indication
- Freedom of movement throughout labor
- Continuous labor support
- No routine interventions
- Non supine positions for birth
- No separation of mother and baby after birth with unlimited opportunity for breastfeeding

c) **Bradley*:* Robert Bradley** (*Husband Coached Childbirth,* 1965), the Bradley method has objectives of drug free childbirth, active participation of husband, relaxation and deep breathing. Dr. championed getting husbands into the delivery room.(http://www.bradleybirth.com)

d) **Le Boyer Method*:* Frederick Le Boyer** - French obstetrician -childbirth without violence; believed that the harsh environment of the traditional delivery room caused psychological trauma to the infant. In the Le Boyer method, the infant is delivered in a dimly lit, quiet room and placed on the mother's abdomen until the umbilical cord stops pulsating whereupon it is placed in a warm bath.

e) **Birthing from Within (BFW):** childbirth classes divided into three parts:

(1) Multi-sensory activity such as learning from Birth Art or singing lullabies;

(2) Building a pain-coping mindset through BFW pain-coping practices, such as Non-Focused Awareness or Coyote Circle;

(3) Practical information, such as "How to Push Your Baby Out" or "What to Do For Back Labor."

f) **Hypnobirthing: relaxation techniques are emphasized.**

b. Factors that influence the perception of pain and choices for pain relief in labor

- Physical
- Psychological
- Environmental
- Cultural

> ***Midwife Message:*** *"Comparable stimuli in different people do not produce the same intensities of pain (McCaffery, 1999)."*

1) **Physical factors related to pain** and pain perception in childbirth

a) Age, parity, and general condition of parturient

(1) Older woman may have longer labors; younger age and lower education associated with more pain

(2) Cervix less sensitive in multipara, stronger contractions in late active phase in multipara

b) Condition of the cervix at onset of labor

c) Relationship of the size of infant to birth canal

d) Fatigue, loss of sleep

e) Presence of support person: less pain when husband/partner present

f) History of menstrual disorders

2) **Psychological factors**

a) Fear, apprehension, anxiety versus intense motivation and cultural factors

b) Past experience, e.g., sexual abuse

c) Meaning of pain

3) **Harmful consequences of unrelieved pain**

a) Increase in catecholamines

b) Decreased PaO_2

c) Decreased fetal PaO_2

d) Decreased uterine activity, secondary to catecholamine build up

4) **Midwifery use of pain relief measures in practice** (4,171 respondents)

a) Paced breathing (55%)

b) Activity and position change (42.4%)

c) Narcotics (30%)

d) Epidural (19%)

e) Paced breathing with narcotics was the most frequently used modality

5) **Epidural use in midwifery practice**

a) Rank Order, highest to lowest use

(1) Tertiary hospitals

(2) Community hospitals

(3) Hospital birthing centers

b) Approximately half of CNMs agree with the statement, "Experiencing labor pain is a valuable experience for most women."

c) Respect for woman's choice and marketability influence practice

c. **Birth plans**

1) Structures the discussion between the health care provider and the woman/family.

2) Provides a framework for resolving inconsistencies between the woman's expectations and the risks of her particular pregnancy.

3) Serves as documentation of the agreement between the health care provider and the woman.

d. Assisted delivery techniques

1) Modified Ritgen maneuver

a) Moderate upward pressure is applied to the fetal chin by the posterior hand covered with a towel through the perineum and just in front of the coccyx. Usually done during a contraction when the head distends the perineum approximately 5 cm.

2) ***Forceps***

a) Indications

- Maternal heart disease
- Pulmonary injury or compromise
- Intrapartum infection
- Certain neurological conditions
- Exhaustion or prolonged second-stage labor
- Prolapsed cord
- Premature separation of placenta
- Nonreassuring fetal heart rate pattern

3) Vacuum extraction

- Indications and prerequisites for use same as for forceps

2. **Counseling/preparation of women for external breech version**

a. Breech occurs in 3-4% of all singleton pregnancies

b. External version is a procedure in which the fetus is turned to a cephalic presentation by manipulations through the abdominal wall.

c. ~80% of breeches in late third trimesters will persist at delivery vs. 3% of those who underwent a successful version.

d. ***Usually done between 35 and 37 weeks EGA***

e. Success rate is ~65%

f. Despite version attempts, 37% of women with breeches in late pregnancy will have a CS.

g. **Risks of external version**

1) Maternal mortality
2) Placental abruption
3) Uterine rupture
4) Fetomaternal hemorrhage
5) Isoimmunization
6) Preterm labor
7) Fetal distress
8) Fetal demise

h. **Factors associated with successful version**
    1) Parity
    2) Gestational age (earlier is more successful but also higher rate of reversion)
    3) Adequate amniotic fluid volume
    4) Maternal weight gain within normal limits
    5) Posterior placental location
    6) No cervical dilatation
    7) Breech not in pelvis
    8) Lateral positioning of the fetal spine.
    9) Use of tocolysis

i. Technique for external version (by MD)
    1) Document presentation and position of fetus with sonography
    2) Each hand grasps a fetal pole. The fetal buttocks are elevated from the maternal pelvis and displaced laterally. The buttocks are then gently guided toward the fundus, while the head is directed toward the pelvis.
    3) Frequent fetal heart rate monitoring before, during, and after procedure
    4) Usually done in labor and delivery
    5) Anti-D immune globulin prophylaxis should be given to all Rh negative women

3. **Counseling regarding vaginal birth after cesarean (VBAC)**
    a. Also called TOLAC (trial of labor after cesarean)
    b. 60-80% of TOLAC result in successful vaginal births.
    c. Women who have given birth vaginally before and women whose previous CS was for breech presentation or nonreassuring heart rate have greater success.
    d. While there is no difference in perinatal morbidity or mortality, there are maternal benefits
        1) Shorter hospital stays
        2) Fewer postpartum transfusions
        3) Decreased incidence of maternal fever and infection.
    e. ***The most serious risk with VBAC is uterine rupture;*** continuous intrapartum fetal monitoring is required.
    f. Screening/Diagnosis
        1) Obtain history of the previous CS, specifically the indication; also, details of any other births
        2) Obtain official records of the previous CS
            a) **Confirm that it was a low transverse uterine incision**.
            b) Ensure that the record is available to all care providers.

g. Documentation
   1) Discussion of risks/benefits of VBAC
   2) Indications for prior section
   3) Records from previous pregnancies, including surgical notes

h. Management
   1) Full informed consent
   2) Referral if the woman, with informed consent, wishes repeat CS
   3) Careful documentation (medicolegal risk)
   4) Major controversies at this time regarding augmentation or induction of labor with oxytocin/prostaglandins as well as ACOG statements about recommendation for immediate availability of an operative birth. Has caused many CNMs/CMs to change birth sites to tertiary care settings or otherwise impacted their practices in this area.
   5) Article in 2001 had large impact on VBAC policies (*Risk of Uterine Rupture during Labor among Women with a Prior Cesarean Deliver, Lydon-Rochelle M., Holt V. L., Easterling T. R., Martin D. P. N Engl J Med 2001; 345:3-8, Jul 5, 2001)*
      a) Reviewed women who had one CS and then attempted VBAC. **VBACs were most successful for women who had:**
         (1) Spontaneous onset of labor
         (2) Previous vaginal birth
         (3) ***NO** use of prostaglandins for induction or augmentation*
   6) ACOG (2002) Committee Opinion: **do not use prostaglandins for cervical ripening or induction in women with previous uterine surgery, including CS.** They did not discourage VBAC for appropriate women and under appropriate conditions.
   7) **Position Statement from ACNM : Midwifery Care of Women Planning VBAC**

The American College of Nurse-Midwives strongly supports the practice of vaginal birth after cesarean delivery (VBAC) for women who are appropriately selected, counseled and managed. This position is consistent with current research which reports that successful VBAC results in significant benefits and fewer risks for women and infants than repeat cesarean delivery.

Midwives are qualified to manage care during pregnancy, labor and birth for a woman planning a vaginal birth after cesarean if appropriate arrangements for medical consultation and emergency care are in place. Labor support and the care offered by midwives increase the chances of a successful vaginal birth after cesarean section and lower cesarean rates in general.

Rupture of the uterus is the major risk for women laboring after a prior cesarean section. The incidence ranges from 0.4-1.2%. The incidence of uterine rupture in women laboring after prior cesarean is similar to other sudden obstetric emergencies such as placental abruption, cord prolapse and unexplained severe fetal heart rate decelerations. The occurrence of this rare, but potentially catastrophic, event is minimized with appropriate patient selection and labor management.

Care of the woman who desires a vaginal birth after a cesarean section should include informed consent as well as heightened surveillance of fetal heart rate patterns according to established high-risk criteria in labor. Well established and on-going communication between midwifery and obstetric providers to facilitate transfer of care and surgical intervention is essential to promoting optimal outcomes.

Source: Board of Directors, Approved by the ACNM Board of Directors: October 1992, Revised: August 1997, December 2000

4. **Infant nutrition (includes breast and bottle feeding)/parenting skills** (for specifics about breast and bottle feeding, including techniques and management of problems, see Chapter V, Newborn)

   a. **Breast feeding: parents should be given the following information based on recommendations of the American Academy of Pediatrics,** Section on Breastfeeding. Breastfeeding and the Use of Human Milk. Pediatrics 2005;115;496-506. accessed at http://www.pediatrics.org/cgi/content/full/115/2/496

      1) **Benefits for the child** (compared to formula feeding)

         a) Human milk is species-specific; ideal nutrient for human babies
         b) Exclusive breastfeeding is the norm; alternative feeding methods are measured against it when evaluating growth, health, development, and other long and short term outcomes
         c) Premature infants have less infection and improved development
         d) Decreased incidence and/or severity of a wide range of infectious diseases, including bacterial meningitis, bacteremia, diarrhea, respiratory tract infection, necrotizing enterocolitis, otitis media, urinary tract infection
         e) Post neonatal infant mortality rates are reduced by 21%
         f) Decreased rates of sudden infant death syndrome (SIDS) in the first year
         g) Reduction of Type 1 and Type 2 Diabetes Mellitus, lymphoma, leukemia, Hodgkin disease, overweight and obesity, hypercholesterolemia, and asthma in older children and adults
         h) Slightly better performance on tests of cognitive development
         i) Analgesia during painful procedures, e.g., heel stick for newborn screening

2) **Benefits for the mother**
   a) Decreased postpartum bleeding
   b) More rapid uterine involution
   c) Decreased menstrual blood loss
   d) Better child spacing with lactational amenorrhea
   e) Earlier return to prepregnancy weight (according to some studies)
   f) Decreased risk of breast and ovarian cancer
   g) Possibly decreased risk of hip fractures and osteoporosis in the post menopausal period
3) **Benefits to the community**
   a) Potential for decreased health care costs
   b) Decreased costs for public health programs, e.g., Women, Infants, and Children (WIC)
   c) Decreased parental employee absenteeism and loss of family income
   d) More time with siblings and family because of decreased infant illness
   e) Decreased environmental burden for disposal of formula containers
   f) Decreased energy use for production/transport of artificial feeding products
   g) (Above would be offset somewhat by costs of physician and lactation consultants' time, cost of breast pumps and other breast feeding paraphernalia)
4) **Contraindications to breastfeeding**
   a) Infant has classic galactosemia
   b) Mother has active untreated tuberculosis
   c) Mother is human T-cell lymphotropic virus (HTLV) type I or II positive
   d) Mother is receiving diagnostic or therapeutic radioactive isotopes or has been exposed to radioactive material (as long as radioactivity in the milk)
   e) Mother is receiving antimetabolites or chemotherapeutic agents (or several other medications) until the milk is clear
   f) Mother is using illicit drugs of abuse (street drugs)
   g) Mother has herpes simplex lesion on breast (use other breast until healed)
   h) Mother is HIV positive (in the US)
5) Specific conditions that **do not preclude breastfeeding**
   a) Mother is HBsAg positive
   b) Mother has hepatitis C
   c) Mother is febrile (unless the cause is listed above in 4)
   d) Mother exposed to low level environmental chemicals

e) Mother is CMV carrier; freezing can reduce the CMV load in breast milk

f) Tobacco smoking (though mother should be encouraged to quit, and avoid smoking in the home)

g) Alcohol can inhibit milk production; small amounts at special occasions are acceptable; wait 2 hours to breast feed

h) Baby is jaundiced (most of the time); rarely, breastfeeding needs to be interrupted briefly

b. Bottle (formula) feeding (specific directions in Chapter V, Newborn):

1) If the mother chooses to formula feed (or must do so because of a previously listed contraindication), she should be supported in a nonjudgmental manner
2) Use of commercial formula is safe as long as it is prepared and stored properly
3) Formula companies strive to replicate the content of human milk in artificial formulas
4) Parents should still hold the baby for feeding to prevent risk of aspiration, ear infection, and tooth decay

c. Parenting skills

1) Parents should be encouraged to attend classes to prepare for childbirth and parenting if appropriate and available, and referred to current and accurate sources of information when they are ready; specific attention can be given to the following by the midwife prenatally:
2) Inquire about preparations for the newborn; is there a place for the baby to sleep, are there diapers and clothing available, facilities for washing clothing and baby items, clean water, warmth, etc
3) Evaluate support system for emotional and physical assistance
4) Car seat and other safety information
5) Basics of baby care and danger signs
6) Circumcision counseling
7) Anticipatory guidance regarding changing family dynamics, e.g., sibling rivalry, pets, how will the partner be involved
8) Explore plans for returning to work
9) Refer to La Leche League if appropriate
10) Assist the family in selecting a compatible pediatrician
11) Keep in mind the developmental tasks of pregnancy; unless the woman asks about newborn care earlier, she will probably not be ready to learn about it until the third trimester.

H. Assessment and management of deviations from normal pregnancy; indications for referral

1. Hypertensive disorders

a. National High Blood Pressure Education Program (2000) definitions

1) **Gestational Hypertension** (Pregnancy induced Hypertension, or PIH)

a) **BP ≥140/90** for first time without proteinuria is "transient hypertension" <u>if</u> preeclampsia does not develop <u>and</u> the blood pressure has returned to **normal by 12 weeks postpartum**

b) Final diagnosis made postpartum

2) **Preeclampsia**

a) ***BP ≥140/90 after 20 weeks gestation with proteinuria***

(≥300 mg/24hr or persistent 30mg/dL[1+ on urine dipstick])

3) **Eclampsia**

a) Clonic Tonic seizures before, during, or up to 10 days postpartum that are not attributable to other causes

4) **Superimposed preeclampsia**

a) ***New-onset proteinuria in hypertensive women but no proteinuria before 20 weeks gestation.***

b) Sudden increase in proteinuria or blood pressure, or platelet count <100,000/mm^3 in women with hypertension and proteinuria before 20 weeks gestation.

5) **Chronic hypertension**

a) BP ≥140/90 before pregnancy and/or

b) ***≥140/90 before 20 weeks gestation and/or***

c) ≥140/90 persists long after delivery

6) **HELLP Syndrome**-hepatic involvement as evidenced by

- **H**emolysis, **E**levated **L**iver enzymes, and **L**ow **P**latelets.

b. Hypertension risk factors

1) Nulliparous

2) New father

3) Medical history of cardiovascular disease, chronic hypertension, preeclampsia in prior pregnancy, diabetes, collagen vascular disease, chronic renal disease

4) Family history of preeclampsia (mother, sister)

5) Current pregnancy occurrences: Multiple gestation, hydatidiform mole, fetal hydrops

6) Race

7) Obesity

8) Age >35 years

c. **Inconclusive research on these factors as risk**

1) Age <19 years
2) Lower socioeconomic status
3) Poor nutrition
4) Poor weight gain

d. **Signs and symptoms of hypertensive disorders**

1) Signs: hypertension and proteinuria (note: edema was deleted in the NHBEP report because it occurs so often in normal pregnancy)
    a) Hypertension (BP≥140/90)
    b) Proteinuria (30 mg/dL random; 1-2+ on dipstick; > 300 mg/24 hr)
2) Thrombocytopenia
3) Headache (usually frontal; resistant to ordinary analgesics)
4) Visual disturbances
5) Decreased urine output
6) Epigastric pain/right upper quadrant
7) Hyperreflexia may precede a convulsion but is not diagnostic
8) Edema may be generalized and severe, but is not diagnostic of preeclampsia; eclampsia may occur in the absence of edema.

e **Development of management plan (in consultation with physician)**

1) Educate, assess for signs/symptoms each visit
2) Early, mild hypertension—home care
    a) Left lateral bedrest: 2 hours in morning and afternoon
    b) Daily blood pressure checks
    c) Daily weight
    d) Daily urine dipsticks for protein
       Teach woman to do above
    e) Daily phone consults
    f) Twice weekly office visits
    g) Daily fetal kick counts
    h) Diversional activity counseling
    i) Consult with physician
    j) Education regarding signs and symptoms of worsening disease

3) **Pre-eclampsia—in-patient care**

a) Bed rest

b) Decreased environmental stimulation

c) 24 hour intake and output

d) Labs: 24 hour urine for protein and creatinine clearance

e) Blood for liver function tests

f) High protein diet

g) Daily fetal kick counts

h) NSTs twice weekly

i) Sonogram if <36 weeks EGA to assess IUGR

j) Daily weights

k) Blood pressures q 2-4 hours; routine vital signs and FHTs otherwise

l) Education and support

m) Deliver at term

n) Above in consultation with and collaborative management with MD

4) **Eclampsia**

a) Call for help; notify MD stat

b) Observe seizure, but don't stop

c) Prevent injury (side rails up, turn to left side if possible, do not restrain)

d) Magnesium Sulfate if patent IV

e) After seizure:

- Clear airway; suction; place soft airway until conscious
- Oxygen via face mask at 8 liters/minute
- Electronic fetal monitoring
- Evaluate contractions and labor
- Examine for injury
- Evaluate maternal blood gases, electrolytes, and serum
- Magnesium levels

2. **Cytomegalovirus (CMV)**

a. ***Herpesvirus family***

b. Most common congenital virus in US—approximately 30,000-40,000 cases annually

c Risk factors

1) Multiple sex partners

2) Exposure to infected sexual partner

3) Young age

4) Exposure to infected child

5) Low socioeconomic status

6) Overcrowding with poor sanitation

d. Fetal transmission can occur at any point
   1) 1st trimester (and perhaps early 2nd) more serious—e.g. microcephaly
   2) 3rd trimester—more likely fetal hepatitis and thrombocytopenia
   3) Transmission is usually primary (30-40%), although it can be recurrent (0.2-2.0%)

Long Term Sequelae	Asymptomatic Mother	Symptomatic Mother
Primary Infection	10%	90%
Recurrent Infection	<1%	5-10%

e. Clinical signs of CMV if woman is symptomatic
   1) Adenopathy
   2) Mononucleosis type symptoms
   3) Rare fever or hepatitis
   4) Symptoms more severe if immunocompromised
f. Neonatal signs of CMV
   1) Symptomatic (15% mortality)
      a) Small for gestational age, microcephaly, thrombocytopenia, petechiae, jaundice, retinitis, hyperbilirubinemia, splenomegaly
      b) Long term sequelae
         (1) Hearing Loss (most common cause of nonfamilial hearing loss)
         (2) Various neurological symptoms
         (3) Mental retardation
         (4) Retinitis
         (5) Developmental delay
g. Diagnosis of CMV
   1) Maternal
      a) IgM not reliable
      b) CMV-IgG: baseline, at exposure and convalescent at 3-4 weeks after exposure
   2) Fetal
      a) Ultrasound
         (1) Cerebral calcifications
         (2) Microcephaly
         (3) Hyperechoic bowel
         (4) Hydrops/ascites
      b) Amniocentesis for fluid culture: the amount of virus does not correlate with severity of disease

h. No specific therapy for CMV although trials with antivirals (e.g. Gancyclovir) and vaccines are currently being conducted

i. Prevention is primary: e.g., handwashing, CMV negative blood for transfusions

3. **Toxoplasmosis**

a. Caused by Toxoplasma Gondii

1) Parasite, unicellular protozoan

2) Oocytes shed in cat feces and found active in feces/soil for several months

b. Incidence

1) 3,000 cases of congenital infection annually in US

2) Approximately 30% of US women are IgG positive

3) ***Rare exposure/seroconversion in pregnancy—less than 0.5%***

c. ***Risk Factors for toxoplasmosis***

1) Exposure to cat feces

2) Undercooked infected meat

3) Exposure to contaminated soil

d. Transmission of toxoplasmosis

1) More likely to have transmission as pregnancy increases—but severity is less e.g., 1st trimester 15% transmission; 2nd trimester 25%, 3rd transmission 60%

e. Clinical signs and symptoms of toxoplasmosis

1) Maternal

a) Most are asymptomatic

b) If symptomatic, lymphadenopathy, mononucleosis type symptoms, rare encephalitis

c) If immunocompromised, more severe symptoms

d) Slight increase in stillbirths and abortions

2) Neonatal

a) 75% asymptomatic

b) If symptomatic, 10-12 % mortality

c) IUGR, retinitis, jaundice, hepatosplenomegaly, pneumonia, fever, adenopathy, anemia, thrombocytopenia

d) Long term sequelae: seizures, mental retardation, hearing loss, visual impairment

f. Diagnosis of toxoplasmosis
  1) Maternal: IgM
  2) Fetal: Ultrasound shows hydrops, ascites, microcephaly, ventriculomegaly, intracellular calcifications, hepatomegaly, growth restriction
    a) Amniocentesis
    b) PUBS Culture and IgM

g. Treatment of acute infection with toxoplasmosis: Pyrimethamine, folic acid and sulfadiazine

h. Prevention of toxoplasmosis
  1) Avoid eating raw meat
  2) Avoid handling cat litter
  3) Hand washing, washing food contaminated from soil (e.g. root vegetables), wearing gloves when gardening

4. Varicella (chickenpox)

a. Varicella Zoster Virus (VZV) is a Herpes Virus

b. Incidence
  1) 95% occur in children
  2) 90-95% of adults are immune

c. Transmission
  1) Aerosolized virus, highly contagious
  2) Infectious 48 hours prior to symptoms and until lesions dry
  3) Incubation 10-12 days
  4) Perinatal transmission is usually within 1st 20 weeks

d. Clinical signs and symptoms of varicella
  1) Fever, chills, cough
  2) Rash
  3) Starts as maculopapular on trunk, progresses to vesicles and crust
  4) Adults are more likely to develop pneumonia--and varicella pneumonia has high risk of national mortality
  5) Increased risk of preterm birth
  6) Zoster (shingles)
    a) Not associated with intrauterine infection
    b) Maculopapular rash over dermatome distribution
    c) Headache, fever, malaise, burning

e. Fetus (congenital infection)
   1) ***Greatest risk at 13-20 weeks***
   2) Skin scarring
   3) Microcephaly and micro-ophthalmia
   4) Limb reduction
   5) Growth restriction
   6) Polyhydramnios
   7) Dextrocardia
f. ***Newborn may have 30% mortality rate if maternal infection near birth***
g. Diagnosis of varicella
   1) Maternal
      a) Tzanck smear—intranuclear inclusion bodies and giant cells
      b) Viral culture
      c) Varicella serology (ELISA)—VZV IgM
   2) Fetal: amniocentesis for viral culture and PCR—but does not correlate with severity
h. Treatment for varicella (refer to MD)
   1) If exposure for nonimmune woman
   2) Check VZV serology
   3) If negative, VZIG (IgG passive immunity) within 96 hours
   4) No data that it prevents fetal infection
   5) If symptomatic infection without complications, palliative treatment. Add acyclovir if immunocompromised
   6) If symptomatic infection with complications, hospitalization with IV acyclovir
i. Prevention; VZV vaccine (since 1995) for nonpregnant women

5. **Human Parvovirus** B 19 (fifth disease)
   a. Only human parvovirus
   b. 50%-60% of women already immune
   c. Transmission of fifth disease
      1) Maternal
      2) Especially common among women who work in day care centers and schools
         a) Aerosolized virus
         b) Infectious 7-12 days after inoculation
      3) Perinatal information is not well established, estimated at 33% transmission

d. Clinical signs and symptoms of fifth disease
   1) Maternal
      a) 25% are asymptomatic
      b) Erythema infectiosum
      c) Red cheeks ("slapped cheek" sign) – more common in children
      d) Rash in multiple sites
      e) Malaise, headache, fever pharyngitis
      f) 80% of adults have joint involvement that can continue for up to 8 months, especially wrists, hands, knees and ankles
      g) Aplastic crises (transient acute anemia, especially without rash)
      h) Chronic bone marrow suppression
      i) Neurologic involvement
   2) Fetus
      a) Possible teratogen
      b) Anemia, hydrops, thrombocytopenia
      c) Hepatic dysfunction
      d) Myocarditis
      e) CNS abnormalities

e. Diagnosis of fifth disease
   1) Maternal
      a) Must look at both IgG and IgM parvovirus B 19

Specific for Parvovirus B19	Negative IgG	Positive IgG
Negative IgM	Nonimmune	Past infection, Immune
Positive IgM	False positive or recent infection (retest in 2 weeks)	Recent infection

      b) High MSAFP may provide high index of suspicion
   2) Fetus
      a) Ultrasound abnormalities usually within 6-8 weeks.
      b) If hydrops and maternal infection, PUBS for serologic testing and hematocrit and reticulocyte count

f. Treatment of fifth disease is aimed at saving the fetus: intrauterine transfusion if anemic (raise Hct to 45%); >90% recover within 6-12 weeks

6. Rubella

a. Togavirus

b. Incidence

1) Rare now that vaccination is common

2) Less than 200 cases annually in US

c. Risk factor: contact with unvaccinated persons

d. Transmission

1) 14-21 day incubation

2) Usually through nasopharyngeal secretions

3) No documented congenital defects after 20 weeks gestation

4) First trimester exposure results in 20-80% congenital abnormalities (more likely the earlier the pregnancy)

e. Clinical signs and symptoms of rubella

1) Maternal

a) 1/3 asymptomatic

b) Lymphoadenopathy, fever arthralgias

c) Maculopapular rash beginning on face and spreading to trunk and extremities

2) Fetal

a) Fetal growth restriction, cataracts, congenital heart disease, bone lesions, hepatosplenomegaly, congenital deafness, petechiae, anemia, microcephaly

b) Late sequelae

(1) Mental retardation

(2) Diabetes

(3) Thyroid disease

(4) Visual damage

(5) Encephalitis

> **Remember**
> Even if a woman has rubella in early pregnancy, her infant may be shedding the virus at term birth

f. Diagnosis of rubella

1) Maternal

a) Rubella IgM (appears within 7 days of infection, disappears in 4-5 weeks)

b) Titer > 1:8 indicates immunity (some use 1:10)

c) IgG is negative if acute/convalescent/positive after vaccination

2) Fetal

a) Ultrasound revealing heart disease, growth restriction, microcephaly

b) IgM on percutaneous umbilical blood sampling (PUBS)

g. Treatment is palliative

h. Prevention of rubella

1) Vaccination of children and susceptible women of childbearing age

a) 95% long term protection

b) Not recommended in pregnancy, but no congenital anomalies reported with inadvertent immunization

7. Thyroid disease in pregnancy

a. Changes in pregnancy

1) Moderate thyroid enlargement due to increased vascularity and growth of glandular tissue (~15% enlargement) due to decrease in plasma iodide levels

a) Fetus uses maternal iodide

b) Increased maternal renal clearance of iodide

2) Elevated estrogen levels in early pregnancy stimulate hepatic synthesis of thyroxine-binding globulin (TBG), resulting in higher serum total triiodothyronine (TT_3) and total thyroxine (TT_4)

a) Free T_4 (FT_4) may rise first trimester, but still within the normal range

b) TSH does not change in pregnancy

3) During first trimester, fetus is dependent on maternal T_4

a) By 20 weeks, fetal thyroid is independent of maternal thyroid status

b) TSH does not cross placenta: small amounts of T_4 and T_3 do cross

c) Thyrotropin releasing hormone (TRH), iodine, TSH receptor immunoglobulins cross placenta

d) Propylthiouracil (PTU) and methimazole cross the placenta

b. Clinical management

1) Significant increase in size of thyroid, goiter or nodule need evaluation

a) ***ACOG (2002) recommends TSH as initial test for screening and evaluation of symptomatic thyroid disease***

b) If hypothyroidism or hyperthyroidism suspected, measure TSH and FT_4

c) Measure free T_3 (FT_3) in thyrotoxicosis with suppressed TSH but normal FT_4 levels; elevated FT_3 indicates T_3 toxicosis, which may occur before FT_4 is elevated.

2) Routine measurement of thyroid function is not recommended for hyperemesis gravidarum unless there are overt signs of hyperthyroidism

3) Thyroid storm is a medical emergency; extreme hypermetabolic state with risk of maternal heart failure; signs/symptoms are fever, tachycardia, changed mental status, vomiting, diarrhea, cardiac arrhythmia. Obtain medical assistance immediately.

4) Any thyroid nodule in pregnancy should be evaluated by a physician; because they are associated with thyroid cancer
5) Test women with personal history of thyroid disease or symptoms of thyroid dysfunction. Asymptomatic women with slightly enlarged thyroid do not need screening; significant goiter or nodules should be evaluated by physician.
6) Notify pediatrician of maternal thyroid disease
7) Women with thyroid dysfunction in pregnancy should be managed in collaboration with a physician.

Thyroid Function Tests in Pregnancy and Thyroid Disease (ACOG 2002)

Maternal status	**TSH**	**FT_4**	**TT_4**	**TT_3**
Pregnancy	No change	No change	Increased	Increased
Hyperthyroidism	Decreased	Increased	Increased	Increased or no change
Hypothyroidism	Increased	Decreased	Decreased	Decreased or no change

TSH: thyroid stimulating hormone; **FT_4**: free thyroxine; **TT_4**: total thyroxine; **TT_3**: total triiodothyronine

> **Midwifery Memo**
> - TSH is the lab test to use for initial evaluation of thyroid function in pregnancy
> - Significant thyromegaly or nodules should be evaluated, even with normal lab values

8. Multiple gestation

a. Types of twins

1) **Dizygotic (or multizygotic for higher order multiples)**
   a) 70% of twins
   b) "Runs in families"
   c) Spontaneous occurrence is more likely among African American women than Caucasians
   d) Risk factors
      (1) Race
      (2) Increased maternal age
      (3) Family history
      (4) Multiparity
      (5) Pharmaceutical agents for ovulatory stimulation (e.g. Clomid, Pergonal)
   e) Physiology
      (1) ***Multiple ova fertilized by different sperm***
      (2) ***Two placentas and separate membranes***

2) Monozygotic (identical)

a) 30% of twins

b) Usually no predictable risk factors

c) Some data suggest small increase with ovulatory stimulants

d) Relationship of number of placenta/membranes depends upon timing of division – may be monoamniotic and monochorionic, diamniotic and monochorionic, diamniotic and dichorionic; conjoined twins.

b. Fetal/Neonatal risks

1) Both types risk higher mortality and morbidity due to preterm labor and birth

2) Monozygotic also more likely to have vascular anastomoses, umbilical cord accidents, conjoining, fetal anomalies

c. Sonography and multiples

1) Can help with early diagnosis

2) Difficult to evaluate chorionicity before 10 weeks

3) 10-12 gestational weeks to assess number of gestations and FHTs

d. Maternal risks

1) Hypertension (10-25%)

2) Abruption (2-6%)

3) Postpartum hemorrhage (10-20%)

4) Preterm birth (25-50%)

e. Fetal risks

1) Growth restriction

2) Preterm birth

3) Discordance (less than 10% expected singleton weight or more than 20% discordance between twins)

4) Demise of one twin (more common with monozygotic twins)

a) "Vanishing twin"

(1) Early in pregnancy

(2) No risk to living twin

b) Fetus papyraceous

(1) Midtrimester loss, not expelled

(2) Minimal risk to living twin

c) Late demise

(1) Small maternal risk of disseminated intravascular Coagulopathy (DIC)

(2) Risk to other twin if vascular communication

5) ***Twin to twin transfusion***
   a) Only monochorionic gestation
   b) ***Blood shunts from donor to recipient twin*** (usually arterial to venous via vascular anastomosis)
   c) Suspect it if one twin has edema/other not; macrosomia/growth restriction; etc.
   d) Earlier developed in gestation, poorer the prognosis
6) Other fetal abnormalities (rare)
   a) Acardiac twin
   b) Conjoined twins
   c) Stuck twins via sonographic diagnosis (one does not move with maternal positional changes)

f. Midwifery management for multiple gestation

1) Large for dates
2) Elevated MSAFP with good dates
3) Leopold findings confusing
4) Manage collaboratively with physician once diagnosed

9. Sexually transmitted diseases (STD)

a. Sexually transmitted diseases/infections are extensively elsewhere in this book. The following table summarizes some of the most important implications for pregnancy of common STDs.

Condition	Etiology	Maternal, Fetal Concerns	Treatment (if different in pregnancy)
Genital Warts Condylomata Acuminata Cervical dysplasia secondary to HPV	Human Papilloma Virus (HPV)	Potential lesions on vocal chords or in upper airway and can result in rare respiratory papillomatosis	Podophyllin & podofilox are contraindicated; imiquimod is pregnancy class B in some publications (CDC does not recommend) Attempt to avoid laser treatments or surgical incision because of increased bleeding
Herpes simplex	Herpes Simplex Virus, usually type II	Neonatal infection	CS if active lesion or prodromal symptoms at onset of labor in order to reduce risk of neonatal infection Consider prophylaxis with oral acyclovir in last month of pregnancy
Gonorrhea	*Neisseria gonorrhea* (bacterium)	Neonatal blindness due to ophthalmia neonatorum at birth	Neonatal eye prophylaxis at birth
Chlamydia	*Chlamydia trachomatis* (bacterium)	Ophthalmia neonatorum (not linked to blindness); neonatal pneumonia Maternal treatment during pregnancy may decrease neonatal pneumonia	Tetracycline, doxycline contraindicated Azithromycin commonly although long term data is lacking Neonatal eye prophylaxis at birth

Condition	Etiology	Maternal, Fetal Concerns	Treatment (if different in pregnancy)
Syphilis	*Treponema pallidum* (bacterium)	Congenital syphilis including, cataracts, microcephaly, Hutchinson's teeth, snuffles, rhinorrhea, hepatosplenomegaly. Treat as soon as possible to minimize fetal/neonatal effects, optimally in first trimester	Generally treat as latent (3 injections of benzathine penicillin; one each week for 3 weeks) If woman is penicillin allergic, desensitize as erythromycin is a macrolide with poor placental crossing; woman may be treated but not fetus. Penicillin has good fetal and maternal coverage
Human Immunodeficiency Virus; Acquired Immune Deficiency Syndrome (AIDS)	HIV (retrovirus)	Maternal course usually not affected during pregnancy Perinatal transmission may occur, especially with vaginal birth or breastfeeding	Antiretroviral therapy during pregnancy and neonatal period CS recommended No breastfeeding (developed countries, including US)

b. **Bacterial vaginosis (BV)**

1) Controversial; evidence linking BV and preterm labor has been contradictory.

2) CDC 2002 guidelines suggest treating asymptomatic women at high risk in pregnancy.

10. Bleeding in early pregnancy

a. Vaginal bleeding is neither uncommon nor always ominous in early pregnancy. However, not only can it be abnormal, but also in some cases, such as ectopics, it can be life threatening. The key to management appears to be first obtaining a complete database so that the correct diagnosis may be made and appropriate management may be individualized. ***Approximately 25% of women in 1st and 2nd trimesters will experience bleeding, about half of those will miscarry (abort).***

b. Differential diagnosis

1) **Threatened abortion**

a) Continuation of pregnancy is in doubt

b) Does not always culminate in abortion

c) Usually pain is absent or minimal; if present, it is an ominous sign

d) The cervix is closed and uneffaced

2) **Inevitable abortion**

a) Termination of pregnancy is in progress

b) Usually characterized by dilated cervix with accompanying pain, bleeding, or rupture of membranes

c) Inevitable abortion usually proceeds to complete or incomplete abortion

3) **Complete abortion**
   a) All products of conception have been passed
   b) After the uterus is empty the bleeding lessen
   c) Most frequently these women are early in pregnancy and do not need surgical intervention
4) **Incomplete abortion**
   a) Products of conception protrude through the cervical os
   b) Bleeding is apt to be more severe than other types of abortions, often necessitating a dilation and evacuation (D&E)
5) **Missed abortion**
   a) Fetal death occurs but the products of conception are not expelled for several weeks. Bleeding may or may not occur, and may be light if it does.
   b) Uterus is smaller than expected; no viable embryo/fetus
6) **Blighted ovum (anembryonic pregnancy)**
   a) Diagnosis of unknown etiology
   b) Usually a gestational sac develops, but embryo does not develop
   c) Usually treated as an inevitable or incomplete abortion
7) **Ectopic pregnancy**
   a) Pregnancy outside the uterine cavity
   b) Most often tubal in location
   c) Usually associated with pain, irregular bleeding and possible adnexal mass or fullness on one side
8) **Gestational trophoblastic disease** (also gestational trophoblastic neoplasia; hydatidiform mole; molar pregnancy)
   a) Abnormal chorionic villi that form grape-like vesicles; may occur with fetus (incomplete mole) or in the absence of a fetus (complete)
   b) Incomplete may be result of fertilization with diploid sperm; complete is composed of only paternal genetic material, possibly from 2 sperm fertilizing an ovum with no maternal genetic material
   c) Uterus large or small for dates; no FHT if complete mole
   d) Associated with early preeclampsia, hyperemesis gravidarum, and very high serum hCG levels.
   e) May progress to invasive mole or choriocarcinoma (the latter may also follow a normal pregnancy or abortion)
9) **Septic abortion:** Products of conception become infected during abortion process.

10) **Recurrent abortion:** ***2 or more successive pregnancies result in spontaneous abortion.*** (Note: various criteria for number and sequence; Williams Ob 22nd ed defines as 3 or more.)

11) **Lesions/others**
    a) Remember just because the bleeding is below the waist, do not assume it is uterine
    b) With cervical eversion in pregnancy, postcoital or post Pap smear bleeding is common; chlamydia causes cervical friability
    c) Constipation associated with pregnancy may culminate in Valsalva straining and rectal fissures or bleeding hemorrhoids
    d) Vaginal/perineal lesions
    e) Cervical cancer is associated with irregular vaginal bleeding, as is a cervical polyp (particularly post coital bleeding)
    f) Domestic violence and genital trauma

12) Other rare causes, e.g., uterine tuberculosis

c. **Diagnosis for bleeding during early pregnancy:**

1) History
2) Pelvic Exam
    a) Cervical changes (abortion)
    b) Blood in vault (to ascertain amount/character of bleeding)
    c) Presence of tissue in vagina/cervix (inevitable abortion)
    d) Adnexal fullness (ectopic)
    e) Cervical motion tenderness (pelvic inflammatory disease, ectopic)
    f) Uterine size (Gestational trophoblastic disease, missed abortion)

3) Wet Smear/cultures
    a) If the bleeding is thought to be cervical, look for trichomonas, chlamydia or other STDs
4) FHT with Doppler
5) **Quantitative serum β hCG**
    a) Positive 7-10 days post ovulation
    b) **Doubles about every 48 hours (2 days) until about week 8**
    c) Rises slowly until 10 weeks
    d) Plateaus at 24 weeks

6) Quantitative serum β hCG and ultrasound
   a) With gestational sac >10 mm, yolk sac should be visible
   b) Gestational sac >18 mm should contain embryo
   c) Embryo >5mm should have cardiac activity
   d) Gestational sac visible transvaginally if hCG >2000 mIU/mL
   e) Gestational sac visible abdominally if hCG >6500 mIU/mL
7) **Conditions**
   a) ***Ectopic:* β hCG does not double in 48 hours as normal pregnancy up to level of 100,000**
   b) ***Gestational trophoblastic disease:* β hCG higher than expected**
   c) ***Complete abortion:* hCG < 5 mIU/mL or less; may take several weeks to go down**
8) Hematocrit/Hemoglobin if heavy bleeding
9) Ultrasound
   a) Gestational sac by 6 weeks; fetus and cardiac activity by 7 weeks
   b) Snowstorm pattern suggests gestational trophoblastic disease
   c) With ectopic, no pregnancy in uterus but may or may not be able to see mass elsewhere
   d) According to Enkin et al. (2000) there are no definite signs of inevitable abortion, even with decreased amniotic fluid, diminished fetal activity and/or large intrauterine hematomas.

> A gestational sac that is 18 mm (6.9 weeks) by transvaginal ultrasound or 2.5 cm by abdominal sono should always contain an embryo

10) Draw blood type, Rh, and antibody screen if transfusion is anticipated or blood type and Rh not known;
    a) If mother is Rh negative order Anti D serum (*RhoGAM*)
11) Serum progesterone levels if suspect ectopic or abortion at less than 7 weeks pregnancy
    a) If ≥25 ng/mL, 95% are viable pregnancy
    b) If <10 ng/mL, probably nonviable

11. Bleeding in late pregnancy

a. Incidence 4% of all pregnancies

b. Usual causes

   1) **Placenta Previa (20%)**

2) **Placental Abruption** (30%); includes abruptions caused by domestic violence and motor vehicle accidents
3) Other causes (50%)
    a) Marginal placental separation difficult to define
    b) Preterm labor
    c) Genital tract infection

c. Obtaining information to help make the diagnosis
1) Bleeding characteristics
    a) Amount
    b) Color (dark is oxygenated and more likely old)
    c) Associated factors
        (1) Pelvic, abdominal, or back pain
        (2) Contractions
        (3) Foul vaginal discharge
        (4) Rupture of membranes
        (5) Recent examination
        (6) Abdominal or pelvic trauma
        (7) Intercourse
2) Fetal movement
3) Previous ultrasounds (especially helpful to rule out placenta previa)
4) Examination
    a) Blood Pressure and pulse
        (1) Vital signs often normal despite significant bleeding
    b) Abdominal exam
        (1) Pain on palpation
        (2) Palpable contractions
        (3) Hypertonic uterus (more likely to be abruption, remember board like uterus)

    c) Fetal monitoring
        (1) External fetal monitor for FHT
        (2) Tocodynamometry for contraction monitoring
    d) Radiology: transvaginal ultrasound
        (1) Placental location (best method for identifying previa)
        (2) Placental abruption (inconsistently identifiable)

e) **Pelvic examination only if no placenta previa**

(1) Remember, if there is active bleeding in the third trimester—***rule out placenta previa with ultrasound before performing a bimanual exam.***

(2) Once placenta previa is ruled out, bimanual examination can be performed

5) **Labs**

a) Wet prep of vaginal discharge if you suspect vaginitis

b) Nitrazine and ferning if you suspect rupture of membranes

c) Perform cultures as appropriate (e.g. chlamydia, GC, GBS)

d) Emergent management if actively bleeding

e) Hemoglobin/Hematocrit

f) Type and cross 2 to 6 units packed red blood cells

g) Type and cross for platelet transfusion

h) Coagulation studies, including Protime (PT), Partial Thromboplastin Time (PTT), Fibrin split products (Fibrin Degradation Products; D Dimer), Fibrinogen

6) **Management: emergency – consult and obtain neonatal support**

a) **Indications**

(1) Brisk vaginal bleeding

(2) Unstable vital signs

(3) Fetal distress

b) **Immediate interventions**

(1) Maternal oxygen

(2) Trendelenberg position or at least pelvic tilt to relieve pressure from uterus on vena cava

(3) Obtain immediate intravenous access

(a) Two large bore IV (16-18 gauge)

(b) Initiate IV solutions, e.g. Lactated Ringers

(4) Order type and cross 2 units whole blood

7) Remember: **Give RhIG with any prenatal bleeding if the mother is Rh negative.** Dosage should be determined with Kleihauer Betke determination.

12. Post dates/post term pregnancy

a. Definition: **Post term pregnancy is one that lasts 42 weeks or longer since the onset of the last menstrual period**. Assumption is that conception occurred 2 weeks following the menses. A post term pregnancy may or may not produce a baby with postmaturity syndrome. A 41 week or shorter pregnancy might produce a baby with postmaturity syndrome if ovulation occurred much earlier than expected.

b. Incidence

1) True post-dates pregnancy: 2-3%

2) Wrong dates or misdated pregnancy: 10-14%

c. Complications

1) Maternal

a) Birth trauma secondary to macrosomic infant and shoulder dystocia

b) Increased incidence of operative delivery, secondary infection, or hemorrhage

2) Neonatal

a) Meconium aspiration syndrome, polycythemia, hyperbilirubinemia, hypoglycemia, and anoxic organ damage

b) Post dates might also indicate a higher risk of preexisting neonatal complication such as anencephaly

d. Management

1) Accurately determine gestational age as early in pregnancy as possible, with ultrasound if LMP is not known or there are inconsistent physical findings.

2) Stripping (sweeping) membranes after 39 weeks is suggested by some; risks are infection (theoretical), disrupting previously unsuspected placenta previa, accidental rupture of membranes, irregular contractions and discomfort to the woman. Enkin et al (2000) report that stripping the membranes may shorten pregnancy but does not affect the route of delivery (i.e., does not prevent CS).

3) Methods such as use of sexual intercourse or oral or vaginal evening primrose oil have not been proven effective.

4) **When should the pregnancy be terminated?**

a) Cunningham et al (2005) note that there are no adequate studies comparing induction at 41 weeks versus 42 weeks solely due to pregnancy length, and recommend that ***in the absence of other indications for termination, pregnancy is allowed to proceed to 42 weeks.***

b) ACOG (2004) recommendation***: at 42 completed weeks of gestation EITHER antenatal testing OR induction of labor***; there is insufficient evidence to recommend a management strategy between 40 and 42 weeks.

c) ACOG acknowledges that many recommend induction at 42 weeks with a favorable cervix and no other complications.

5) **Fetal surveillance**
   a) ACOG recommends that in spite of a lack of evidence that:
      (1) Monitoring improves outcomes, it is "reasonable" to initiate fetal surveillance between 41 and 42 weeks gestation with **NST and AFI**; they note that no single method is superior.
      (2) **Fetal surveillance is usually performed twice weekly once initiated**
   b) Induction is indicated if there is evidence of fetal jeopardy
   c) Management of the post term pregnancy is in collaboration with MD
6) **Postmaturity syndrome (neonate)**
   a) Underweight due to loss of subcutaneous fat
   b) Long and thin in girth
   c) Skin with patchy areas of desquamation
   d) Skin, long nails may be covered with meconium
   e) Wrinkled hands and feet on ventral surfaces

13. Asthma

a. How does pregnancy affect asthma?
   1) 28% improve
   2) 33% no effect
   3) 35% worsen
b. How does asthma affect pregnancy?
   1) Maternal complications
   2) Few fetal/neonatal complications
   3) Low birth weight with severe disease
c. Maternal complications
   1) Hyperemesis
   2) Preeclampsia
   3) Chronic hypertension
   4) Vaginal bleeding
   5) Preterm labor and birth
d. Historical markers for potentially fatal asthma
   1) Multiple hospitalizations
   2) Admission to intensive care units
   3) Hypoxia as evidenced by seizures, syncope or need for intubation
   4) Systemic steroid therapy more than 4 weeks
   5) 3 Emergency department visits in recent past
e. Midwifery management is in consultation/collaboration with physician

Asthma in Pregnancy

Preconception
- Folic acid
- Optimize health
- Stop smoking
- Determine personal best on pulmonary function tests

Antepartal
- Careful observation of fetal size
- Fetal activity counts
- Since condition can change, educate woman
- Use previous pregnancy as guide
- Continue peak flow diary
- Condition most likely to worsen at 29-36 weeks
- Almost always improves in last 4 weeks of pregnancy
- Avoid beta adrenergics; use $MgSO_4$ (controversial) for PTL

Acute Treatment
If peak expiratory flow is less than 40%, admit
- Keep pa O_2 normal
- O_2 saturation at least 95%
- Continuous pulse oximetry
- Electronic fetal monitoring
- Pulmonary function tests
- Beta adrenergics
- Mortality more than 40% if asthma so severe that intubation is required

14. Gestational diabetes mellitus (GDM)
    a. Pregnancy is diabetogenic state characterized by
        1) Mild fasting hypoglycemia, postprandial hyperglycemia, and hyperinsulinemia
            a) Estrogen, progesterone and human placental lactogen (hPL) involved in process
            b) HPL thought to decrease insulin effectiveness by decreasing tissue sensitivity thereby increasing blood glucose levels for fetus
            c) Progesterone thought to increase basal levels of plasma insulin
            d) Progesterone and estrogen thought to have role in increasing tissue resistance to insulin
        2) Normal pregnancy response to meal
            a) Oral glucose meal→extended hyperglycemia and hyperinsulinemia, with suppression of glucagon (stimulates conversion of glycogen into glucose)
            b) ***In gestational diabetes, the mother cannot produce enough insulin to overcome peripheral insulin resistance***
    b. Risks of diabetes in pregnancy
        1) 4x greater likelihood of preeclampsia
        2) Increased risk of infection, e.g. UTI, monilia
        3) Fetal macrosomia and subsequent complications

c. **Risks to fetus**

1) Neonatal hypoglycemia
2) Birth injury

d. **Long term implications**

1) A significant percentage of women with GDM develop Type 2 diabetes, perhaps 50% in 20 years.
2) Evidence showing obesity and diabetes in offspring of women with GDM

e. **Identification – risk factors**

1) Low risk (no routine blood glucose testing)
   a) Member of an ethnic group with a low prevalence of gestational diabetes
   b) No known diabetes in first-degree relatives
   c) Age less than 25 years
   d) Weight normal before pregnancy
   e) No history of abnormal glucose metabolism
   g) No history of poor obstetrical outcome
   h) NOT a member of racial or ethnic group with a high prevalence of diabetes (e.g., Hispanic, African, Native American, South or East Asian, or Pacific Islands origins)

> **Remember**
>
> Screen for pregestational diabetes on 1st visit if woman has had previous GDM since she may have developed Type II since she had her baby.

2) Average Risk (blood glucose testing at 24-28 gestational weeks)
3) **High risk: blood glucose testing at first visit; repeat at 24-28** weeks if not diagnosed or any time woman has signs or symptoms of hyperglycemia
   a) Marked obesity
   b) Strong family history of type 2 diabetes
   c) Prior gestational diabetes, macrosomic infant or unexplained stillbirth
   d) Glucosuria, signs/symptoms DM

f. **Glucose screening tests**

1) ***Random glucose: If ≥ 130mg/dl, order 1 hour glucose tolerance test (GTT)***
2) 1 Hour GTT: administer 50 g glucose oral load between 24-28 weeks or earlier for high risk women
   a) Last meal and time of day irrelevant
   b) Serum test 1 hour after administration
   c) ≥140 mg/dL requires further testing
   e) Carpenter & Coustan suggested using 130 mg/dL as cut off for diagnostic testing.
   f) ***ACOG suggests if 1 hour screen is ≥ 200 mg/dL, treat as gestational diabetic***
   g) Jelly beans and other sources of glucose not standardized and not recommended by most authors and panels

3) **3 Hour GTT**: administer 100-g oral glucose challenge
   a) **Two or more of the following values must be <u>met or exceeded</u> for diagnosis of gestational diabetes** (Plasma levels)--National Diabetes Data Group values (listed here) are most often used
   b) Carpenter & Coustan levels are acceptable, but not used as widely

NDDG	C&C
Fasting > 105mg/dL	**Fasting > 95mg/dL**
1 hour > 190mg/dL	**1 hour > 180mg/dL**
2 hour > 165mg/dL	**2 hour > 155mg/dL**
3 hour > 145mg/dL	**3 hour > 140mg/dL**

4) WHO recommends the 75 g 2 hour GTT; used more in Europe than U.S.
5) Most, including ACOG, do not recommend universal serum screening. HOWEVER, they acknowledge that it may be difficult in a busy practice to determine who does not need to be screened since the criteria are so broad

g. **How is blood sugar controlled?**

1) **American Diabetes Association (ADA) diet; 2200 calories**

Complex CHO	55-60%
Protein	20%
Fat	<30%
Cholesterol	<300mg/day
Fiber	Up to 50 gm per day

2) **Exercise** – increases efficiency of insulin and blunts appetite
   a) Vigorous walking recommended 4-5X per week
3) **Fetal surveillance for women with GDM:**
   a) Ultrasound for size, amount of fluid, position of placenta
   b) Nonstress testing
   c) Biophysical profile
   d) Fetal kick counts
   e) Contraction stress testing
4) ***The pregnancy with gestational onset or pregestational onset diabetes mellitus is managed in collaboratively with physician***

15. Prelabor rupture of membranes (PROM)

a. **Spontaneous rupture of membranes prior to onset of regular uterine contractions;**

- **PPROM:** If preterm (prior to 37 weeks gestation)

1) PROM associated with complications such as preterm labor, chorioamnionitis, prolapsed cord and malpresentation
2) Associated with 30-40% of all preterm deliveries
3) The earlier in pregnancy PROM occurs, the longer the latent period (time between ROM and onset of labor)

b. **Diagnosis of rupture of membranes (ROM)**

1) Complete history: gush or leaking of fluid-time, circumstances, color, continued leaking
2) External assessment: maternal vital signs, FHTs, Leopold's for presentation and position
3) **Do not perform digital vaginal examination unless labor is obvious**
4) **Sterile speculum exam**
   a) **Pooling of fluid in vagina**
   b) **Nitrazine test** (blood or cervical mucus may give false positive)'
   c) **Ferning test** (obtain fluid from vaginal pool rather than cervix. Cervical mucus may produce false positive fern; semen may alter results)

c. **Etiology of PROM**

1) **Infection**
   a) Bacteria release proteases that weaken collagen in membranes and initiate prostaglandin synthesis that stimulates contractions
   b) Common organisms: BV, trichomonas, GC, GBS, chlamydia

d. **Associated risk factors for PROM**

1) Chorioamnionitis
2) Polyhydramnios
3) Twins
4) Breech presentation
5) Incompetent cervix
6) Antepartum hemorrhage
7) Previous cervical lacerations
8) Cerclage
9) Smoking
10) History of PROM

e. **Management**: induction versus expectant

1) **Induction**

a) Shortens latent period in effort of avoid infection

b) Risk of prolonged labor, increased cesarean section, infection

c) Avoid unnecessary vaginal exams

d) Assess for signs and symptoms of infection

(1) Warmth of vaginal walls

(2) Color and odor of fluid

(3) Maternal vital signs

(4) Fetal tachycardia

2) **Expectant management**

a) The longer the latent period the greater the chance of infection

b) ***70% of women will go into spontaneous labor within 24 hours and almost 90% within 48 hours.***

c) Labor is shortened, CS is reduced

d) Assessment of mother and fetus

(1) Sterile speculum exam, GBS culture (induce if positive)

(2) Temperature every 4 hours

(3) Assess for uterine tenderness daily

(4) Fetal movement counts

(5) NST and /or BPP every 2 days to weekly

(6) BPP < 6 may indicate amnionitis

(7) Pelvic rest

(8) WBC every other day, watch for shift to left

f. **Preterm ROM**

1) Amniocentesis to detect infection and assess fetal lung maturity

2) Studies showed that active management causes more harm than expectant management in cases of preterm PROM

3) Antibiotic therapy

4) Administration of corticosteroids (see preterm labor)

5) Plan is generally to prolong pregnancy as long as possible in the absence of infection, labor, fetal distress

g. Consultation and referral: **All cases of PROM require consultation**. Management arrangements depend on practice agreements.

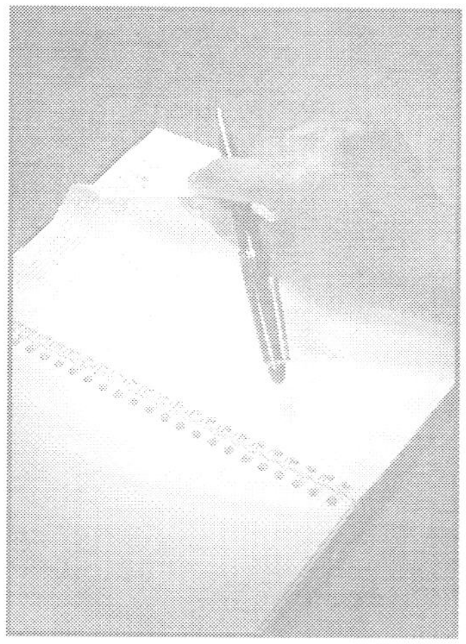

Chapter III

Intrapartum Care

III. Intrapartum Care (25%-35%)

- **A. Physiology/Pathophysiology of labor**
- **B. Assessment for admission to labor**
  1. Update personal history and health status
  2. Vital signs
  3. Physical examination to determine labor status
  4. Fetal status
     - a. Auscultation/initial monitoring of fetal heart rate
     - b. Presentation
     - c. Position
  5. Diagnosis of rupture of membranes
- **C. Fetal monitoring**
  1. Manual
     - a. Palpation
     - b. Auscultation
  2. Electronic
     - a. Uterine activity
     - b. Fetal heart rate
     - c. Indications/techniques for internal monitoring
     - d. Interventions for fetal distress
- **D. Labor support**
  1. Nonpharmacologic support techniques and measures
  2. Analgesia
  3. Anesthetic techniques
     - a. Epidural (co-management)
     - b. Paracervical
     - c. Pudendal
- **E. Labor management**
  1. Assessment and management of progress in labor—first stage
  2. Assessment of woman's physical response to labor
  3. Assessment of fetal status following artificial rupture of membranes (AROM)
  4. Assessment and management of second stage labor
- **F. Monitoring/co-management of woman receiving pharmacologic therapy during labor**
  1. Cervical ripening/induction agents
  2. Group B streptococcus prophylaxis
  3. Tocolytics
  4. Magnesium sulfate

G. Management of the perineum

1. Perineal preparation and support
2. Local anesthetic techniques (including pudendal)
3. Episiotomy

H. Conduct of delivery

1. **Hand maneuvers/mechanisms of labor**
    a. Occiput anterior
    b. Occiput posterior
    c. Nonvertex presentations
2. Maternal position at delivery
3. ***Management of the umbilical cord (including nuchal cord)***
4. ***Shoulder dystocia***

I. Third stage labor

1. **Determination of placental separation**
2. Delivery of the placenta
3. Inspection of the placenta (includes cord vessels)

J. Fourth stage labor/immediate postpartum period

1. Examination of cervix, vagina and perineum
2. Repair of episiotomy or laceration
3. Diagnosis of hemorrhage/estimated blood loss
4. ***Control of hemorrhage***

K. Assessment and management of deviations from normal labor and delivery; indications for consultation, co-management, referral or transport

1. **Management of labor dystocia (Friedman)**
2. **Bleeding in late pregnancy**
3. **Chorioamnionitis**
4. **Umbilical cord prolapse**
5. **Meconium stained amniotic fluid**
6. **Deep transverse arrest**
7. **Cephalopelvic disproportion**
8. **Uterine rupture**
9. **Uterine inversion**
10. **Maternal mortality – Safe Motherhood**
11. **Intrapartum care of women with HIV**
12. **Hypertension in pregnancy**

NOTES

III. Intrapartum Care (25%-35%)

A. Physiology/pathophysiology of labor

1. Review of physiology of parturition

a. Current evidence exists that oxytocin, estrogens, progesterone, prostaglandins, corticotropin releasing hormone, relaxin, and other factors are involved with the onset and maintenance of parturition in a complex interplay of fetal (fetus, placenta, and membranes) and maternal (myometrium, decidua) influences.

b. **We still do not understand all the complexities of the initiation of human parturition**

1) Progesterone withdrawal (or an increase in estrogen: progesterone ratio) may be a major factor

2) Estriol has been studied as indicator of fetal well-being—but also mimics fetal adrenal activity; increased fetal adrenal activity prior to onset of labor is a common link in mammalian parturition

> **Bottom Line**
> No one knows the cause of labor
> Oxytocin and Prostaglandins play a role, but probably do not initiate it
> The fetus also plays a role

c. Myometrium

1) Four muscle layers

a) Inner layer is a circular spiral, perpendicular to the long axis of the uterus

b) Middle layer muscle fibers are shaped like a figure of eight

c) Outer layers are parallel to the longitudinal axis of the uterus

2) The smooth muscle is in a matrix of collagen and ground substance

3) Biological and molecular events involved in contractions are similar to any smooth muscle

a) **Control of smooth muscle tone is usually electromechanical** (increasing intracellular calcium through changes in the membrane potential) **or receptor mediated** (binding of an agonist to a receptor so there is an ultimate increase in intracellular calcium)

b) Gap junctions use electromechanical method; allow synapses to occur across them and excite the muscle. Oxytocin receptors are an example of receptor mediated control

c) High levels of cAMP (cyclic adenosine monophosphate) inhibit contractions by increasing calcium in sarcoplasmic reticulum (outside the cell)

d) Uterus has both sympathetic and parasympathetic innervations and different neurotransmitters

(1) alpha adrenergic receptors

(2) beta adrenergic receptors

(3) all the receptors are subject to influences of agonists or antagonists

(4) Pharmacologic examples include

- *$alpha_1$ adrenergic agonists* include ergot alkaloids (to stimulate uterine contractions)
- *beta adrenergic agonists* are used as tocolytics (to decrease uterine contractions) by increasing cAMP that inhibits actin and myosin, moves calcium out of the cell and causes smooth muscle relaxation; beta adrenergic drugs can be subdivided into
    - $beta_1$ has strong cardiac stimulation
    - $beta_2$ tend to affect the uterus and lung more

ACTION	AGENT
Uterine Stimulation	Oxytocin Alpha adrenergic drugs (e.g. ergots) Prostaglandins
Uterine Relaxation	Ethanol Magnesium Sulfate Prostaglandin Synthesis Inhibitors $Beta_2$ Adrenergic Drugs Calcium Channel Blockers Aminophylline

B. Assessment for admission to labor

1. Update health history, pregnancy history and interval history

a. Current interview and review of prenatal record (Focus on OB history in multiparas)

1) Age, gravidity and parity, LMP, EDD
2) Length of previous labors
3) Years since last birth
4) Delivery method for previous births
5) Complications of previous births
6) Size of previous babies
7) Current pregnancy prenatal complications/treatments/diagnostic tests
8) Past medical, surgical, family history
9) Drug allergies, blood transfusions, drug, alcohol or tobacco use
10) Current signs and symptoms of labor
    a) Time, onset, frequency, intensity, location, and duration of contractions
    b) Presence of bloody show (early sign of labor)
    c) Status of membranes-time, color of fluid
    d) Fetal movement

ABCs of Labor Assessment

Amniotic fluid leakage
Bleeding vaginally
Contractions
Dysuria
Evidence of preeclampsia
Fetal movement

2. Vital signs

a. Blood pressure (BP)

1) Expect rises during contractions-systolic 15 mmHg; diastolic 5-10mmHg

2) Elevated BP rule out preeclampsia chronic hypertension, pain response/anxiety, drugs of abuse, e.g., amphetamines, cocaine

3) Low BP rule out hemorrhage, shock

b. Temperature

1) Expect slight elevation throughout labor, highest during and after birth

2) Elevated temperature rule out infection, dehydration

c. Pulse

1) Expect slightly higher pulse than pre-labor

2) Elevated pulse rule out infection, anxiety, hemorrhage, drugs of abuse

d. Respirations

1) Expect slight increase in rate in normal labor

2) Elevated respiratory rate rule out hemorrhage, anxiety, pulmonary problems etc

3. Physical examination to determine labor status

a. Vital signs

b. Head and eyes

1) Inquire about visual changes, headache, and dizziness

2) Ophthalmoscopic examination as indicated, e.g., woman with severe preeclampsia

c. Mouth and throat

d. Neck

1) Palpate thyroid, lymph glands

e. Cardio-respiratory

1) Inquire about cardiac or breathing difficulties

2) Auscultation of heart and lungs, noting that functional systolic murmurs in pregnancy are quite common (e.g., systolic ejection murmur Grade 1-II/VI)

f. Breasts

1) Inspection and palpation of breasts

g. Gastrointestinal including abdominal examination

1) Inquire about epigastric pain, vomiting

2) Abdominal examination

a) Leopold's maneuvers for engagement, lie, presentation, position, attitude, variety

b) Fundal height

c) Fetal heart tones

d) Fetal movement

e) Estimated fetal weight

f) Abdominal scars

h. Urinary

1) Signs and symptoms of UTI

2) CVAT

i. Genital

1) Inspect mons, vulva, perirectal area for lesions, discharge, fluid, blood

2) Pelvic examination (IF no undiagnosed bleeding or premature rupture of membranes)

a) Position of cervix, effacement, dilation

b) Presenting part: molding, caput succedaneum

c) Station, lie, presentation, position, variety, synclitism/asynclitism

d) Status of membranes: sterile speculum exam if rupture is suspected

e) Evaluation of perineum

f) Evaluation of bony pelvis

j. Endocrine

1) History of known disease/diabetic screening

k. Musculoskeletal

1) Skeletal deformities

l. Vascular

1) Edema, varicosities, Homan's sign

m. Central nervous system

1) Deep tendon reflexes (DTR)/clonus

n. Skin

1) Color, rashes, lesions, jaundice, lice, scars, tattoos, piercing, shaving

4. Fetal status

a. Auscultation of fetal heart tone (FHT) rate

1) May use fetoscope or Doppler (ultrasound). There is no scientific evidence identifying the most effective method of fetal heart rate assessment, including frequency or duration of fetal surveillance.

2) ***Standard for first stage of labor- every 30 minutes in low risk pregnancies, every 15 minutes in high risk pregnancies (ACOG 1995)***

3) ***Standard for second stage of labor, every 15 minutes in low risk pregnancies and every 5 minutes in high risk pregnancies***

4) **Indications for additional FHT assessment**
   a) Rupture of membranes
   b) Sudden change in contraction pattern
   c) Before and after maternal medication and at peak of medication
   d) Any indication of complication
5) **Listen to FHT through contraction**
   a) Consider electronic fetal monitoring if periodic changes noted (refer to fetal monitoring section for further information)

b. Presentation

1) ***Presentation*** is the part of the fetus that lies over the inlet
2) ***Presenting part*** is the most dependent part of the fetus, lying nearest the cervix -- the area that the finger contacts during a vaginal exam
3) ***Longitudinal lies***
   a) **Cephalic presentation**

      Presenting part may be

      - Vertex
      - Brow
      - Face

   b) **Breech presentation**
      (1) Complete (flexion at both hips and knees)
         - Presenting part is buttocks

      (2) Frank (flexion at hips, extension at knees)
         - Presenting part is buttocks

      (3) Footling (extension at hips and knees)
         - Presenting part is foot, feet

      (4) Kneeling (extension at hips, flexion at the knees)
         - Presenting part is knees

   c) **Transverse or oblique lie**
      (1) Shoulder (some texts say acromion process) is presenting part

c. ***Position:*** relationship of the denominator to the front back or sides of the maternal pelvis

1) **Possible fetal relationships to the maternal pelvis**
   a) Cephalic (flexed, vertex) presentation, occiput is the denominator
      - Left occipital anterior (LOA)
      - Left occipital transverse (LOT)
      - Left occipital posterior (LOP)
      - Right occipital anterior (ROA)
      - Right occipital transverse (ROT)
      - Right occipital posterior (ROP)

b) Face (deflexed, extended) cephalic presentation; mentum (chin) is the denominator
- Left mentum anterior (LMA) (mentum at 1o'clock)
- Left mentum transverse (LMT)
- Left mentum posterior (LMP)
- Right mentum anterior (RMA)
- Right mentum transverse (RMT)
- Right mentum posterior (RMP) (mentum at 7 o'clock)

c) Breech presentation; sacrum is the denominator
- Left sacrum anterior (RSA)
- Left sacrum transverse (LST)
- Left sacrum posterior (LSP)
- Right sacrum anterior (LSA)
- Right sacrum transverse (LST)
- Right sacrum posterior (RSP)

d) Shoulder presentation; acromion is the denominator
- Left acromion anterior (LAA)
- Left acromion posterior (LAP)
- Right acromion anterior (RAA)
- Right acromion posterior (RAP)

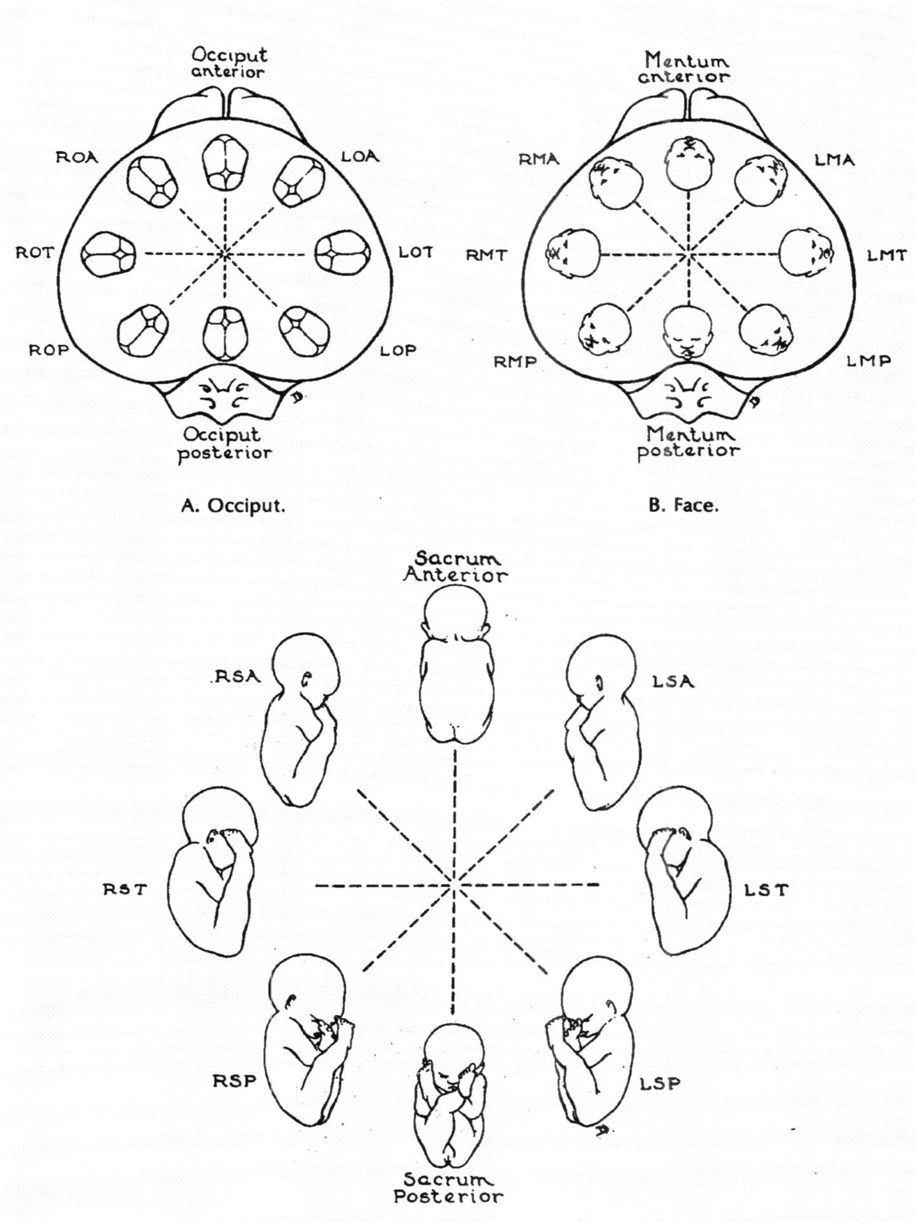

From Oxorn and Foote

5. Diagnosis of rupture of membranes

a. Sterile speculum examination

1) Fluid visualized pooling in the posterior fornix; most definitive diagnosis

2) Nitrazine paper test detects alkaline pH by turning blue

a) ***pH of amniotic fluid is 7.0to 7.5; pH of vagina 4.5 to 5.5***

b) Obtain specimen sample with sterile cotton swab in pool of fluid in posterior fornix and touch to paper; or if using sterile nitrazine swab, put the swab in the pool in the posterior fornix and observe for color change

c) Maintain sterility

d) Not completely reliable due to presence of mucus, blood, and secretions that cause false positive results

3) Fern test-based on fern-like crystallizations of NaCl in amniotic fluid

a) Apply fluid to slide and allow to dry thoroughly

b) Microscopic examination reveals fern-like pattern

4) Digital examination-contrasting smooth, slick sensation of membranes versus irregular and possibly coarseness of fetal hair; hour glassing or bulging of membranes.

C. Fetal monitoring

1. Manual

a. ***Palpation*** (contractions start in the fundus and move downward toward the cervix)

1) Until contractions reach 40 mm Hg in intensity, the uterine wall can be depressed with one finger

2) Using pads of finger tips, assess contractions at the fundus

3) Assess frequency, duration, and intensity

4) Frequency is from the beginning of one contraction to the beginning of the next

5) Duration is the time from start of the contraction to end of the contraction

6) Intensity is the firmness of the uterus to palpation; may be expressed as mild, moderate or firm; may also use numbers to express, e.g., 1+, 2+ etc

b. ***Auscultation***

1) Fetoscope

2) Doppler

3) Evaluate both during and between contractions

4) Start listening between contractions and continue listening through and after the next contraction

5) More frequent counting of FHT for several consecutive short periods of time is most reliable way to detect abnormal or periodic changes

6) Fetoscope is adequate and safe for low-risk

7) Doppler is equivalent to fetoscope but has advantage of detecting FHT that are difficult or impossible to hear with a fetoscope

2. Electronic

a. ***Uterine activity***

1) Intensity of uterine contractions in early labor approximately 25mm Hg and increases to 50 mm Hg for each contraction by the end of labor.

2) According to Caldeyro-Barcia and Poseiro, clinical labor commences when uterine activity reaches 80-120 Montevideo units; approximately 3 contractions in 10 minutes, each 40 mm Hg in intensity
3) External tocodynamometer records frequency and approximate duration of contractions. Not reliable for intensity. Must use manual palpation for intensity and resting tone.
4) ***Intrauterine pressure catheter (IUPC) provides the only electronic method of measuring uterine resting tone and intensity/strength of contractions objectively.***
   a) IUPC-recorded resting tone usually ranges from 5-15 mm Hg. Brands may vary, need to check manufacturer's guidelines.
   b) Nullipara may have higher resting tone and contraction strength than multipara
   c) **Uterine hyperstimulation:** ***> 5 contractions in 10 minutes or > 7 contractions in 15 minutes, contractions lasting longer than 60 to 90 seconds, or nonreassuring FHR***
   d) May be associated with an elevated resting tone and non-reassuring fetal heart rate

b. ***Fetal heart rate***

1) External ultrasound transducer lacks precision of internal electrode, though newer monitors with "auto-correlation" feature may accurately record FHR variability. External transducers tend to add the appearance of variability, so a FHR without variability on external monitoring will probably also lack variability with internal monitoring.
2) ***Internal fetal spiral/scalp electrode (FSE): advantage is in measuring beat to beat variability*** (unless monitor is newer model, see above)

FETAL HEART RATE TRACING INTERPRETATION
(National Institute of Child Health and Human Development Research Planning Workshop Guidelines, 1997)

Baseline: Approximate mean FHR rounded to increments of 5 bpm during a 10 minute segment, excluding periodic changes, periods of marked variability, and segments of the baseline that differ by greater than 25 bpm. In any 10 minute window, the minimum baseline duration must be at least 2 minutes or the baseline for that period is indeterminate. If the baseline FHR is less than 110 bpm, it is termed bradycardia; if the baseline FHR is greater than 160 bpm, it is termed tachycardia

Variability: The most important heart rate characteristic in predicting the status of the fetus. It is defined as fluctuations in the baseline FHR of 2 cycles per minute or greater. These fluctuations are irregular in amplitude and frequency and are visually quantified as the amplitude of the peak-to-trough in bpm as follows

Absent: Amplitude range undetectable
Minimal: Amplitude range greater than undetectable, but 5 bpm or less
Moderate: Amplitude range 6-25 bpm
Marked: Amplitude range greater than 25 bpm

Early deceleration: A visually apparent gradual decrease and return to baseline FHR associated with a uterine contraction. The decrease is calculated from the most recently determined portion of the baseline. In most cases, the onset, nadir, and recovery of the deceleration are coincident with the beginning, peak and ending of the contraction, respectively.

Late deceleration: A visually apparent, gradual decrease and return to baseline FHR associated with a uterine contraction. The decrease is calculated from the most recently determined portion of the baseline. The deceleration is delayed in timing, with the nadir of the deceleration occurring after the peak of the contraction. In most cases, the onset, nadir, and recovery of the deceleration occur after the beginning, peak, and end of the contraction, respectively

Variable deceleration: A visually apparent, abrupt decrease in FHR below the baseline. The decrease is calculated from the most recently determined portion of the baseline. The decrease is ≥ 15 bpm, lasting ≥ 15 seconds, and less than 2 minutes from onset to return to baseline. An atypical feature of a variable is an overshoot. An overshoot is an acceleration of the FHR following a moderate or severe variable deceleration. They are generally smooth in appearance, last more than 20-30 seconds, are non-reassuring in nature and are associated with fetal hypoxia.

Prolonged deceleration: A visually apparent decrease in FHR below the baseline. The decrease is calculated from the most recently determined portion of the baseline. The decrease is ≥ 15 bpm, lasting ≥2 minutes, but < 10 minutes. A prolonged deceleration of ≥10 minutes is considered a baseline change.

Preterminal pattern: Synonymous with agonal or ominous, it is one that precedes fetal death. It is usually characterized by absent FHR variability and atypical patterns.

Acceleration: A visually apparent abrupt increase in FHR above the baseline. The increase is calculated from the most recently determined portion of the baseline. The acme is ≥15 bpm above the baseline and it lasts between 15 seconds and 2 minutes. Before 32 weeks gestation, accelerations are defined as having an acme of ≥10 bpm and a duration of ≥10 seconds. A prolonged acceleration lasts 2-10 minutes. An acceleration of ≥10 minutes is a baseline change

Reactivity: A clinical judgment that allows the interpreter to state whether or not the tracing is adequate and reflects fetal well-being. Reactivity is defined as two or more FHR accelerations above the baseline in a twenty-minute period. The accelerations must be at least 15 bpm above the baseline and last at least 15 seconds from beginning to end.

c. Indications/techniques for internal monitoring

1) *Indications for internal monitoring*

a) Inability to monitor externally

b) Fetal distress

c) High risk pregnancy

d) Meconium stained fluid

2) ***Must have the following to monitor internally***

   a) Ruptured membranes

   b) Cervical dilation

   c) Accurately identified presenting part

3) ***Contraindications internal monitoring***

   a) Scalp sampling, scalp electrode and IUPC increase the risk of perinatal transmission of HIV and other infections

4) ***Possible causes of fetal tachycardia (FHR ≥160 x 10 minutes)***

   a) Mild: 161 to 180 bpm

   b) Severe: greater than 180 bpm

   c) Causes

      (1) Fever

      (2) Infection

      (3) Medications (beta sympathomimetic, e.g., terbutaline; atropine)

      (4) Chronic fetal hypoxia

      (5) Cardiac problem

      (6) Reaction to a hypoxic event, e.g., maternal hypotension related to epidural anesthesia

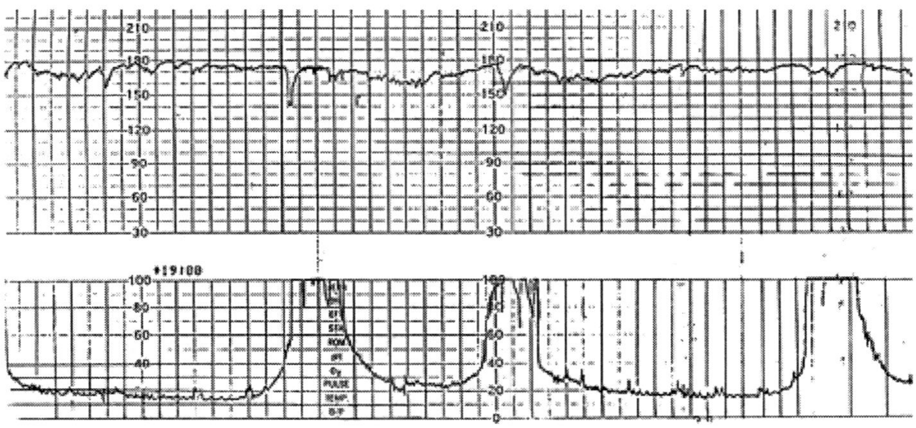

FHR tachycardia with moderate beat to beat variability

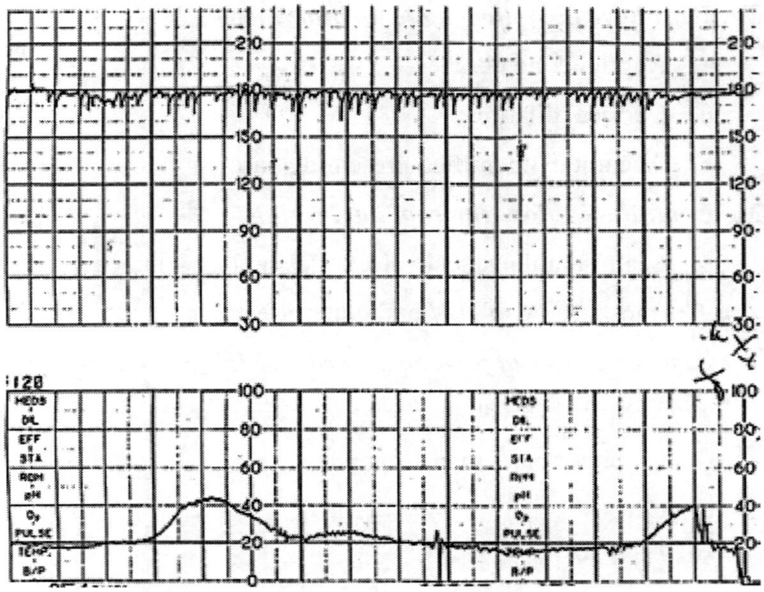

FHR tachycardia with possible arrhythmia

5) ***Possible causes of fetal bradycardia (FHR<110 x 10 minutes)***
   a) Mild: FHR 100-110 bpm
      (1) Not associated with fetal compromise, more likely positional
   b) Moderate: FHR 80-100 bpm
   c) Severe: FHR <80 bpm for 3 minutes or longer
   d) Possible causes
      (1) Anesthesia
      (2) Vagal stimulation (i.e. head compression with posterior positions)
      (3) Cord compression
      (4) Placental insufficiency
      (5) Medications (beta blockers)
      (6) Cardiac problem
      (7) Terminal fetal condition
6) **FHR variability**
   a) Short-term and long-term are assessed together not separately
   b) Normal variability consists of two cycles or more in a minute and 6-25 bpm change
   c) Possible causes of changes
      (1) Fetal sleep
      (2) Fetal hypoxia/acidemia when accompanied with decelerations
      (3) Medications (CNS depressants; opioids [e.g., meperidine, butorphanol]; sedatives; magnesium sulfate)

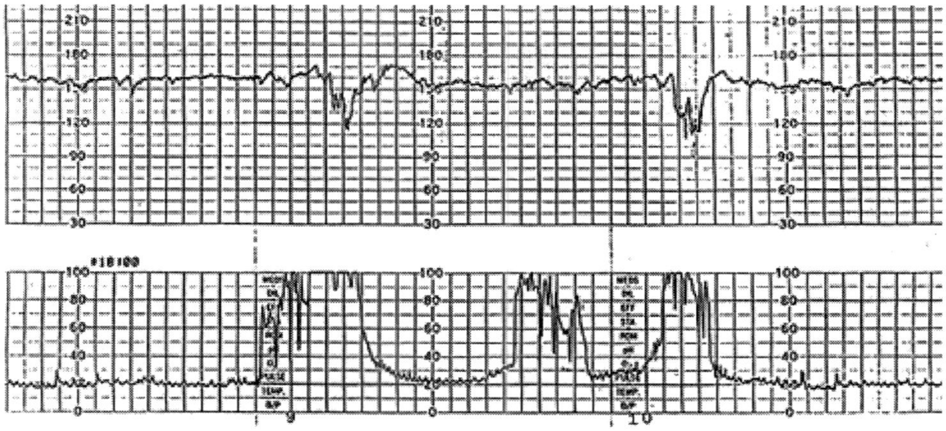

Normal baseline rate, moderate variability, variable decelerations

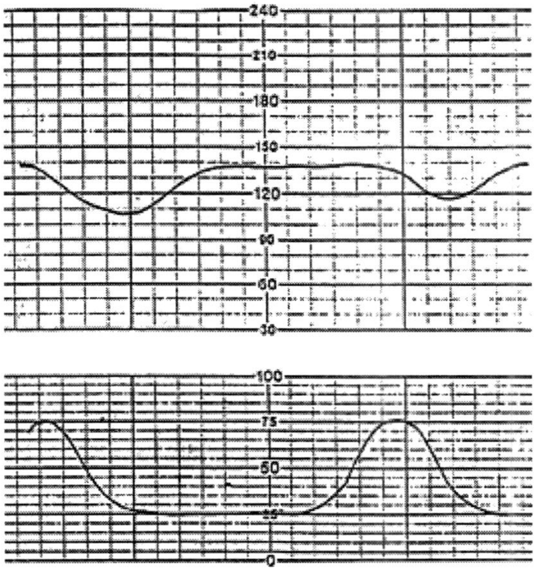

Normal FHR baseline rate, absent beat to beat variability and late decelerations

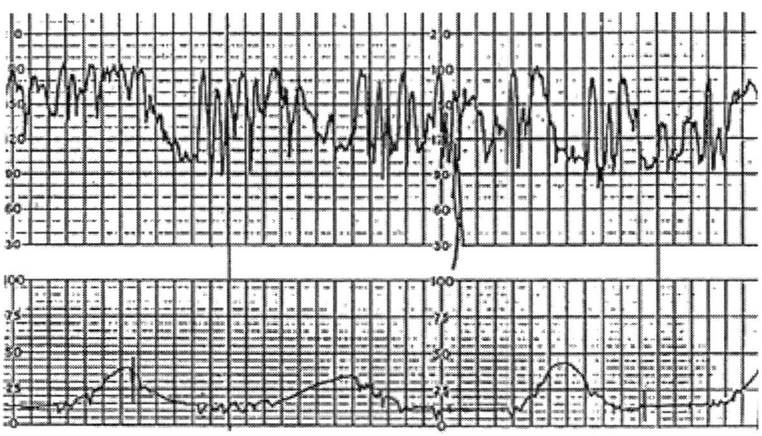

Saltatory FHR (marked beat to beat variability); possibly caused by cord compression

7) Possible causes of early decelerations

a) Head compression

b) Vagal stimulation

c) Reduced carotid artery blood flow with decreased oxygen to the brain

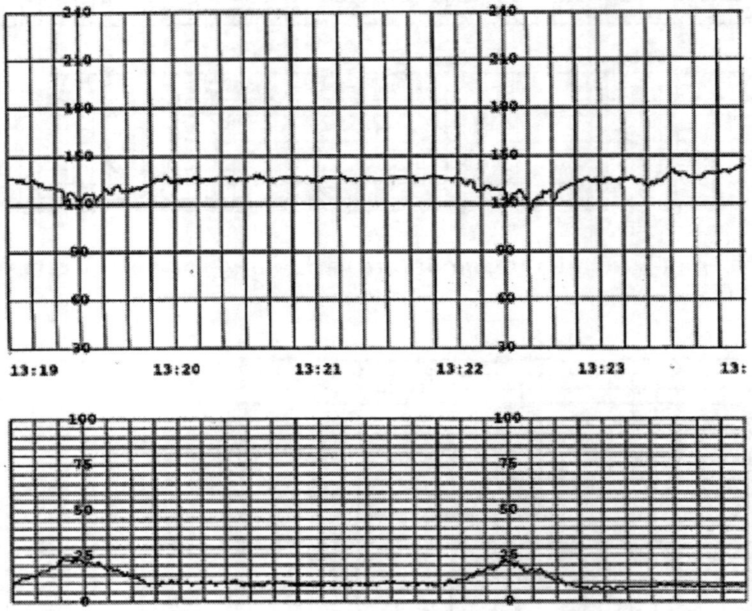

Normal FHR baseline rate, minimal variability, and early decelerations

8) Possible causes of late decelerations

a) Uteroplacental insufficiency

b) Fetal hypoxia

c) Maternal hypotension

d) Blood loss

e) Medications

f) Uterine hyperstimulation

g) Abruption

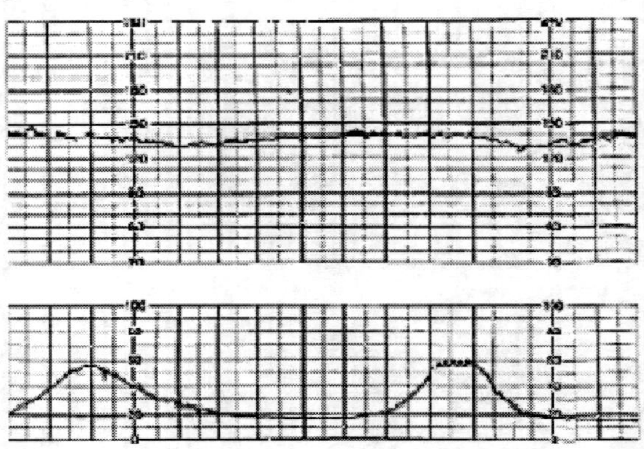

Normal FHR baseline rate, reduced beat to beat variability, and late decelerations

9) Possible causes of variable decelerations

a) *Most common deceleration pattern seen during labor*

b) Probably caused by umbilical cord occlusion, which raises fetal blood pressure and stimulates baroreceptors to reduce FHR

c) ACOG deems variable decelerations "significant" when the nadir is <70 bpm and the deceleration lasts >60 seconds (Williams Ob 22nd ed).

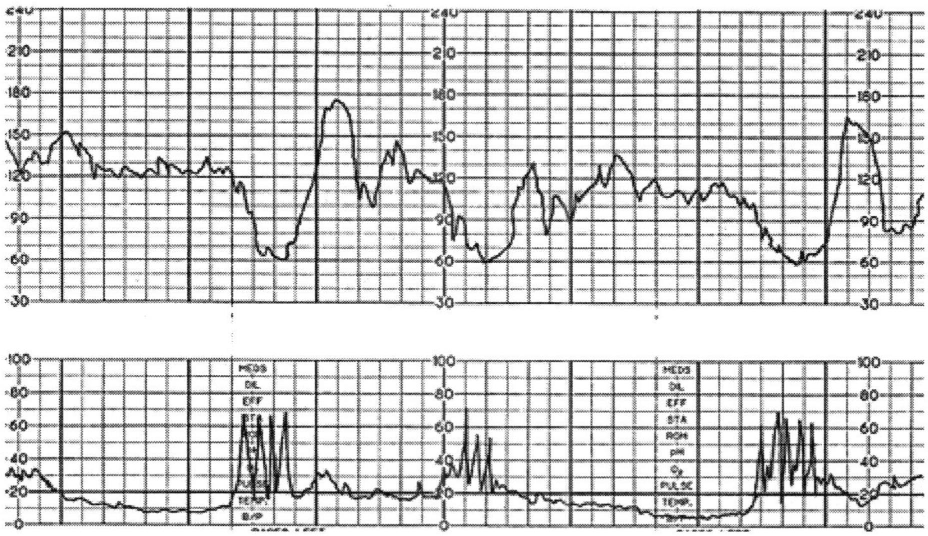

Normal FHR baseline rate, moderate variability, and severe variable decelerations

10) Possible causes of sinusoidal patterns

a) True sinusoidal pattern occur with severe fetal anemia (e.g., from hemolysis due to Rh isoimmunization, ruptured vasa previa, fetomaternal hemorrhage, etc). The appearance is a smooth, undulating baseline with a normal rate. There are 2 to 5 cycles per minutes, with an amplitude of 5-15 bpm; no beat to beat variability; no reassuring signs, such as FHR accelerations.

b) "Pseudosinusoidal" FHR patterns may be seen after maternal administration of narcotics and narcotic agonist/antagonists; there are other reassuring signs, such as accelerations.

c) Intrapartum patterns not usually associated with fetal compromise

d) Fetal sucking, umbilical cord occlusion, and oxytocin usage have been associated with pseudosinusoidal patterns.

e) Pathophysiology is not well understood

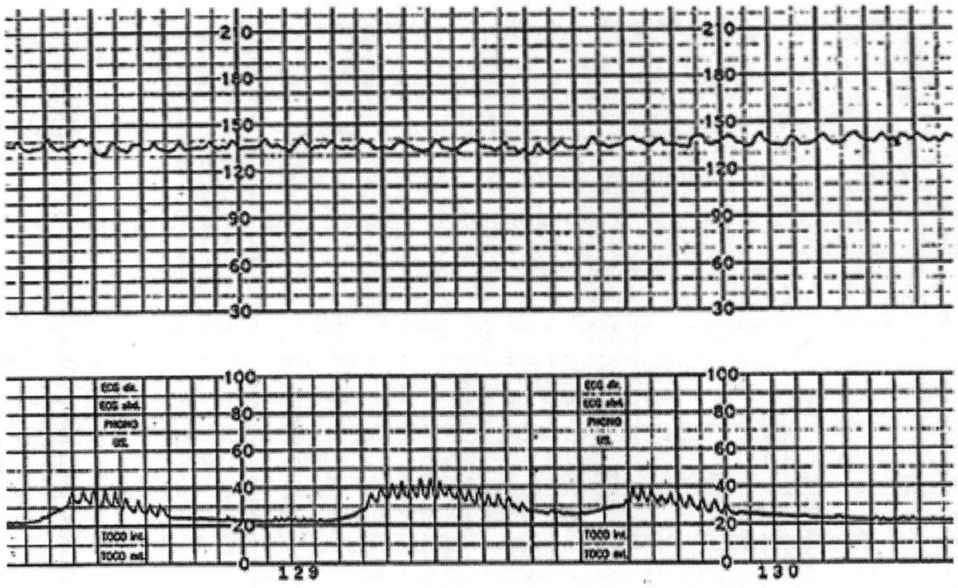

Pseudosinusoidal FHR pattern

d. Interventions for nonreassuring FHR patterns or fetal distress

1) ***Maternal position change***. Relieves aortocaval compression and may relieve cord compression
2) ***Administration of intravenous fluids***. Relieves hypotension related to epidural anesthesia, hemorrhage etc
3) ***Reduce uterine activity*** by discontinuing oxytocin or administering a betamimetic ***(0.25 mg terbutaline subcutaneously or intravenously)***
4) ***Amnioinfusion for severe variable decelerations***
    a) Indicated to relieve umbilical cord compression
    b) *Evidence is not consistent* that amnioinfusion reduces meconium aspiration syndrome by flushing out thick meconium.
    c) Evidence demonstrates significant reduction in persistent variable decelerations, reduced rate of cesarean section (CS) and decreased incidence of postpartum endometritis.
5) ***Maternal oxygen administration***
    a) No scientific evidence of efficacy, but commonly done
6) ***Vaginal examination*** to determine proximity to delivery and rule out cord prolapse
7) ***Notify anesthesia, nursing staff, and obstetrical consult*** of possible need for emergency delivery; notify pediatrics when delivery is imminent
8) ***Continuously monitor*** fetal heart rate

*****Remember: Consult as appropriate and prepare for delivery**

INTERPRETATION OF FETAL HEART RATE TRACINGS (NIH, 1997)

Reassuring Components

A normal tracing is defined as

- Normal baseline rate
- Moderate variability
- Presence of accelerations
- Absence of decelerations

Non-reassuring Components

Includes any pattern that may indicate fetal stress, fetal hypoxia or lead to hypoxia if it continues.

- Late decelerations
- Tachycardia
- Bradycardia
- Absent variability
- Repetitive variable decelerations

FREQUENCY OF ASSESSMENT AND DOCUMENTATION IN LABOR (AWHONN and ACOG STANDARDS)

Low-Risk Patients	High-Risk Patients
First Stage	First Stage
q 1 hr. in latent phase	q 30 min. in latent phase
q 30 min. in active phase	q 15 min. in active phase
Second Stage	Second Stage
q 15 minutes	q 5 minutes

D. Labor support

1. Nonpharmacologic support techniques and measures

a. Hydrotherapy (evidence from scientific studies is lacking)

b. Lamaze/prepared childbirth

1) Relaxation

2) What works

a) Breathing techniques

b) Certification of instructors

c) Approach to use of medication

d) Timing

c. Biofeedback

1) A method to educate women to recognize signals of internal physiological events

a) Once she recognizes relaxation, she can seek it through patterning her

d. Hypnosis

1) Based on relaxation, rarely try to gain anesthetic level

2) May be related to guided imagery; such phrases as "safe place", prenatal preparation of safety, comfort in the mind; reinforcement of safety and comfort during labor

e. Transcutaneous electrical nerve stimulation (TENS)

f. Acupressure

g. Acupuncture

h. Therapeutic touch

1) Based on laying on of hands

i. Chakras

1) Some practitioners of therapeutic touch also use chakra and meridian systems as used in Eastern Cultures

2) Little data available about use in pregnancy and birth

j. Maternal movement and position changes

1) Women prefer to select their own positions

2) Positional changes alter the center of gravity, and the relationship of powers, passenger and passage; may alter pain perception

3) Studies lacking but hands and knees and lunging can maximize pelvic width and assist in rotating a fetus in the OP position.

Maternal Positions in Labor

Position	*Contribution to Comfort*
Walking, Standing	-Contractions usually less painful -Provides new environment and distractions
Leaning on partner, bed or other object	-Relieves backache -Good position for backrub
Swaying (also known as "slow dancing")	-Allows pelvic tilt to decrease backache/discomfort -Less exhausting than walking
Sitting/Semi sitting	-Less exhausting than walking -Can relax perineum if woman complaining of pressure
Hands and Knees	-Good position for backrub -Relieves backache
Kneeling	-Same as hands and knees, but less pressure on hands and wrists
Side Lying	-Less exhausting than walking -Easier to relax between pushing efforts
Squatting/Supported squat/Dangle	-Difficult to maintain squat for long time -Promotes expulsion -Perineal outcome may suffer

Adapted From Simkin, P. (1995). Reducing pain and enhancing progress in labor A guide to nonpharmacologic methods for maternity caregivers. Birth, 22(3), 161-171

k. Massage and other techniques

1) **Counterpressure**

a) Anecdotally effective, especially for occiput posterior labors

2) **Bilateral hip pressure**
   a) Pressure with both hands on gluteal muscles pressing toward the center of the woman's pelvis
3) **Knee press**
   a) Facing a seated woman, provider cups each of the woman's knees in his/her hands and presses the knees straight back toward the woman's hip joints during a contraction

l. **Intradermal injections of sterile water**
   1) Reported for use in first stage back pain. Four 0.1 cc injections with 25 gauge needle form small eruptions in the skin. Two sites are over the posterior superior iliac spines; the other two are located 2 or 3 cm below and 1 to 2 cm medial to the first points
   2) Mechanism of action unknown – possibly increased endorphins, or Gate Control Theory
   3) Minimal risk

m. **Doula**
   1) A birth attendant whose sole function is to support the woman

n. **Music therapy**
   1) Women reported fewer pain responses during their labor while music was played

o. **Yoga**

p. **Herbal treatments**
   1) FDA does not monitor safety/efficacy of "dietary supplements"
   2) Herbals cannot claim health care results
   3) Major difficulty surrounds purity of the product
   4) Little in the literature about herbal pain relief for labor, although kava potentiates interactions with sedatives

q. **Homeopathy**
   1) Aconite (Monkshood and Arnica (Leopard's Bane) have been suggested for labor pain, although the latter seems more to be used postpartum, including in sitz baths

<u>Cardinal Principles of Homeopathy</u>

Most diseases are caused by an infectious disorder called the psora, which literally translates to "itch"

Life is a spiritual force (vitalism) which directs the healing of the body

Remedies can be discerned by noting the symptoms that substances produce in overdose and applying them to conditions with similar symptoms in highly diluted doses (Law of Similia or Similars)

Remedies become more effective with greater dilution (Law of Infinitesimals) and become more dilute when containers are tapped on the heel of the hand or a leather pad (potentizing)

2. Analgesia

a. Opioids

1) Morphine-like action; agonists and agonist/antagonists; natural and synthetics

a) Agonists: morphine, meperidine (*Demerol®*), fentanyl (*Sublimaze®*), codeine

b) Agonists/Antagonists: butorphanol (*Stadol®*), nalbuphine (*Nubain®*), pentazocine (*Talwin®*)

c) Antagonist: naloxone (*Narcan®*)

Receptor	The component of the organism with which the chemical agent interacts
Agonist	Drugs that mimic the action of endogenous compounds when interacting with a receptor
Antagonist	Compounds devoid of intrinsic pharmacologic activity but cause effects by inhibition of action of a specific agonist, by competition for agonist binding site

2) Effects of opioids

a) Dose-dependent and receptor mediated

b) Depress CNS

c) Depress respirations by decreasing sensitivity to CO_2

d) Urinary retention

e) Diaphoresis

f) Decreased gastric motility

g) Nausea and vomiting

3) Physiologic response

a) Reduce pain without loss of consciousness

b) Can produce physical dependence

4) Mechanism of action

a) Receptor mediated effects in the CNS and other tissues

b) Multiple receptor theory introduced by Martin in 1976

(1) μ (mu) mediates supraspinal analgesia, respiratory depression, euphoria, physical dependence

(2) K (kappa) spinal analgesia, sedation, little respiratory depression

(3) Δ (delta) alterations in affective behavior, no clear data-spinal analgesia

(4) Σ (sigma) dysphoria, hallucinations, respiratory and vasomotor stimulation

Comparison of Commonly Used Analgesics

BRAND NAME	DEMEROL	STADOL	NUBAIN
Generic Name	**Meperidine**	**Butorphanol**	**Nalbuphine**
Receptor	mu and delta agonists	partial mu, (agonist/antagonist), sigma/kappa agonists	mu antagonist; K and sigma agonist
Dose	25-100 mg IM IV	1-2 mg IM IV	10 mg IM IV
Onset	20 minutes IM immediate IV	10-30 minutes IM immediate IV	15 minutes IM immediate IV
Peak	40-50 minutes IM 10-15 minutes IV	60 minutes IM	30 minutes IM
Duration	2-4 hours IM 2-3 hours IV	may be longer	3-6 hours
Effect on Labor	None in active phase	None in active phase	None in active phase
Maternal Side Effects	Dry mouth, nausea and vomiting, hypotension, diaphoresis, sedation	Vertigo, nausea, headache, diaphoresis, respiratory depression, (ceiling effect), more restlessness	Same; less GI side effects
Fetal Side Effects	Decreased FHR variability, respiratory depression, metabolites, abnormal neurological behavioral exams May be reversed with naloxone	Possible sinusoidal pattern, less respiratory depression (ceiling) May be reversed with naloxone	Very little respiratory depression May be reversed with naloxone
Contraindications	Allergies MAO inhibitors	Substance abuse	Substance abuse
Cost	$.36 (50 mg)	$2.50 (2 mg)	more expensive than Stadol

5) **Considerations for decision making**
   a) Availability, cost and experience
   b) Difference in Apgar scores is not significant
   c) Reversibility by naloxone (Narcan®) for all
   d) Order of administration --administer meperidine before butorphanol, not the other way
   e) Effect on labor is none
   f) Effect on breastfeeding
      (1) Male infants and infants born to primigravidas who had analgesia longer than 1 hour before birth had later initiation of breastfeeding
         (a) The drug to delivery interval was an important factor.
      (2) When demographic factors and delivery outcome are controlled, with women birthing in a hospital with a supportive breastfeeding program, there is no difference among women who had intrapartum analgesia versus those who did not in breastfeeding continuation and success.

> **Midwifery Message**
> Absorption of local anesthetic agents in the maternal circulation occurs in 10-15 minutes regardless of site of injection, perineal and pudendal administration included

3. Anesthetic techniques

> **Pharmacologic properties of local anesthetic agents**
> Concentration of drug used is proportional to the density of the block
> All are potent vasodilators; Degree of absorption related to vascularity of the area
> The greater the lipid solubility the greater the potency
> The greater the protein binding the greater the duration of action
>
> **Bupivacaine (*Marcaine*®)**
> Most widely used agent for 1st stage epidurals
> High affinity for maternal proteins
> Less affinity for fetal proteins than xylocaine
> Cardiac toxicity associated with concentration of .75%
>
> **Xylocaine (*Lidocaine*®)**
> Quicker onset than bupivacaine
> Duration of action (60 min. with epidurals)
> Ion trapping in the fetus (especially for acidotic fetus)
>
> **Local anesthesia toxicity**
>
> **Etiology**
> Accidental intravascular administration
> Accumulation of local anesthetic over time
>
> **Signs and symptoms**
> Tingling of extremities
> Metallic taste
> Confusion, uneasy feeling
> Convulsion (0.03-0.5% incidence)
>
> **Prevention**
> Aspiration
>
> **Neurobehavioral effects of anesthetic agents on the neonate**
> All medication passes through the placenta to some degree
> Fetal effects have been reported
> Most minimal
> Support critical for facilitating maternal infant bonding and breastfeeding initiation

a. Epidural (co-management)

1) Increased incidence of malposition (e.g. OP)
2) Increased length of labor, both 1st and 2nd stage
3) Increased incidence of maternal hyperthermia
4) Increase in assisted vaginal births
5) Potential increase in CS rate
6) Potential complications
    a) Hypotension
    b) Anesthesia toxicity
    c) Post-dural headache
    d) Backache (controversial)

b. Paracervical block

1) Use for 1st stage labor pain
2) Major side effect is fetal bradycardia
3) Minimize fetal bradycardia by
    a) Decreasing volume of anesthetic to less than 10 mL/side
    b) Use 2%-chloroprocaine (very short-acting) instead of 1% xylocaine
    c) Use shallow injections

c. Pudendal block

1) Regional anesthesia which blocks the pudendal nerve
2) Anesthetizes the perineum and entire vulva and rectum
3) It does not affect contractions
4) Very safe, as long as the local is not injected into a vessel
5) Xylocaine 1% is most common agent, given 10 mL per side
    a) Duration of action 90 minutes
    b) Maximum safe dose is 500mg

E. Labor management

1. Assessment and management of progress in labor—***first stage usually starts at 3-4 cm dilation and ends with complete dilation***

Average length 7 hours in nulliparous women and 4 hours in multiparous women

a. Data base for well-being in the first stage of labor
    1) Continuing evaluation of any significant findings from the initial history and physical
    2) Evaluation of progress
    3) Evaluation of woman's response to labor and her support persons
    4) Evaluation of fetal presentation, position, variety, and adaptation to the pelvis
    5) Evaluation of fetal heart tones every 30 minutes in low risk women; auscultate during and after a contraction
    6) Evaluation of maternal physiologic changes
    7) Continued screening for signs and symptoms of abnormality
    8) Contractions become more frequent, longer, and more intense.
        a) They reach a uterine pressure of 25 mm Hg in early first stage to 50 mm Hg in late first stage.
        b) By end of active phase, contractions are usually every 2-3 minutes, lasting 60-90 seconds, and firm (e.g. ~55 mm Hg).
        c) Woman becomes increasingly apprehensive, more serious, and may be frightened of being alone and less confident of her ability to cope.
    9) Transition usually is end of active stage (deceleration phase in Friedman)

b. Continuing evaluation of labor progress

1) Effacement, dilation, and station

a) The cervix is approximately 2 inches long prior to effacement

(1) 50% effaced is approximately 1 inch

(2) 75% effaced is approximately ½ inch

b) Dilation in centimeters or fingertip if <2 cm.

c) Station: there are 2 methods of reporting station. The most current is to report the location of the leading edge of the presenting part as the number of centimeters above or below the level of the ischial spines. Stations above the level of the ischial spines are MINUS 1-5; at the plane of the spines is 0; below the plane of the spines is PLUS 1-5.

2) **Synclitism/asynclitism/molding/caput**

a) Synclitism occurs when the sagittal suture is midway between the pubis and the sacrum

b) Asynclitism occurs when synclitism is not maintained

(1) In *posterior* asynclitism the sagittal suture is closer to the symphysis pubis (the *posterior* parietal bone presents)

(2) In *anterior* asynclitism, the sagittal suture is closer to the sacral promontory (the *anterior* parietal presents)

(3) Either may be normal as the fetal head negotiates the pelvis.

c) Molding is overlapping of the bones of the fetal skull; frontal and occipital bones pass under the parietal bones

d) Caput succedaneum is localized swelling of the scalp resulting from obstruction of venous return due to cervical pressure on the fetal scalp. Varies with position of the vertex. With OA positions the caput forms on the vertex and to the right (LOA) or to the left (ROA) of the sagittal suture. It disappears within 24 to 36 hours after birth

e) Cephalhematoma is hemorrhage under the periosteum caused by prolonged pressure, forceps, manual rotation, or rapid compression/decompression. Limited to individual bones; does not cross suture lines. Lasts for weeks.

3) Contraction pattern frequency, duration, intensity

4) Position of location of maximum intensity of fetal heart tones

a) Generally auscultated through the fetal back with vertex and breech presentations; through the fetal thorax with face presentation

b) Location of maximum intensity of FHT varies with descent and presentation

c) Midway between umbilicus and symphysis in cephalic presentations

d) Above umbilicus with breech or transverse presentations

5) Maternal behavior changes

6) Signs and symptoms of transition and impending second stage

7) Bladder status

8) General condition, e.g., hydration, fatigue, coping ability

c. First stage management decisions

1) Frequency and indications of vaginal examinations for normal labor

a) On admission to verify presentation, position, station, status of membranes and cervical assessment

b) Before deciding on pain medication

c) To verify complete dilation (i.e., encourage or discourage pushing)

d) After spontaneous rupture of membranes, to check for a prolapsed cord

e) FHR abnormalities (fetal distress)

2) Artificial rupture of membranes (amniotomy; AROM)

a) To attach an internal fetal scalp electrode

b) Birth is imminent

c) Need to stimulate labor, or to facilitate fetal descent, or to reduce the possibility that a sudden, strong rupture of the membranes will cause a cord prolapse

d) Early amniotomy will not impede labor IF the presenting part is well applied to the cervix (may shorten labor by 30 minutes to 2 hours)

3) Ambulation

a) Ambulation is safe and provides women with more control and options for comfort than confinement to bed.

b) Women should not labor in the supine position (i.e., lying flat on their backs)

4) Food and fluids

a) There is no way to ensure that a laboring woman has an empty stomach or to increase gastric pH above 2.5.

b) Fasting, antacids and mechanically emptying the stomach are only partially effective.

c) Although pregnancy and labor slow the emptying of the GI tract, opioid analgesia that has the greatest impact on slowing the emptying of the GI tract.

d) In labor when allowed to consume oral intake, most women will choose fluids and light intake (e.g. gelatin, soup).

e) Aspiration is rare and some studies have documented no increase in aspiration when women consumed up to 150 milliliters of fluid within 2 hours of anesthesia for elective surgery

5) Types of graphic analysis of labor

a) **Partogram**: A labor graph used by WHO to monitor labor progress (i.e. cervical dilation and fetal descent)

(1) Labor is divided into a latent phase and an active phase beginning at 3 cm.

(2) A 4 hour wait (lag time) is recommended before intervention or when active phase is slow.

b) **Friedman curve**: A graphic analysis of labor that plots cervical dilation and fetal descent.

c) Friedman's 2 phases of first stage

(1) Latent phase

Mean length latent phase

- Nullipara = 6.4 hrs
- Multipara = 4.8 hrs

(2) Active phase

(a) Acceleration

(b) Maximum slope

(c) Deceleration

Mean length active phase

- Nullipara = 4.6 hrs
- Multipara = 2.6 hrs

(3) Minimum (NOT average!) rates of normal dilation

- Nullipara.= 1.2 cm/hr
- Multipara= 1.5 cm/hr

(4) Second stage (mean length)

- Nullipara = 50 min
- Multipara = 20 min

d) ABNORMAL labor progress (according to Friedman)

(1) Latent phase length

- Nullipara = > 20 hr
- Multipara = >14 hr

(2) Active phase

- Nullipara = >11.7 hr
- Multipara = > 5.2 hr

NOTE: Friedman reported 8-9 cm. as the end of active phase for these timing purposes

e) Clinical features of Friedman's functional divisions of labor

(1) Preparatory division

(a) Coordinating contractions; preparing cervix

(b) Disorder: Prolonged latent phase

(2) Dilational division

(a) Actively dilating cervix

(b) Phase of maximum slope

(c) Disorders

i. ***Protracted active phase***

ii. ***Secondary arrest of labor***

iii. ***Prolonged deceleration phase***

> **Midwifery Message**
> If you have a question on progress in labor (and odds are you will) remember the difference between Friedman's <u>average</u> lengths of normal labor and lengths for <u>abnormal</u> labor. It is easy to confuse the two

(3) Pelvic division

(a) Negotiating pelvis, mechanisms of labor, fetal descent, delivery

(b) Disorders

i. ***Protracted descent***

ii. ***Arrest of descent***

2. Assessment of woman's physical response to labor

a. Effacement and dilation are the hallmark physical signs of true labor and first stage labor progress

1) True labor

a) Intensified by walking

b) Pain located across the uterus, moving from the fundus to the back

2) Active stage (from beginning of cervical change, e.g. 3-4cm, until complete)

3) Physical signs of transition (8-10 cm dilation, just before complete)

- Beads of perspiration on the upper lip
- Shaking, chattering, hiccupping, belching/burping
- Thirst
- Nausea
- Restlessness
- Irritable abdomen
- Difficult to rouse
- Toe curling
- Severe backache
- Increased bloody show
- Rectal pressure/bulging
- Grunting
- Loss of modesty

3. **Assessment of fetal status following artificial rupture of membranes**
   a. Fetal assessment should be performed before and after amniotomy (and after spontaneous rupture of membranes). Remove hook but keep vaginal hand in place through another contraction to assure that there is no prolapsed cord and that the presenting part is filling the pelvis.
   b. Note cervical dilation, effacement, station, presentation and position
   c. Note amount, color, and odor of fluid
   d. Note FHR as soon as possible after amniotomy or spontaneous rupture of membranes.
   e. Scalp electrode can be applied immediately following amniotomy if internal monitoring is indicated; may monitor FHT by Doppler continuous or intermittent or intermittently by fetoscope if normal.
   f. Meconium stained fluid usually is an indication for more frequent monitoring, perhaps even continuous
4. **Assessment and management of second stage labor**
   a. ***The second stage of labor begins when the cervix is fully dilated and ends with the baby's birth.*** Median time in nulliparous women is 50 minutes and 20 minutes in multiparous women (no epidural)
   b. Data base for well being for the second stage of labor
      1) Continuing evaluation of significant findings from history, physical, pelvic examinations, labs
      2) Continuing evaluation of labor progress, specifically descent
      3) Continuing evaluation of fetal well being every 15 min. in low risk women and every 5 min. in high risk women
      4) Continuing evaluation of laboring woman and support with pushing as needed
      5) Continuing observation for signs of complications
   c. **Physiologic changes**
      1) Uterine action
         a) Contractions are often stronger and longer except in the case of epidural anesthesia. Fetal descent provides an endogenous stimulus for oxytocin release (Ferguson reflex)
         b) Continued, progressive contraction and retraction of upper uterine segment
         c) Contractions become increasingly expulsive as pressure exerted on pelvic floor
      2) Membranes often rupture spontaneously
      3) Pressure on the fetal axis increases flexion of head
      4) Maternal urge to push
      5) Pain migrates from lower back to around the rectum and perineum

6) Use of secondary powers of expulsion by contracting abdominal muscles and diaphragm

d. Signs of beginning of second stage

1) Expulsive uterine contractions
2) Rupture of forebag
3) Dilation and gaping of rectum, perineal bulging
4) Appearance of presenting part
5) Increased bloody show
6) Congestion of the vulva
7) Maternal need to have a bowel movement
8) Maternal statement, "baby's coming"

e. Confirming second stage

1) Confirm, when necessary, by vaginal examination
2) Evidence suggests that vaginal delivery may be more likely in women with epidural anesthesia if pushing is delayed for 1-2 hours after complete dilation (delayed pushing or "laboring down")

f. The mechanisms of labor that culminate during the second stage are called the cardinal movements of labor. The fetus turns slightly to take advantage of the widest available space in each plane as it descends through the pelvis.

1) **Descent**
    a) Often begins before onset of labor
    b) First stage labor aids descent
    c) After rupture of membranes and complete cervical dilation, maternal efforts speed progress
2) **Flexion**
    a) Increases throughout labor
    b) Increased flexion results in smaller presenting diameters
    c) With flexion, the occiput becomes the presenting part
3) **Internal rotation**
    a) With contraction, the occiput is pushed onto pelvic floor
    b) Resistance is an important determinant of rotation
    c) Rotation may be delayed in women with epidural anesthesia due to relaxation of pelvic floor muscles
    d) In well flexed vertex presentation, the occiput rotates 45 degrees
    e) ***Upon completion of internal rotation, the occiput lies under symphysis***

f) ***If flexion is maintained, the suboccipitobregmatic diameter distends the vaginal orifice***

4) **Extension**

a) Once crowning occurs, the fetal head extends, pivoting around the pubic bone

b) Sinciput, face, and chin sweep perineum and fully extend

5) **Restitution**

a) Slight untwisting of neck-occiput moves 45 degrees toward side from which it started

6) **External rotation**

a) As shoulders rotate into the anteroposterior diameter, the fetal head rotates 45 degrees further

b) The fetal head now is transverse, with the occiput on the left or right

7) **Expulsion**

a) Lateral flexion with birth of shoulders and body

g. Duration of second stage

(Friedman's data)

1) Second stage (means)

Nullipara = 50 min

Multipara = 20 min

2) Parameters of normal length second stage

a) Nullipara

- No epidural ≤2 hours
- Epidural ≤3 hours

b) Multipara

- No epidural <1 hour
- Epidural <2 hours

c) Time limits for length of second stage have been challenged

(1) De-emphasize defined time limit

(2) Doesn't mean you can't continue to labor the woman, but should take measures to document fetal well-being when parameters are exceeded

h. Management of second stage labor

1) Evaluation of fetal well being fetal heart rate changes every 15 minutes for low risk women and every 5 minutes for high risk women.

2) Pushing

a) Physiologic approach

(1) Based on response to Ferguson's reflex (stimulation of receptors in pelvic floor in response to pressure of fetal head as it descends past ischial spines)

(2) Wait for maternal spontaneous urge to bear down

(3) Involuntary bearing down pressures accompanied by exhalatory or "open glottis" pushing efforts

(4) Mothers less likely to have episiotomies, second or third degree laceration

3) Traditional pushing technique

a) Directed, strong sustained pushing with contractions

b) "Hold breath and push as long and hard as you can for 10 seconds"

c) Closed glottis or Valsalva maneuver

d) Prolonged bearing down efforts may have negative outcomes

(1) Maternal fatigue

(2) Increased intrathoracic and abdominal pressure

(3) Produces vasoconstriction and decreased cardiac output

(4) Decreases fetal cerebral oxygenation and blood volume

(5) Nonreassuring fetal heart rate tracings

(6) Increased risk of cesarean delivery

e) Implications of epidural anesthesia

(1) Longer second stage

(2) Higher incidence of operative vaginal and cesarean birth

(3) Women may have more difficulty pushing

(4) Decreased bearing down reflex

(5) Decreased efficacy of pushing efforts

(6) To avoid prolonged labor, may resort to directed, sustained pushing

f) Delayed pushing with epidural anesthesia

(1) "Laboring down"; "rest and descent"

(2) Allowing 1-2 hours of rest at complete dilation before onset of pushing

(3) Results in shortened periods of pushing, lower incidence of FHT decelerations, less maternal fatigue

F. Monitoring/co-management of woman receiving pharmacologic therapy during labor

1. Cervical ripening/induction agents

a. Commonly used method of assessment for induction of labor is the Bishop Score

Bishop Score

Factor	Score			
	0	1	2	3
Cervical Dilation (cm)	Closed	1-2	3-4	5+
Cervical Effacement (%)	0-30	40-50	60-70	80+
Fetal Station	-3	-2	-1,0	+1, +2
Cervical Consistency	Firm	Medium	Soft	
Cervical Position	Posterior	Mid	Anterior	

From Bishop, E. (1966). American Journal of Obstetrics and Gynecology, 24, 266

b. Scores 0-4 usually are associated with a failure rate of greater than 20%; scores greater than 9 have <1% failure rate. ***Most inductions are performed with scores of 6 or higher when possible***

   1) Note that original research was performed with multiparous women, and has not been validated with nulliparous women. Dr Bishop's purpose was to predict the success of induction by amniotomy for multiparas.

c. Several uterotropins have been recognized -- agents that break down the collagen matrix of the cervix, softening it and thus making it more suitable to induction

   1) Herbs: there is lack of adequate research to support their use

      a) Evening primrose oil
      b) Raspberry leaf
      c) Black cohosh
         (1) Overdose can cause cardiotoxicity
      d) Blue cohosh --papoose root or squaw root
         (1) Side effects tend to be fetal, as in increased meconium, fetal tachycardia, fetal distress
      e) Castor oil
         (1) Triglyceride and ricinoleic acid stimulate the bowel
         (2) Onset of action is 1-6 hours
         (3) Usual dosage is 60 mL per hour for up to 5 times

Nonpharmacologic Approaches to Cervical Ripening and Induction

Sexual orgasm	Not included in standard medical texts, although several studies in literature, most researching preterm labor Biologically plausible Female—mechanical stimulation of orgasm on uterus Male—addition of prostaglandins from ejaculate
Nipple and breast stimulation	Effective means (as documented in history); RCT's do not demonstrate efficacy Potential hyperstimulation is concern: limit to healthy pregnancies Minimize hyperstimulation by gentle stimulation of one breast at a time, with stimulation stopped during a contraction
Herbal remedies	Primarily anecdotal, particularly *Evening primrose oil* and *black cohosh tincture*
Homeopathic solutions	Most commonly recommended remedy is Caulophllus or *Caulophyllum thalictroides (Blue cohosh)*: Up to 6 doses of 30C strength
Castor oil	Theorized to stimulate prostaglandin release Effects may be most pronounced among primigravidas Best taken 1-2 hours before a woman usually arises, not at end of day No evidence that it is linked to meconium in fetus
Warm water	Suggested that warmth may help augment labor via increased firing of neurons, relaxation and pain relief (decrease in catecholamines)
Enemas	Never well established for initiation or even augmentation
Acupuncture	*San Yin Chiao* (Sp 6) and *Ho Ku* (L4) have been used Some studies found very favorable results (e.g. 21/31 women induced by acupuncture of these sites), but studies are limited.
Sweeping (stripping) membranes	Increase in prostaglandin production; RCT's show reduction in inductions for post-term May increase cervical ripening Often uncomfortable for woman Obviously contraindicated if previa, bleeding Potential problems with infection and accidental rupture of membranes
Balloon catheters	#16 Foley catheter with 30 cc of saline in the bulb, passed through the cervical os produced cervical ripening after 12 hours
Laminaria	Desiccated stems of cold water seaweed (*Laminaria japonicum)* Also can use synthetic osmotic dilators (up to 24 weeks) Most commonly used with second trimester abortions
Amniotomy	Most successful with ripe cervix Commits to delivery Usually will reduce length of labor by approximately 30 minutes Best done 4 centimeters or more

From Summers, L. (1997). Methods of cervical ripening and labor induction. Journal of Nurse-Midwifery, 42(2), 71-85.

2) Other pharmaceuticals for ripening, induction

a) **Dinoprostone** (PGE_2 gel, *Cervidil®, Prepidil®*); FDA approved for cervical ripening

(1) Gel (*Prepidil®*): One syringe of gel (0.5 mg/ 3 ml gel) in cervical os

(a) Repeat every 6 hours up to 3 doses in 24 hours

(b) Wait 6-12 hours before starting pitocin

(2) Tape (*Cervidil®*): Insert around cervix in posterior fornix

(a) Repeat every 12 hours

b) **Misoprostol** (PGE_1, *Cytotec®*); NOT FDA approved for cervical ripening

(1) Insert 25 to 50 microgram tablet intravaginally

(2) Repeat every 4-6 hours as needed

(3) Major controversy since manufacturer sent letter around country noting that the agent is not FDA approved for cervical ripening. Recent studies have shown prostaglandins should not be used for cervical ripening in women with a previous cesarean section.

c) ***Major complication of prostaglandin ripening agents is hyperstimulation***

(1) Cochrane Library suggests not to use misoprostol due to lack of studies and propensity for hyperstimulation

(2) If there is hyperstimulation, consider giving terbutaline .25 mg SQ

(3) If Dinoprostone (*Cervidil*®) was used, remove it from vagina

(4) If Misoprostol (*Cytotec*®) was used, irrigate vagina

(a) Use normal saline via 100 cc Syringe (no needle)

(b) Repeat several times until pill fragments are recovered

d) **Oxytocin (*Pitocin*®)**

(1) Preparation usually is *Pitocin*® in IV fluid

(2) Dosage regimen, e.g., high versus low dose, depends on institutional guidelines; commonly used dilutions (know how to calculate, as there are <u>many</u> variations):

- *Pitocin* 10 units in 1000 mL IV fluid (10 mU/mL)
  - ❖ 6 cc/hr = 1 mU/min
- *Pitocin* 20 units in 1000 mL IV fluid (20 mU/mL)
  - ❖ 3cc/hr = 1 mU/min

(3) Monitoring: continuous electronic monitoring of uterine activity and FHR is usually employed

(a) If intrauterine pressure catheter (IUPC) is used, may calculate Montevideo units (MVU) to quantify labor

(b) Adequate contraction pattern indicators

- Uterine pressure >50 mmHg per contraction
- MVU 200-300 (total heights of uterine contractions in mm Hg minus baseline tone per 10 minutes)
- Progress in labor

(4) Complications

(a) **Fetal distress**

(b) Hyperstimulation/tetanic contractions : *> 5 contractions in 10 minutes, >7 contractions 15 minutes, contractions lasting longer than 60 to 90 seconds, or nonreassuring FHR*

(c) Management includes discontinuing or decreasing oxytocin (depending upon severity of contractions)

(d) Oxygen for woman, lateral position and fluid bolus may be given, though there is little evidence of efficacy

(e) Consultation/referral with physician

(f) According to Enkin, there is evidence linking oxytocin induction with an increased risk of neonatal hyperbilirubinemia

2. Group B streptococcus (GBS) prophylaxis

a. Group B Streptococcus infection (CDC, 2002)

1) Leading cause of life-threatening infection (meningitis, sepsis) in newborns.

2) May be transmitted to infant during labor and delivery if mother is colonized.

a) Newborn might appear healthy at birth, then suddenly develop fever, lethargy, and respiratory distress; then meningitis, sepsis, or pneumonia and, in extreme cases, death. If the baby survives, child may develop hearing loss, vision loss, or mental retardation years later. In the pregnant woman, GBS can cause urinary tract infection, pre-term birth, and miscarriage. Postpartum, may cause endometritis.

b) Incidence is 0.6 cases/1000 live births; approximately 7,500 GBS cases annually in newborns; death in ~ 5%

c) Disease rates are higher in African Americans of all age groups and Caucasian women under 20 years of age

3) 10-30% of women are colonized with GBS bacteria. The natural reservoir for the organism is the GI tract. Most women show no symptoms.

4) Risk factors

a) Previously delivered infant with GBS infection

b) GBS in urine during antepartum course or positive GBS culture this pregnancy

c) Delivery less than 37 weeks

d) Rupture of membranes ≥ 18 hours

e) Intrapartum temperature ≥ 100.4° F (38.0° C)

f) ***In presence of any of the above risk factors give intrapartum antibiotic prophylaxis (IAP)***

5) Prevention

a) In 2002, CDC recommended universal screening (i.e. all pregnant women)

(1) Culture rectal and vaginal areas at 35-37 gestational weeks. Culture results are good for 5 weeks; if negative at 35 weeks and she goes past 40 weeks, consider reculturing. If positive, consider her GBS positive.

(2) IAP for women who are positive or have preterm birth

(3) IAP for women with previous affected baby (don't need to culture with current pregnancy)

(4) IAP for women with GBS bacteriuria (and treat prenatally if symptomatic)

(5) No IAP for positive culture in previous pregnancy with unaffected baby and negative screen with current pregnancy

(6) IAP only for risk factors identified above if GBS status is unknown

b) For premature rupture of membranes (PROM) when gestation < 37 weeks and no labor, obtain cultures and begin IAP until culture results are obtained. If negative discontinue IAP; OR wait for culture results before beginning antibiotics

c) **Treatment regimens for IAP**

(1) Penicillin G 5 million units IV; 2.5 million units IV every 4 hours until birth (preferred as it is less broad spectrum than ampicillin, thus causing less development of antibiotic resistant strains)

(2) Ampicillin 2 grams IV; 1gram IV every four hours until delivery

(3) Penicillin allergic

(a) Clindamycin 900 milligrams IV every 8 hours until birth OR

(b) Erythromycin 500 milligrams IV every 6 hours until birth

Source: http://www.cdc.gov/mmwr/preview/mmwrhtml/rr5111a1.htm

Did you know GBS is transmitted at birth and IAP is not indicated for a planned CS birth?

But even women planning to deliver by CS should participate in universal screening since they may go into spontaneous labor before their due date

3. **Tocolytics**

a. ***Preterm labor (PTL): labor that commences between the 20th to the 37th gestational week or delivery at or before 36 weeks gestation (<37 weeks)***

1) ***Regular uterine contractions (often painless) accompanied by cervical change with dilation 2cm or greater and cervical effacement of 80% or more*** (exact parameters are not standard). Presenting symptoms may be mild or nonspecific and include:

a) Dull backache
b) Suprapubic pain or pressure
c) Pelvic pressure/fullness
d) Vaginal discharge, spotting, bleeding

2) Risk Factors

a) History
- **Previous preterm birth**
- Several abortions
- Low pre-pregnancy weight
- Cervical trauma
- DES exposure
- Hemoglobinopathies (e.g., G6PD)
- Short interval between pregnancies

b) Current Pregnancy
- SROM (spontaneous rupture of membranes)
- Amniotic fluid infection
- Fetal anomalies
- Fetal death
- Cervical incompetence
- Uterine anomalies
- Retained intrauterine contraceptive device (IUD)
- Faulty placentation
- Serious maternal disease
- Hypertension
- Multiple gestation/overdistention of the uterus
- Poor weight gain

c) Demographic/life style risk factors
- Lower socioeconomic status
- Age < 17 years
- African American
- Unmarried, low education
- Smoking/substance abuse

3) While previous preterm birth is the factor most highly predictive of preterm labor and birth, any woman with signs or symptoms of preterm labor with or without predisposing factors should be seen immediately.

a) Perform history and physical exam to rule out infection (UTI, vaginitis, cervicitis, viral or bacterial).

b) Pelvic exam is performed AFTER collection of fetal fibronectin specimen, if appropriate.

c) If rupture of membranes is suspected, perform a sterile speculum exam and omit the bimanual exam.

d) Lab tests may include:

(1) Microscopic and/or dipstick urinalysis

(2) Urine culture and sensitivity

(3) Wet mount of vaginal discharge

(4) Fern and nitrazine tests

(5) With premature rupture of membranes, add a CBC with differential

(6) **Fetal fibronectin**: obtain specimen from posterior fornix BEFORE cervical examination. May obtain specimen and save it until the assessment is complete. If indicated it can be sent to lab. If not indicated, dispose. False positive more likely if test is done within 24 hours of pelvic examination or vaginal intercourse.

4) Diagnosis of PTL

a) Cervix

(1) Exact dilation not established

(2) Sonographic determination of shortening of cervix has been found to be useful as predictor

b) Fetal fibronectin

(1) Level in cervicovaginal secretions is associated with preterm labor and birth; > 50 nanograms/mL at 24-34 weeks gestation is associated with preterm delivery

(2) Greatest use is negative predictive value (if negative 99.5% will not deliver in 2 weeks)

(3) Helps midwives determine which women need referral

5) Non-pharmaceutical management of PTL

a) Identification of women at risk for preterm labor

b) Bed rest and limitation of physical activities are widely used; however, research does not support. Benefits, if any, do not outweigh risks. Bed rest does not change the incidence of preterm birth.

c) Social support, home visiting may improve outcomes by reducing stress, but does not change the incidence of preterm birth.

d) Hydration decreases uterine irritability, but does not change the incidence of preterm birth.

e) Advise against sexual intercourse with internal ejaculation because of theoretical risk of inducing labor with seminal prostaglandins. If the patient continues to have sexual intercourse, the use of condoms is strongly encouraged.

f) Education on the signs and symptoms of preterm labor

g) Home uterine monitoring for early recognition of contractions (not recommended by ACOG because evidence does not support)

h) Nutritional counseling (continues to be debatable, but it cannot hurt)

6) Tocolysis for PTL

a) Tocolytic: drug that inhibits uterine contractions

(1) Most work by stimulation of cAMP that inhibits actin/myosin, moves calcium out of the cell and culminates in relaxation of myometrium

(2) Since initiation of labor is not well understood it is not illogical that tocolytics are not well understood

(3) Large number of drugs proposed to be used as tocolytics

(4) No study has convincingly demonstrated an improvement in survival, long-term perinatal morbidity or mortality, or neonatal outcome with the use of tocolytic therapy alone

b) Tocolytic therapy may offer short-term benefit in the management of preterm labor by delaying delivery to administer corticosteroids.

(1) 1994 NIH Consensus Panel recommended broad use for women at risk for preterm delivery

(2) Corticosteroids enhance pulmonary maturity, reduce the severity of neonatal respiratory distress syndrome, and reduce the risk of intraventricular hemorrhage.

(3) *No more than one complete course of corticosteroids should be administered. Adverse neonatal outcomes are suggested with multiple courses of treatment:*

(a) Lower birth weight

(b) Potentially increased mortality

(c) Prolonged adrenal suppression

(d) New controversy that corticosteroids even in one dose may be harmful

> In spite of the fact that there is a large body of scientific evidence that tocolytic agents prolong pregnancy only by 24-48 hours at best, these agents often are used. The choice of the agent seems to be determined regionally or by the institution. ***Often they are chosen to provide time to administer steroids***

c) Delay can permit transfer of woman to a tertiary care center.

d) ***Tocolytic therapy also has potential for maternal complications, in particular pulmonary edema***

(1) Contraindications to tocolysis include nonreassuring fetal heart rate tracing, eclampsia or severe preeclampsia, fetal demise (singleton), chorioamnionitis, fetal maturity and maternal hemodynamic instability.

(2) Criteria for initiating tocolytic therapy vary by institution. Regular uterine contractions and cervical change (effacement or dilatation) appear to be the most widely used criteria. Dilation of at least 3 cm is associated with less effective treatment results.

Typical Dosing Regimens of Selected Tocolytics

Drug	Initial Dose	Maintenance	Maximum
Ritodrine (Yutopar)*	0.1 milligrams/min IV Increase 0.05 milligrams/min Every 10 min	Continue IV for 12 h after cessation of contractions, then 10 milligrams PO every 2 h for 24 h; then 10-20 milligrams every 4 – 6 h	120 milligrams over 24 h
Terbutaline (Brethine, Bricanyl)	2.5 micrograms/min IV Increase by 2.5 mcg every minute until contractions cease or maximum dose attained	250 mcg SQ every 3 h	20 mcg per min IV
Magnesium Sulfate ($MgSO_4$)	6 g in 10% solution over 15 min, followed by infusion rate of 2 g/h Increase by 1 g/h until contractions are less than 1 in 10 min	Continue IV for 12-24 h Wean at 1 g/h every 30 min Stop when rate is at 2 g/h PO use – magnesium oxide or magnesium gluconate 1 g every 2-4 h	4-5 g per h
Nifedipine (Procardia)	10 mg PO or SL Repeat every 20 min for two or three doses	10-20 mg every 4-6	40 mg in an hour
Indomethacin (Indocin)	50 milligrams PO or 100 milligrams rectally	25 mgr every 6 h for 2-3 days	50 mg in an hour

*only drug that is FDA approved for treatment of preterm labor

Complications Associated with Various Tocolytics

Magnesium Sulfate	Beta Adrenergic Agents (e.g. Terbutaline, Ritodrine)	Nonsteroidal Anti Inflammatory Drugs (e.g. Indomethacin)	Calcium Channel Blocker (e.g. Nifedipine)
Pulmonary edema Profound hypotension Profound muscular paralysis Maternal tetany Cardiac arrest **Respiratory depression at toxic level**	Hypokalemia Hyperglycemia Hypotension Pulmonary edema Arrhythmias Cardiac insufficiency Myocardial ischemia Maternal death	Renal failure with toxic level Hepatitis with toxic level Gastrointestinal bleeding if chronic use	Transient hypotension

4. **Magnesium sulfate ($MgSO_4$)**

a. Anticonvulsant for prophylaxis and treatment of seizures in eclampsia (also used as tocolytic; see section above)

b. IV administration for seizure prophylaxis

1) 4-6 g IV over 5-10 minutes; then 1-2 g/hour

c. IV+IM administration

1) 4 g 20% solution IV over 5 minutes

2) 10 g 50% solution deep IM

3) 5 g 50% solution deep IM every 4 hours thereafter

(1) IF DTRs, respirations, and urine output are normal

d. Usually discontinue 24 hours post delivery

e. Monitor for toxicity

1) Hourly deep tendon reflexes and respiratory rate

2) Monitor magnesium levels

3) *For magnesium overdose/toxicity*

Calcium gluconate in 10% solution 10 mL (1 g) IV

Magnesium Levels	
6-8 mEq/L	**Ideal therapeutic level**
8-10 mEq/L	Decreased DTRs
13-15 mEq/L	Respiratory paralysis
>15 mEq/L	Cardiac conduction affected
>25 mEq/L	Cardiac arrest

G. **Management of the perineum**

1. Perineal preparation and support to prevent tears, lacerations and need for episiotomy

a. Factors associated with protection of the perineum (research evidence):

1) Prenatal perineal massage

2) Parity

b. Other measures that may promote perineal integrity

1) Warm compresses at birth

2) Flexion/counterpressure to slow delivery

3) Birth positions other than lithotomy

4) Avoidance of the use of forceps

5) Avoidance of oil and lubricants at birth

(1) A recent study by Albers in JMWH found that three techniques -- massage with lubricants, hands off or warm compresses as applied by experienced midwives -- were equally effective in maintaining perineal integrity. Mothers randomized to massage with lubricant more often asked that the intervention be stopped.

6) Non valsalvar pushing

c. The primary cause for third and fourth degree perineal lacerations is an episiotomy

2. Local anesthetic techniques (including pudendal)

a. Pharmacologic properties of local anesthetic agents

1) Concentration of drug used is proportional to the density of the block

2) All are potent vasodilators. Degree of absorption related to vascularity of the area

3) The greater the lipid solubility the greater the potency

4) The greater the protein binding the greater the duration of action

b. Bupivacaine (*Marcaine*)

1) Most widely used agent for 1st stage epidurals

2) High affinity for maternal proteins

3) Less affinity for fetal proteins than lidocaine

4) Cardiac toxicity associated with concentration of .75%

c. Lidocaine (*Xylocaine*®)

1) Quicker onset than bupivacaine

2) Duration of action 60 min. with epidurals

3) Ion trapping in the fetus (especially problematic for acidotic fetus)

d. To administer a local anesthetic

1) Use a small bore needle

2) Insert needle into laceration/episiotomy or intact perineum along anticipated tract of episiotomy incision if planned

3) Aspirate to ensure the needle is not in a blood vessel.

4) Inject local anesthetic as needle is withdrawn

5) Anesthesia is very rapid

6) Repeat as needed within the range of normal dosage

e. Pudendal aesthesia is regional anesthesia, which blocks the pudendal nerve

1) Anesthetizes the perineum and entire vulva and rectum; it does not affect contractions

2) Very safe, as long as the local is not injected into a blood vessel

3) *Xylocaine 1% most common agent with 1 0mL per side as usual dose*

a) Duration is approximately 90 minutes

b) Maximum safe dose is 500 mg (50 mL of 10 mg/mL solution)

4) To administer a pudendal

a) Locate the pudendal nerve by first locating the ischial spine and insert the needle in guide; position the tip immediately beneath and medial to the inferior medial border of the spine

b) Insert the needle through the guide and aspirate

c) Some advocate rotating the needle180 degrees and aspirate again; this ensures the bevel is not against the wall of a blood vessel

d) If no blood return, inject. If blood return, remove and begin again

f. Local anesthesia toxicity

1) Accidental intravascular administration

2) Accumulation of local anesthetic over time

3) Signs and symptoms

a) Tingling of extremities

b) Metallic taste

c) Confusion, uneasy feeling

d) Convulsion (0.03-0.5% incidence)

4) To prevent toxicity,

a) Aspirate prior to administration

b) Do not inject more than the maximum dosage

3. Episiotomy

a. Incision into the perineum (area of skin between the vagina and the anus) to enlarge the opening.

b. Types of episiotomies

1) ***Midline*** cuts through the central tendinous point of the perineum, separates the bulbocavernosus and superficial transverse muscle. With deeper cuts, the deep transverse muscle is separated

2) **Mediolateral** cuts to the left or right on a slant, starting at the mid-fourchette. Cuts into the central tendinous point of the perineum, through the bulbocavernosus and the superficial transverse muscle and into the levator ani, particularly the pubococcygeus muscle

> **Tip**—know the muscles that are cut with an episiotomy.

H. Conduct of delivery

1. Hand maneuvers/mechanisms of labor

a. Occiput anterior (OA)

1) Mechanism of labor

a) Six cardinal movements (mechanism of labor) exist that describe the passage of the fetus through the pelvis and vagina. The average labor begins with a fetus in either a transverse position or one of the anterior positions, i.e. the occiput is in the forepelvis. The following table summarizes how the fetus follows the pelvic curve (Curve of Carus) and is born

Mechanism of Labor for Occiput Anterior Presentation

Descent	Engagement occurs when the widest portion of the presenting part has passed through the pelvic inlet. In a cephalic presentation, the widest portion is the biparietal diameter (BPD); when the BPD passes through the pelvic inlet, the lowermost part of the head is usually at the plane of the ischial spines (0 station). Primigravidas usually engage before entering labor, Multiparous women frequently do not.
Flexion	Usually the fetus is in a position of partial flexion since this is the natural "attitude" of the term intrauterine conceptus. Flexion changes the diameters of the head so that the presenting diameter is smaller. The more resistance from the pelvic floor, the more flexion.
Internal Rotation	The purpose of this action is to rotate the head into the anteroposterior diameter so that it can be born. Although it may occur in early labor, it usually is not complete until the head reaches the pelvic floor, in second stage.
Extension	The flexed head continues its descent and the occiput passes slowly through the outlet until the nape of the neck pivots under the pubic arch. Then the sinciput quickly sweeps along the sacrum, followed by the bregma, forehead, nose, mouth and chin.
Restitution	Allows the head to return to be in line with the shoulders that are in the oblique diameter.
External Rotation	Outward manifestation of shoulder internal rotation.
Expulsion	Birth of the body

Think of the pelvis as a cylinder. It is round or oval shaped at the top (inlet), wider than it is deep. In the middle (mid pelvis, at the level of the ischial spines), it is round, and at its smallest diameter. At the bottom (outlet), it is deeper than it is wide. Therefore, the head enters the pelvis in a transverse or oblique diameter and the occiput rotates to the widest part of the pelvis for expulsion – either anteriorly or posteriorly, depending on the shape of the pelvis.

2) **Hand maneuvers**

a) ***Keep the head flexed with pressure on the occiput (downward if the mother is recumbent and baby is OA) and control speed of delivery.***

b) ***Perineal support (no evidence).***

c) ***Let the head gradually emerge*** until it completely extends and the chin sweeps the perineum.

d) ***Check for nuchal cord***

e) ***Suction mouth and then nose if indicated with bulb or DeLee catheter***

f) ***"Sandwich" the head with your fingers to the face*** to minimize pulling too hard and causing injury to the neck or tentorial tears.

g) ***Gently guide the baby in the curve of Carus*** by directing the head away from the pubis (downward if the mother is recumbent) until the anterior shoulder delivers, then toward the pubis (upward if the mother is recumbent) to guide the posterior shoulder over the perineum.

h) ***Maintaining control*** over the upper part of the baby's body with one hand cradling the head and holding the shoulder, slide the other hand down the body and grasp the baby between the legs.

i) ***Place baby on mother's abdomen,*** in her arms, on the bed, or in a football hold as appropriate and indicated by the mother's wishes and the baby's condition.

Anterior and Transverse Positions of the Occiput: Mechanism of Labor				
Onset of Labor	**LOA**	**ROA**	**LOT**	**ROT**
Descent and Flexion	LOA	ROA	LOT	ROT
Internal Rotation	OA	OA	LOA, OA	ROA, OA
Extension	OA	OA	OA	OA
Restitution	LOA	ROA	LOA	ROA
External Rotation	LOT	ROT	LOT	ROT

b. **Occiput posterior (OP)**

1) OP positions are less common than anterior, but still occur relatively frequently. It is estimated that they may occur in 25% of labors. More commonly ROP than LOP.
2) Posterior positions may rotate either long arc (and culminate in an occiput anterior for birth) or short arc (and culminate in an occiput posterior for birth; sometimes called sunny side up; or--in the UK--face to pubis).
3) Clinical signs/symptoms
   a) Severe back pain (so called "back labor")
   b) Dip at the umbilicus upon inspection of the abdomen
   c) Inability to locate the fetal back easily on Leopold maneuvers
4) ***Women with anthropoid type pelvises (or android) are more likely to have a posterior position***. Since African American women have a higher incidence of an anthropoid hindpelvis, some texts may indicate that they have a higher risk of having a fetus in an occiput posterior position.
5) Most of the time an occiput posterior will deliver vaginally. However, sometimes it necessitates an operative intervention, for which the midwife would consult.
   a) Cesarean section if an arrest occurs.
   b) Forceps rotation or delivery as persistent OP
   c) Manual rotation should be performed carefully, moving the head in the normal arc and facilitating internal rotation.

6) Head enters the pelvis in OT or OP position. Internal rotation may be short arc to OA or long arc to OP. Head may not be well flexed

Posterior Positions of the Occiput: Mechanism of Labor				
Onset of Labor	**LOP Long arc**	**ROP long arc**	**LOP short arc**	**ROP short arc**
Descent and Flexion	LOP	ROP	LOP	ROP
Internal Rotation	LOP-LOT LOT-LOA	ROP-ROT ROT-ROA	OP	OP
Extension	OA	OA	OP	OP
Restitution	LOA	ROA	LOP	ROP
External Rotation	LOT	ROT	LOT	ROT

7) Hand maneuvers are similar to those used for an OA, except to keep the head flexed, pressure on the occiput should be directed toward the pubis (up if the mother is recumbent). Caution should be exercised as the head extends, since it can do so quickly and cause anterior and perineal damage.

c. Nonvertex presentations

- Malpresentation is a term used to describe the unusual incidences wherein the fetus is not in an occiput position, be it anterior, transverse or posterior. These include face, brow, breech and shoulder/transverse presentations.
- Malpresentations are associated with fetal-pelvic disproportions.
- Other etiologies include problems with the passage/powers (uterine fibroids, lax abdominal muscles for multiparous women, uterine abnormalities, placenta previa) or the passenger (multifetal pregnancy, fetal anomalies, hydramnios, fetal attitude of extension instead of flexion, macrosomia).
- Breech presentations are more common for the preterm infant than the term infant

> For malpresentations, make certain you could identify one from a description of FHT location, Leopold's findings, and pelvic examination. Know which ones deliver by extension and which deliver by flexion

- ***Clinical signs often include unusual placement of fetal heart tones (e.g. above the umbilicus), strange curvature of the abdomen, inability to feel the sagittal suture on vaginal examination and unusual findings upon Leopold maneuvers***
- **Note that in several of these presentations, the baby is born via <u>flexion</u>, not extension**

1) **Face presentation is unusual, < 1 % of all births.** Predisposing factors include infants with neck injuries, thyroid tumors, multiple coils of nuchal cord, anencephaly and prematurity. Occasionally a woman with a large pelvis has a small infant who fits incompletely into the pelvis and a malpresentation such as a face presents.
   a) Vaginal exams need to be particularly gentle because of proximity to the orbits and soft facial tissues
   b) Spiral electrodes are contraindicated for face presentation.
   c) Hand maneuvers generally include perineal support and little if any direct pressure on the presenting part until the head has totally emerged.

> **Quick tip**
> If the mentum presents anterior, vaginal birth is possible. If it is posterior arrest and an operative birth must follow. **("Ma can, Pa can't")**

Face Presentation: Mechanism of Labor				
Onset of Labor	**LMA**	**LMT**	**LMP long arc**	**LMP short arc**
Descent and Extension	LMA	LMA	LMP	LMP
Internal Rotation	MA (MA can)	MA (MA can)	LMT-LMA-MA (MA can)	LMP-MP Arrest (Pa can't)
Flexion	MA	MA	MA	
Restitution	LMA	LMA	LMA	
External Rotation	LMT	LMT	LMT	

2) **Brow presentations are even less likely to occur than faces**. The presenting diameter is the longest AP diameter of the fetal head (the verticomental diameter). Most brow presentations are *secondary*, that is, they occur after labor begins. Few are *primary*, or occur prior to labor. Most frequently brow presentations convert—with flexion to vertex or with extension to face presentations
   a) Etiology is essentially the same as a face, as is the clinical picture.
   b) Hand maneuvers are essentially the same as for occiput, if progress occurs
   c) Mechanism of labor may include flexion with descent if conversion to vertex presentation, or extension if conversion to face presentation.
   d) Spontaneous delivery as brow presentation is rare, and can occur only if there is a large pelvis, strong contractions, and small baby.

Brow Presentation: Mechanism of Labor (Fr=frontum)				
Onset of Labor	**LFrA**	**RfrA**	**LFrT**	**RFrT**
Descent and Extension	LFrA	RfrA	LFrT	RFrT
Internal Rotation	FrA	FrA	LFrA-FrA	RFrT-FrA
Flexion	FrA	FrA	FrA	FrA
Restitution	LFrA	RfrA	LFrA	RFrA
External Rotation	LFrT	RFrT	LFrT	RFrT

3) **Breech Presentations are probably the most common malposition (3-4% at term)**. The incidence varies inversely with gestational age. Women with one breech birth are more likely to have a repeat breech, perhaps because of pelvic differences. Tips to remember with breeches

- There is a higher potential incidence of fetal trauma and neonatal morbidity and mortality with a breech--plan the birth site accordingly
- Most CNMs only attend breeches in emergencies (or with the consultant literally at hand)
- There is lack of consensus of criteria for elective vaginal breech birth, but recent data suggests vaginal route is more complicated for mother and infant, and abdominal route better
- Often it is an emergency situation (e.g. undiagnosed, or arrival at birth site when completely dilated)
- Make certain the woman is completely dilated before she pushes; complete dilation for the body may be less than the 10 cm necessary for the head. Incomplete dilation may allow the cervix to trap the after coming head
- Have adequate anesthesia, since intervention may be needed, such as Piper's forceps
- PATIENCE--never pull or tug; apt to cause the baby to raise the arms and compound complications; the general rule of thumb is hands off until the umbilicus appears
- **Warm towel (not hot, not cold) for the torso as it emerges allows provider to grasp the slippery baby better, but extremes of temperature may cause infant to attempt to gasp in utero**
- ALWAYS KEEP THE BACK UP--do not allow baby to rotate to the chest up position
- Pull down loop of cord when torso emerges
- Have someone else "follow" the head down and give suprapubic pressure to keep the head flexed

> Questions on a breech might involve the concepts of keeping the back up and having an assistant follow the head down to keep it flexed.
> **Back up, head flexed!**

➢ Remember that you need to think of breech as 3 overlapping mechanisms of labor: one for sacrum/limbs, one for shoulders and one for head.

Breech (RSA): Mechanism of Labor			
Sacrum	**Buttocks and Lower Limbs**	**Shoulders**	**Head**
RSA	Descent	--	---
RSA	Flexion (at the waist)	---	---
RSA-RST	Internal Rotation	Anterior Position	---
RST	Birth of Buttocks by Lateral Flexion	---	---
RST-RSA	Feet Born	Engage in Oblique	Directly Face Down
RSA	---	Descent	--
RSA-RST	Rotate to facilitate shoulders	Internal Rotation	Descent and Engagement Head enters the pelvis
RST	--	Birth of Shoulders by Lateral Flexion	Head in the pelvis
RST-RSA	Rotate to facilitate head	Shoulders in Oblique	Flexion
RSA-SA	Rotate to facilitate head	Shoulders in Transverse	Internal Rotation
SA	Position for birth of head	Shoulders in Transverse	Birth of the Head by Flexion

Breech Presentations: Mechanism of Labor						
Onset of Labor	**RSA**	**LSA**	**RST**	**LST**	**RSP***	**LSP***
Descent and Flexion	RSA	LSA	RST	LST	RSP	LSP
Internal Rotation	RSA-RST	LSA-LST	RST	LST	RSP -RST	LSP -LST
Extension	RST	LST	RST	LST	RST	LST
Restitution	RST-RSA	LST-LSA	RST-RSA	LST-LSA	RST-RSA	LST-LSA
External Rotation	RSA-SA	LSA-SA	RSA-SA	LSA-SA	RSA-SA	LSA-SA

* Keep the back up after the buttocks are born

a) ***Mauriceu-Smellie-Veit Maneuver***: The index and middle finger of one hand are applied over the maxilla to flex the head, while the fetal body rests upon the palm of the hand and forearm. The forearm is straddled by the fetal legs. Two fingers of the other hand are hooked on either side of the fetal neck and while grasping the shoulders, downward pressure is applied. This allows the baby to be securely held and facilitates the chin sweeping over the perineum and allowing the infant to breathe

4) **Transverse lie is rare and today is a clear indication for a cesarean section birth.**

5) **Compound Presentation usually is a hand with the head**. Most often it is simply alongside the head; rarely does it present before the head. The mechanisms of labor continue as usual, however arrest is more likely since the diameters are larger.

6) **Funic presentation indicates that the cord (funis) presents first**. This rarely occurs, and even more rarely can it be diagnosed before the membranes have ruptured and a prolapse has occurred. Usual treatment is a cesarean section birth. If prolapse has occurred, remember to:
   a) Raise the presenting part (frequently a breech) off the cord
   b) If you have to transport (e.g. in clinic and have to move to hospital)
      (1) TALK to her and family
      (2) Shift her toward a hip if possible to prevent supine hypotension
      (3) Some sources have suggested filling the bladder with fluid to keep the presenting part off the cord
      (4) Trendelenburg position may relieve pressure on the cord

Effects of Pelvis Type on Labor

Pelvis	Gynecoid	Android	Anthropoid	Platypelloid
Effect on Labor	• Posterior asynclitism is common. • OA is most common. • Wide pubic arch reduces tears.	• Engages in transverse or posterior. • Extreme molding • Deep transverse arrest as OP • Narrow pubic arch leads to tears (if able to deliver vaginally)	• Engages in AP or oblique • Often OP • Less likely to arrest than android • Most likely to deliver OP (if vaginally)	• Tries to engage in transverse • Marked asynclitism • Usually will not engage at all and arrests at inlet (brim) unless the AP diameter is deep

2. Maternal position at delivery

a. Historically, women labored upright and also delivered upright, squatting or sitting using birthing chairs
   1) ***Horizontal, semi-Fowler, and lithotomy are disadvantageous for mothers, babies***
      a) Slow descent of fetus into pelvis
      b) May restrict movement of lower sacrum and adaptation of pelvic structure to accommodate fetus
      c) Associated with greater need and use of episiotomy
   2) Use of stirrups may cause nerve damage and lower extremity thrombosis related to the non-anatomic alignment and pressure exerted

b. Squatting position may be best position for second stage (anecdotally).
   1) Knees and hips are flexed, hips and thighs pressed against abdominal wall
   2) Uterus elevates, directing fetal presenting part toward outlet, enhancing descent

c. Other position options for birth

1) Dorsal
2) Side lying
3) Standing
4) Knee-chest
5) Hands-knees
6) Birth stool
7) Birth chair
    a) Decreased use of episiotomy
    b) Increase in 2nd degree tears, and increase in blood loss
8) Birth cushion
    a) Decreased tears, and decreased use of forceps or vacuum
    b) Episiotomy prevalence unchanged and postpartum hemorrhage unchanged
    c) Less abnormal FHR decelerations
9) Consideration for anticipated complications such as postpartum hemorrhage or shoulder dystocia
    a) Position woman in lithotomy for best possible visualization and room to function

3. Management of the umbilical cord (including nuchal cord)

a. Nuchal cord (cord around the neck) may be anticipated by variable decelerations, particularly during descent.
    1) At birth, the midwife should check for the cord immediately after the head has emerged.
    2) **If the cord is:**
        a) Loose, slip it over the head (cord reduction)
        b) Too tight to slip over the infant's body but not tight around the neck, slip it over the shoulders as the baby's body is born and deliver the baby through the cord
        c) Too tight to slip back over the shoulders, but has a little give to it, somersault the baby as described by Schorn and Blanco
            (1) Slowly deliver both shoulders with minimal cord manipulation
            (2) Flex the infant's head as the shoulders emerge so the neonatal face is proximate to the woman's thigh.
            (3) Maintain the newborn's head next to the perineum while the rest of the body is born.
            (4) After the baby is born, uncoil the cord from around the baby.

(5) The somersault maneuver does not require any special equipment and thus can be performed any site, any time.

(6) It does place some stress on the cord, which is why is it best when there is some slack in to the cord

d) **Too tight and no give, clamp the cord with two instruments (e.g. Kelly clamps) and cut between the clamps. Be careful.**

b. Cord presentations

1) Cord prolapse

a) 1 in 300 births the umbilical cord prolapses, causing serious jeopardy to the fetus due to constriction of circulation

b) In most cases, if the fetus is viable, an emergency cesarean section is performed.

c) While awaiting the operative birth the midwife should use her fingers to lift the head off the cord if necessary.

(1) There is some data that filling the bladder with fluid and placing the woman in Trendelenburg position may be particularly valuable if transport is need (e.g. from an ambulatory setting to a hospital)

d) If the cervix is fully dilated and birth is imminent, a vaginal birth may be possible

2) Funic presentation

a) Documented less often than cord prolapse, although probably every cord prolapse first has a cord, or funic presentation

b) Estimated 1-2 per 1,000 births (probably for those with a finding by sonography or clinical examination of the umbilical cord interposed between the leading part of the fetus and the internal cervical os while the membranes remain intact.) Thus, cord prolapse is assumed if the membranes rupture.

c) Management is controversial for funic presentation with a closed cervix, no labor and no fetal distress.

d) Much more is known about umbilical cord prolapse than about funic presentation, since the former is a dramatically apparent clinical diagnosis and the latter is usually diagnosed coincidentally by sonography in the asymptomatic patient.

> Many midwives conceptualize the typical cord prolapse in conjunction with a small breech baby. Although the risk is much higher for a fetus in a nonvertex presentation (e.g. 3-10%), since 96-98% of babies are born in a vertex position, even the risk of less than 1% means the "typical" baby with a cord prolapse is vertex. So never relax your guard for a careful exam and caution when performing an amniotomy

3) Risk factors for cord presentations

- Malpresentation (breech and transverse)
- Polyhydramnios
- Maternal pelvic deformities
- Uterine abnormalities such as myomata, multiple gestation
- Low-lying placenta or marginal placenta previa
- Prematurity

4. Shoulder dystocia (SD)

a. Definition

1) No single definition available

2) Few would disagree if there is difficulty delivering the shoulders *and* fetal injury results, shoulder dystocia occurred

b. Incidence: It is estimated at less than 1%; probably around 0.3% (3 in 1,000 births)

c. Significance of shoulder dystocia:

1) Potential obstetrical catastrophe

2) Not only trauma to infant, but also to mother

3) Major cause of litigation

4) Essentially has replaced breech presentation as the major cause of fetal/neonatal injury and, thus, malpractice suit

d. Management

- Recognize conditions that may predispose a woman to having a SD (fetal macrosomia, maternal diabetes or obesity)
- Prompt diagnosis
- Know what to do if SD is encountered; memorize steps and mentally review them prior to every birth
- Act quickly

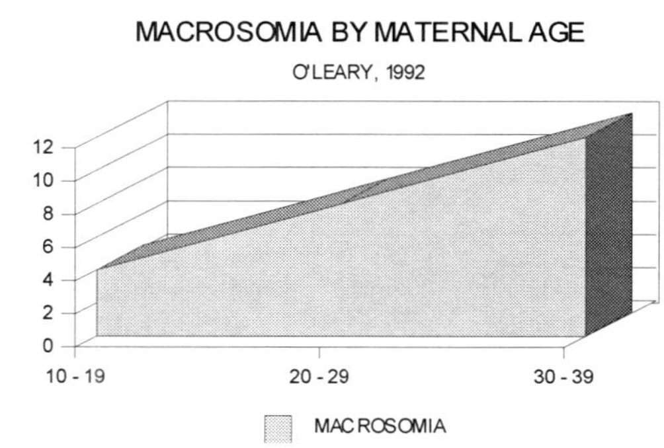

1) Risk factors for shoulder dystocia

a) Macrosomia (ill defined but generally considered birth weight exceeding the 90th percentile. At 39 weeks it is 4000 g; at 42 weeks it is 4400 grams.) The most current ACOG definition is 4500 grams or more at birth, but often 4000 grams is used in local institutions. Not all infants who have SD are macrosomic; *up to one half of cases of shoulder dystocia do not involve a macrosomic baby*, according to Gabbe, 4th ed.

b) Confounding variable is the increased incidence of CS births

c) Authorities agree that shoulder dystocia cannot usually be predicted. Macrosomia may be somewhat more predicable, but there is still no 100% accurate method of estimating fetal weight.

d) Risk factors for macrosomia

   (1) Maternal birth weight: fetal macrosomia may be 'familial', 'constitutional' or 'benign'

   (2) Previous history of macrosomia

   (3) Maternal age and parity

      (a) Macrosomia and/or SD tends to occur more often among mature women

      (b) Mature women frequently are multiparous, heavier, and more likely to have diabetes; it is not a cause and effect

   (4) Obesity

   (5) Maternal diabetes (especially preexisting in the presence of obesity): Class A, B and C diabetes. More severe diabetes may actually be associated with growth restriction because of vascular problems.

   (6) Maternal weight gain during pregnancy, especially if >40 pounds

   (7) Postdatism: the longer the baby stays in the uterus, if well nourished, the bigger it grows.

e) Intrapartum factors for shoulder dystocia: none are absolute

- Prolonged second stage
- Protracted descent
- Arrest of descent
- Failure of descent
- Macrosomia by estimated fetal weight, especially if diabetic mother
- Abnormal first stage (prolongation)
- Marked molding, especially at high station
- Transverse arrest

f) Other risk factors for SD

   (1) ***Previous history of SD--one of the most important factors***

   (2) Pelvic structure--especially platypelloid pelvis

   (3) Short maternal stature

g) Intrapartum management

(1) Good review of history and prenatal course

(2) Rule out risk factors

(3) Pay attention to weight gain and previous estimated fetal weights

(4) Was she screened for diabetes?

(5) Close monitoring of labor: watch for deviations from normal

(6) Verify the pelvis yourself

(7) How is the fetus fitting into the pelvis?

(a) Station

(b) Synclitism

(c) Molding

(8) If you feel she is at risk for SD -- be proactive

(a) Appropriate birth site

(b) Need room

- To move
- To get consultants in (obstetric, anesthesia, pediatric) and for more nurses usually
- May consider "delivery room" instead of LDR, if the former is larger or better equipped

(c) Consider position for birth

- Position for woman--but also for yourself as birth attendant and consultant if needed

(d) Anesthesia

- Good option is pudendal
- Not only anesthetic, but often provides more relaxation so you have room for hands (remember SD is a bony problem, not perineal)

(e) Episiotomy

- Can argue against it from logical standpoint of SD being a bone disorder.
- An argument for episiotomy is from litigation standpoint and fact that provides more space for hands if/when need certain procedures

(f) Empty bladder

- May need to catheterize
- Often overlooked and simple to do
- Also helps to decrease trauma to bladder if major maneuvers needed

(g) Step stool for assistant if suprapubic pressure is needed. Unless assistant is very tall, she will need some height to get the right angle.

2) ***Recognizing shoulder dystocia***

a) Classic picture:

(1) Head is born, and retracts back onto the perineum: ***'Turtle' sign***

(2) Usually assume SD, although could be other problems

(a) Very short umbilical cord

(b) Fetal abnormalities: meningocele, tumors of neck, ascites, organomegaly

3) ***Suggested treatments when SD occurs***

Note that there is no absolute algorithm for the following maneuvers. It is reasonable to proceed from less invasive techniques (positioning and suprapubic pressure) to more invasive techniques (screw maneuvers and delivery of the posterior arm), and then to desperation maneuvers depending on the setting, resources and your experience, and practice guidelines.

- **Call for help**
- **Stay calm**

- **Ensure that the woman is in an advantageous position for birth and you have room to maneuver. Put the head of the bed down and move her hips to the edge. Consider doing an episiotomy.**
- **McRoberts maneuver**
  - Sharply flex the maternal legs onto the abdomen, with the knees toward the chest.
  - Rotates the symphysis pubis upward and decreases the pelvic angle
  - Think of the position as exaggerated lithotomy, or supine squat
- **Suprapubic pressure** may disimpact the anterior fetal shoulder. Some would try this first since it requires only one assistant, or automatically ask for suprapubic pressure in conjunction with McRoberts maneuver.

> **Note:** for most of these, have the woman stop pushing; she may further impact the shoulders based on the fetal position. Once the shoulder is disimpacted, however, a good push may be needed. Get the woman's cooperation.

- **No fundal pressure** (likely to impact the shoulders more)
- **Change maternal position**
  - Put woman on her side and have her pull legs up, particularly if the woman is on a flat surface where there is no room for manipulation
  - Squatting (may be much more difficult for attendant, and impossible for the woman if anesthetized)

- Hands and knees; not mentioned in Williams Obstetrics 22nd ed; Gabbe 4th edition describes this maneuver, but with the caveat that the woman must be mobile, with no significant motor blockade and she should be on a wide and stable enough surface to permit safe transition to the position.

❖ **Screw maneuvers**

Woods: rotation of posterior shoulder toward fetal chest

- Put fingers on scapula and clavicle, **not head**
- Corkscrew back and forth in 180 degrees

Rubin

- Rock fetal shoulders side to side with force on the maternal abdomen
- If unsuccessful, push either fetal shoulder toward the anterior wall of the fetal chest, reducing the shoulder diameter and freeing the impacted anterior shoulder

❖ **Delivery of posterior arm**

- Slide fingers down back of posterior arm elbow and push it toward the chest. If needed, follow lower arm to the wrist. Try to grab the hand/wrist between fingers and sweep the arm across the fetal face and over the perineum. If the arm is extended, try exerting pressure in the antecubital fossa to flex the arm so you can reach the hand/wrist.
- If unable to deliver the anterior should following delivery of the posterior arm, rotate the baby's body with a screw maneuver and repeat delivery of the now posterior arm

❖ **Desperation maneuvers**

- Zavanelli: replacement of fetus into uterus and immediate CS
- Symphysiotomy: not recommended by Williams OB 22nd edition. Gabbe 4th ed. Describes the procedure but does not recommend it.
- Break the clavicle by pressing the anterior clavicle against the pubic ramus. This may be difficult to do in a large fetus.
- Hibbard maneuver: pressure on the fetal jaw and neck toward the maternal rectum with strong fundal pressure as the anterior shoulder is disimpacted (Williams OB 22nd ed.). Most authorities recommend AGAINST FUNDAL PRESSURE.

4) After the baby is born:

a) Prepare for full scale resuscitation; collect cord blood for blood gases.

b) Trauma to baby
   (1) Injury to the brachial plexus (but some good data noting not all brachial plexus injuries are after a difficult birth, suggesting potential intrauterine issue)
   (2) Erb Duchene Palsy
      (a) Fifth and sixth cervical segments
      (b) Causes upper arm to be flaccid and the lower arm to be extended and internally rotated
      (c) Recovery rate reaches 90%
   (3) Klumpke's Palsy
      (a) Rarer
      (b) Eighth cervical and first thoracic segments
      (c) Affects only intrinsic muscles of the hands
      (d) Not as favorable prognosis as Erbs
      (e) From traction to head and neck

> Remember an Erb's is a more favorable diagnosis than a Klumpke's

c) Maternal risks of SD
   (1) Post partum hemorrhage (PPH)
   (2) Vaginal and perineal tears
   (3) Extension of episiotomy

d) Talk to the parents
   (1) Consider telling them what you are doing as you manage the shoulder dystocia

e) Make certain your consultant knows

f) Document accurately and comprehensively

I. Third stage labor

- The average woman loses 250-500 mL of blood during the third stage of labor
- In some ways third stage is the most unpredictable of all. It certainly is not innocuous
  - Retained placenta (1-2% incidence)
  - Primary postpartum hemorrhage (3-4% incidence)
  - Uterine inversion (rare)
- After delivery of the fetus, the uterus continues to contract and retract.
- The placenta separates from the spongiosa layer by one of the following mechanisms
  - **Schultz's mechanism (80%)**
    The central area of the placenta separates first and placenta is delivered like an inverted umbrella so the fetal surface appears first followed by the membranes containing small retroplacental clot. If the placenta remains in the vagina for a prolonged period, the retroplacental clot may be relatively large with a large amount of bleeding. However, normally with a Schultz mechanism there is less blood loss and less risk of retention of fragments
  - **Duncan's mechanism (20%)**
    The lower edge of the placenta separates first and placenta is delivered maternal side first. Compared to the Schultz mechanism, there is more risk of bleeding and retained fragments
- **The 3rd stage is composed of 3 phases**
  - **Placental separation**
  - **Placental descent**
  - **Placental expulsion**

1. **Determination of placental separation**
   a. **Signs of placental separation**
      1) ***Gush of blood***
      2) ***Lengthening of the cord***
      3) ***Change in shape of the uterus as the placenta descends in the vagina and displaces the uterus upward; uterus becomes more globular and rises in the abdomen.***
   b. Brandt Andrews maneuver
      1) Downward suprapubic pressure with simultaneous controlled cord traction: if the cord retracts it suggests separation has not occurred
2. Delivery of the placenta: management of third stage
   a. The Cochrane Library has a large number of studies on third stage. Most of the studies have explored either expectant management (e.g. hands off, no oxytocics) versus active management with oxytocics and controlled cord traction. There appears to be strong, consistent evidence that active management reduces overall blood loss (i.e. cuts the risk of PPH in half and reduces the need for transfusion)
   b. Active management of third stage
      1) Early cord clamping
         a) Results in nonsignificant reductions neonatal jaundice and lower neonatal hematocrits
         b) Delayed cord clamping may be beneficial for preterm babies

2) **Oxytocin**

a) Administering oxytocic either with the anterior shoulder of the neonate or immediately after the placenta reduces postpartum hemorrhage by 60-70%.

(1) This practice does not increase the incidence of retained placenta.

(2) However, it can be a catastrophic intervention if there is an undiagnosed second twin.

(3) Most US practices give oxytocin after the placenta has been expelled

b) Usual dosage is 10 units of *Pitocin®* (1 mL) either intramuscularly or into intravenous fluids..

(1) Studies have not demonstrated clinical differences based upon site of administration.

(2) *Oxytocin should not be given IV bolus*

(3) No firm conclusions on benefits of intra-umbilical vein injection and placental separation, but it may be worth a try if there is retained placenta

3) Nipple stimulation trials fail to demonstrate a reduction in PPH

4) **Controlled cord traction**

a) Associated with lower mean blood loss and shorter 3rd stage

b) No evidence related to incidence of PPH or manual removal of the placenta

c) Controlled cord traction to deliver placenta means a steady gentle pressure on the cord directing it in the curve of Carus.

d) The midwife places a hand on the uterus prior to initiating this maneuver to feel for a second twin and to make sure the uterus is contracting.

5) **After placental expulsion**

a) Massage the uterus until it is firm and bleeding diminishes. Occasionally a clot in the cervix may inhibit normal involution and contribute to bleeding loss. Massage usually expels clots; occasionally a bimanual exam may be needed.

b) If bleeding continues, the midwife should assess for PPH and treat.

6) Retained placenta

a) The normal length of 3rd stage remains undefined. Some sources report the average length of the third stage as 3-10 minutes; others describe the normal third stage as less than 10 minutes, 15 minutes or 30 minutes. For many midwives the time is defined by the institution in which he/she attends births. After the set time (commonly 30 minutes), the undelivered placenta is said to be retained.

b) A retained placenta actually may be separated but undelivered. Often it is in the vagina, but not expelled until gravity or gentle traction intervenes.

c) A partially separated placenta allows the placental site to actively bleed, potentially culminating in a major blood loss. **Aggressive fundal massage before the placenta has separated encourages the organ to partially detach.** Once a placenta is partially separated, it should be removed promptly to decrease the overall blood loss.

d) In case of emergencies, every midwife should know how to manually deliver a placenta (see management of PPH)

e) A placenta that is retained without bleeding enables the midwife to proceed cautiously. The midwife should notify a consultant physician.

(1) Placenta accreta is possible (placental tissue has invaded through the decidua and may be even through the myometrium. They are further described as accreta, increta and percreta, based on the level of invasion).

(2) Placenta accreta may necessitate a hysterectomy.

f) According to the Cochrane Library, there is some evidence that intraumbilical administration of an oxytocic may promote spontaneous expulsion of a placenta. While awaiting obstetrical consultation or before a manual removal of a nonbleeding placenta, the midwife might consider such an intervention

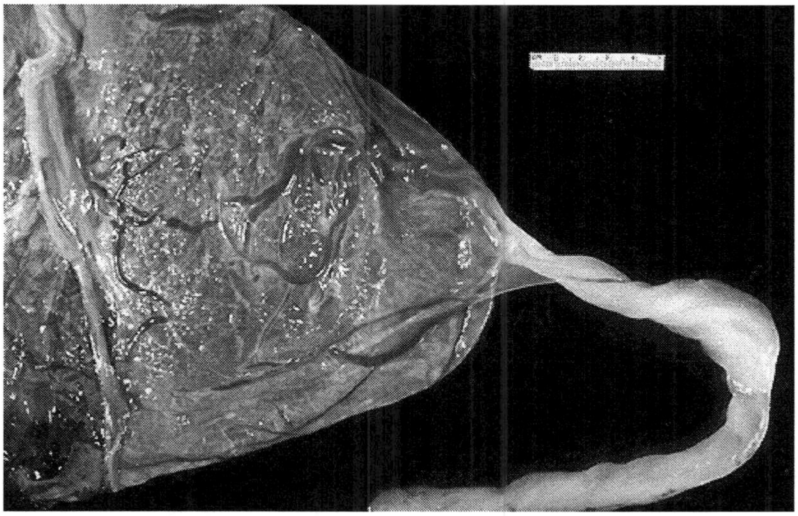

Velamentous insertion--from http://www-medlib.med.utah.edu/WebPath/jpeg2/PLAC009.jpg

3. Inspection of the placenta (includes cord vessels)

a. The purposes of the initial examination of the placenta is to

1) Determine if the entire placenta has been expelled

2) Determine if infection is present (e.g. foul smell) and obtain cultures if suspected

3) Determine if the placenta should be sent to the pathology laboratory.
   a) Many pathologists advocate that a pathologist microscopically assess every placenta. This is not the usual method in most settings.
   b) Perform a careful but rapid assessment of the placenta. If there are no abnormalities it is deemed normal.
   c) Consider sending to pathology:
      (1) Suspected intrauterine infection, abnormalities in size, shape, appearance etc.
      (2) In some tertiary care facilities individual research may be in progress and placentas from women with various conditions may be sent for further investigation. For example, women with DM, preeclampsia, smokers, might have placental changes of interest to scientists and eventually the data may provide information of clinical significance.
      (3) However, there is no single list of which placentas always should be sent to a pathologist or vice versa

Description of Placenta, Variations, and Deviations

Characteristic	Findings	Clinical Significance
Integrity (completeness) of placenta	Intact (all cotyledons present); incomplete (cotyledons missing or velamentous vessels present)	If incomplete, probably retained placenta (e.g. succenturiate lobe, placenta accreta) Retained tissue is associated with hemorrhage and infection
Size of placenta	Normally diameter is ~ 22 cm, thickness 2- 2.5 cm; weight ~ 470 g (1 pound)	If thin (less than 2 cm), suspect placental insufficiency with intrauterine growth restriction If thick (more than 4 cm), consider maternal diabetes, fetal hydrops or intrauterine infections
Shape of placenta	Should be regularly shaped	If irregularly shaped with multiple lobes, consider retained placental fragments as noted above
Surface of placenta maternal	Usually maroon in color and consistent in color and surface throughout	Multiple firm pale or gray areas suggest old infarcts. Dark areas may be fresh infarcts, associated with PIH, lupus and advanced maternal age. Clots (especially toward the center of the placenta) may be suspicious for active bleeding and associated with abruption. Moles or other trophoblastic diseases are very rare and usually resemble grape like clusters of edematous villi.
Surface of placenta fetal	Usually uniformly red	If pale, suspect neonatal anemia, fetal hydrops. If thick ring of membranes this is probably a circumvallate placenta and is associated with prematurity, prenatal bleeding, abruption, and poor outcomes. Tiny whitish nodules may indicate amnion nodosum, associated with oligohydramnios, renal agenesis, pulmonary hypoplasia.
Cord length	Normal length is approximately 40-70 cm	Short cord associated with poorly active fetus (e.g. Down syndrome, fetal malformations); risk of cord rupture, abruption, uterine inversion. Long cord -- increased incidence of fetal entanglement
Wharton jelly	Thick and consistent throughout of approximately 2.0 cm	Thin cord or narrow areas associated with postmaturity, oligohydramnios, torsion, fetal death. Diffusely edematous cord is associated with fetal hemolytic disease, prematurity and preeclampsia. Focal thickening associated with Trisomy 18, omphalocele. Knot in cord may compromise fetal oxygenation.
Insertion of the cord	Usual insertion is in the body of the placenta.	If the cord is inserted through the membranes, it is a velamentous cord insertion; associated with fetal hemorrhage from unprotected vessels, maternal DM, advanced age, smoking, single artery, fetal malformations.
Number of vessels	Normally 2 arteries, 1 vein. Count the vessels >5 cm from placenta, as vessels may be fused at insertion.	One artery is associated with up to a 50% incidence of fetal anomalies. Other thrombosis or clots are associated with fetal compromise.
Color of membranes	Membranes should be translucent, gray and shiny	Green membranes indicate meconium staining, infection or even old blood from an earlier bleeding event.
Odor of placenta	Distinctive smell, not unpleasant	If malodorous, suspect infection. If very sweet, suspect *Clostridium* or *Listeria* infection

J. Fourth stage labor/immediate postpartum period

1. Examination of cervix, vagina and perineum
   a. Fundal assessment and massage
      1) Midline, firm, midway between symphysis and umbilicus
      2) *Right side deviation may indicate a full bladder*

b. Inspection of cervix and vagina
   1) Perform quickly to reduce discomfort
   2) Insert 3-4 fingers full length of vagina
   3) Exert downward pressure away from area to inspect
   4) Place ring forceps with 4x4 in anterior fornix; push in and lift up
   5) May need to grasp posterior lip of cervix with second ring forceps
   6) Small hemostatic lacerations of the cervix are common and need not be repaired. Look for those that are bleeding, and more than 1-2 centimeters long

2. Repair of episiotomy or laceration
   a. Episiotomy repair
      1) Suture techniques to promote healing
         a) Continuous subcuticular technique of perineal repair may be associated with less pain in the immediate postpartum period than the interrupted suture technique. The long-term effects are less clear.
         b) Sterile technique
         c) Remove blood/good visualization
         d) Proper size suture and needle; generally, the smaller the needle and more fine the suture, the less tissue trauma.
         e) Chromic suture dissolves faster than polyglycolic suture material, but causes more tissue reaction and *pain*
         f) Minimize tissue handling
         g) Avoid tissue strangulation
         h) **Use least amount of suture possible**
         i) Close dead space
         j) Hemostasis

3. Diagnosis of hemorrhage/estimated blood loss
   a. Early postpartum hemorrhage (PPH)
      1) Blood loss greater than 500 cc for a vaginal birth in the first 24 hrs postpartum;
      2) **OR** 10% drop in hematocrit between admission and the postpartum period.
      3) Expected blood loss of CS is approximately 1000cc; 1500cc with cesarean hysterectomy.

b. Etiology for postpartum hemorrhage

1) *Uterine atony is the most common cause of immediate PPH*

a) Retained products of conception (more often retained products cause delayed PPH); prolonged third stage; abnormally adherent placenta (e.g., accreta, increta, percreta)

b) Overdistended uterus (e.g. hydramnios, multiple gestation)

c) Multiparity

d) Prolonged or rapid labor

e) Oxytocin induction/augmentation

f) Full bladder

g) Previous postpartum hemorrhage

h) Preeclampsia

i) Infection; chorioamnionitis

j) Uterine relaxing agents (e.g. terbutaline, $MgSO_4$)

2) Other causes of PPH

a) Genital tract trauma (e.g. lacerations, large episiotomy)

b) Coagulopathy

c) Uterine inversion

d) Traumatic delivery

e) Rupture of previous CS or hysterotomy scar

4. Control of hemorrhage

a. Prevention

1) Active management of third stage with prophylactic oxytocic within 2 minutes of baby's birth, immediate cutting and clamping the cord, delivery of placenta by controlled cord traction or maternal effort

2) Versus expectant management; no prophylactic oxytocin, no cord clamping until pulsation ceased, delivery of placenta by maternal effort.

Mnemonic for Your Consideration
Postpartum hemorrhage (PPH) Etiology

TUTUT
Tissue (retained placenta)
Uterine atony
Trauma (traumatic delivery, episiotomy)
Uterine rupture, inversion
Thrombin (coagulation disorders, DIC)

b. Management

1) Early assessment of risk factors

2) Fundal massage; bimanual compression

3) IV access; large bore needle

4) Administer oxytocic

5) Inspect cervix; vagina

6) Blood type and screen; type and cross if appropriate

7) Empty bladder

8) Consult if initial measures do not stop hemorrhage!

c. Note that nipple stimulation or breast feeding does not seem to prevent or treat PPH

d. Pharmacologic management

1) ***Oxytocin (Pitocin®)***

a) 10-20 units in 1000cc IV fluid: almost immediate effect

b) No difference has been found clinically if given IV or IM

c) Do not give IV bolus

d) May be given intramyometrially

e) First line drug

2) ***Methylergonovine (Methergine®)***

a) 0.2 milligrams IM; *do not administer IV*

b) Onset in 2-5 minutes with a duration of 3 hours

c) ***Contraindicated in patients with hypertension***

d) Side effects of ergotism (thirsty, nauseated, coma, seizures)

3) ***Carboprost tromethamine: 15-methyl-prostaglandin $F_{2\alpha}$ (Hemabate®)***

a) Initial: 250 mcg; may repeat at 15- to 90-minute intervals to a total dose of 2 mg (x8)

b) Administer deep I.M.; rotate site if repeat injections are required

c) Do not inject I.V.; may result in bronchospasm, hypertension, vomiting, and anaphylaxis.

d) ***Use with caution with history of asthma, hypotension or hypertension, cardiovascular, adrenal, renal or hepatic disease, anemia, jaundice, diabetes, epilepsy***

4) ***Misoprostol (Cytotec®)***

a) 800 - 1000 mcg rectally

b) Unlike methergine and carboprost, may be given to women with hypertension or asthma.

e. Bimanual compression

1) Insert one hand into vagina and double it into a fist
2) **Place fist into anterior fornix, palmar side up.**
3) Place other hand over the abdomen on top of and behind the uterus.
4) Apply pressure and massage inward and upward with both hands so that the uterus is massaged between the two.
5) Continue until uterus is contracted, while awaiting onset of oxytocic effects

f. Manual exploration of uterus/manual removal of retained placenta

1) Consult; manage hemorrhage and manually remove retained placenta if needed while awaiting MD
2) Implement intravenous access
3) Watchful waiting if no bleeding
4) Manual removal if hemorrhage
    a) Provide analgesia and anesthesia
    b) Empty the bladder
    c) Sterile gloves (gauntlet if available)
    d) Place whole hand including thumb into uterus; follow cord up
    e) Do not go in and out
    f) Grasp uterus with external hand
    g) Assess entire placenta and try to find a separated border
    h) Place back of hand against uterine wall and form cup like position
    i) Establish a line of cleavage between placenta and uterine wall
    j) Use sweeping motion back and forth to peel placenta away
    k) The entire placenta should be in your hand before you remove it
    l) Insure uterus is contracted then inspect the placenta
    m) Uterine exploration after removal is controversial
5) **Uterine exploration**
    a) Empty bladder; medicate as necessary
    b) Wrap a 4 x 4 around 2-4 fingers
    c) Place entire hand into uterus and sweep for fragments
    d) Administer oxytocin and assure uterine contractility
6) **Late postpartum hemorrhage occurs after 24 hours but before six weeks**
    a) Five percent of all deliveries lose over 1000cc of blood (3.9% of vaginal births and 6.4% of cesarean deliveries)
    b) Blood loss greater than 1500cc will show signs and symptoms of shock

c) Roughly, a 500 cc blood loss will result in a 4 point drop in Hct

d) Etiology

(1) **Sub-involution**: a condition in which involution is not occurring as it should (e.g. retained products of conception; infection).

(2) Retained products of conception are a more common cause of late PPH than immediate PPH

e) **Signs and symptoms of late postpartum hemorrhage**

(1) Persistent lochia

(2) Failure of uterus to decrease in size

(3) Painless fresh bleeding

(4) Coagulopathy

(5) Infection

(6) Retained products of conception

f) **Management**

(1) Prevention: ensure that no placental fragments are retained

(2) Methergine 0.2 mg PO every 4 hours for 6 doses

(3) Antimicrobials for infection

K. Assessment and management of deviations from normal labor and delivery; indications for consultation, co-management, referral or transport

1. Labor dystocia (per Friedman)

a. ***Prolonged latent phase***

1) Latent phase >20 hrs. (nullipara) or >14 hrs. (multipara)

2) Etiology

a) Too early use of analgesia or sedatives

b) Onset of labor with unripe cervix vs false labor

3) Management options

a) Therapeutic rest (85% will awake laboring, 10% will stop laboring, and 5% will have ineffective labor)

b) Oxytocin (for the 5% with ineffective labor)

c) AROM may not accelerate latent phase and may exacerbate problem

b. Protraction disorders: slow progress

1) Protracted active phase

a) Maximum slope of dilation is <1.2 cm/hr (nullipara) or <1.5 cm/hr (multipara)

2) Protracted descent

b) Descent of fetal head <1 cm/hr (nullipara) or <2 cm/hr (multipara)

3) Possible etiologies
   a) Malposition
   b) Excessive sedation
   c) Improper anesthesia
   d) Cephalopelvic disproportion (CPD)
4) Management options
   a) Physical and emotional support
   b) Cesarean delivery
   c) Friedman did not mandate oxytocin for protraction disorders, but it is frequently used in modern hospital settings.

3) Arrest disorders
   a) Secondary arrest of dilation
      (1) Active phase stops for more than 2 hours
   b) Prolonged deceleration phase (8-10 cm)
      (1) >3 hr. (nullipara) or > 1 hr. (multipara)
   c) Arrest of descent
      (1) Cessation of descent for > 1 hr
   d) Failure of descent
      (1) Lack of descent during deceleration and 2nd stage
   e) Possible etiologies
      (1) CPD (~52%)
      (2) Hypotonic uterine dysfunction
      (3) Uterine dysfunction
      (4) Excess sedation
      (5) Anesthesia
   f) Management options
      (1) Continue with labor if no CPD
      (2) Oxytocin stimulation
         (a) If post-arrest slope is as good or better than pre-arrest slope, anticipate vaginal delivery.
         (b) If post-arrest slope evolves poorly, anticipate CS

Parameters of Normal Labor		
	Nullipara	**Multipara**
Latent phase	< 20 hours	< 14 hours
Dilation active phase	> 1.2 cm/hr	> 1.5 cm/hr
Descent during second stage	> 1 cm/hr	> 2 cm/hr
Length of second stage	< 2 hr without epidural < 3 hr with epidural	< 1 hr without epidural <2 hr with epidural

2. **Bleeding in late pregnancy**

   a. Incidence of bleeding in third trimester is estimated at 4% of all pregnancies

   b. ***Usual causes fall into three groups***

   1) ***Placenta previa (20%)***

   2) ***Placental abruption (30%) (includes trauma from domestic violence and motor vehicle accidents)***

   3) ***Other causes (50%)***

   a) Marginal placental separation (difficult to define)

   b) Preterm labor

   c) Genital tract infection

   c. Obtaining information to make the diagnosis

   1) Bleeding characteristics

   2) Amount of blood (bloody show is a mucoid discharge and the amount is usually not more than menstrual bleeding)

   3) Color of blood (dark or bright red; dark being oxygenated and more likely old)

   4) Associated factors

   a) Pelvic pain, abdominal pain or back pain

   b) Contractions

   c) Foul vaginal discharge

   d) Rupture of membranes

   e) Recent examination

   f) Abdominal or pelvic

   g) Trauma

   h) Intercourse

   5) Fetal movement

   6) Previous ultrasounds (especially helpful to rule out placenta previa)

   7) Exam

   a) Blood pressure and pulse

   (1) Vital signs are often normal despite significant bleeding

b) Abdominal exam

(1) Pain on palpation

(2) Palpable contractions

(3) Hypertonic uterus (more likely to be abruption, remember board-like uterus)

8) Fetal monitoring

a) External fetal monitor for fetal heart rate

b) Tocodynamometry for contraction monitoring

9) Radiology: abdominal or transvaginal ultrasound

a) Placental location (best method for identifying previa)

b) Placental abruption (inconsistently identifiable)

10) Pelvic examination (**only if placenta previa is ruled out**)

****Remember, if you have active bleeding in the third trimester and do not know the etiology—rule out the placenta previa with ultrasound before you perform a vaginal examination*

11) Lab evaluation

a) Wet prep

b) Nitrazine and ferning if you suspect rupture of membranes; may not be accurate depending on amount of blood in the vagina

c) Perform cultures as appropriate (e.g. chlamydia, GC, GBS)

d) Consider the possibility of fetal bleeding if there are FHR abnormalities

e) Maternal urine for drugs of abuse (cocaine causes placental abruption)

> **Remember:** if woman is Rh negative and the bleeding is large, administer anti D serum (RhoGAM), based on Kleihauer Betke assessment of fetal RBCs in maternal circulation

d. Emergent management if actively bleeding

1) Hemoglobin/Hematocrit

2) Type and cross 2 - 6 units packed red blood cells

3) Type and cross for platelet transfusion

4) Coagulation studies, including Protime (PT), Partial Thromboplastin Time (PTT), Fibrin split products (Fibrin degradation products; D Dimer), Fibrinogen

5) Obstetric, anesthesia, and neonatal consults

6) Immediate interventions

a) *Maternal oxygen*

b) *Trendelenburg position or at least pelvic tilt to relieve pressure from uterus on vena cava*

c) *Obtain immediate intravenous access*

(1) Two large bore IV (16-18 gauge)

(2) Initiate IV solutions, e.g. Lactated Ringers

3. Chorioamnionitis (intra-amniotic infection, amnionitis)

a. Inflammation of the chorion, amnion, and amniotic fluid; usually from ascending bacterial infection

b. ***Most often seen with prolonged rupture of membranes (>24 hours), frequent vaginal examinations, or intrauterine procedures***

c. Effect on mother

1) Poor uterine contractility—may lead to labor dystocia and postpartum hemorrhage

2) Uterus does not respond well to oxytocin

3) Endometritis and wound infection if the mother has cesarean

d. Effect on infant

1) May develop pneumonia or acidosis

2) May have a low APGAR (<7) and hypothermia or may have high APGAR and deteriorate shortly after birth

3) Meningitis, cerebral palsy

e. Signs and symptoms of chorioamnionitis

1) Maternal fever

2) Maternal tachycardia

3) Fetal tachycardia

4) Uterine tenderness

5) Foul-smelling, purulent fluid

6) Increased maternal white blood cell count

f. **Management of chorioamnionitis**

1) **Consult**

2) **Facilitate delivery within 24 hours of diagnosis.** Initiate oxytocin induction or augmentation.

3) **Continuous fetal monitoring:** fetal tachycardia is likely

4) Keep hydrated (D5 Ringer's lactate for intravenous hydration)

5) **Maternal antibiotics**

6) Hourly vital signs

7) Have a pediatric provider at birth

8) At birth, cultures of baby (gastric aspirate, skin, ears) and cord pH

9) May do cultures of uterus, placenta, and umbilical cord

4. Umbilical cord prolapse

a. Frank

1) Cord slips through the cervix into vagina or prolapses outside the vagina

b. Occult

1) Cord slips alongside presenting part, but does not slip through the cervix

2) Danger is fetal hypoxia from cord compression (cord between presenting part and cervix)

c. Possible etiologies

1) Spontaneous rupture of membranes with unengaged head, breech, transverse lie, compound presentation, small fetus, or second twin

2) Amniotomy with an unengaged head

3) Displacement of vertex during fetal assessment (e.g. manual rotation, placement of forceps)

d. Management of cord prolapse

1) ***Place hand in vagina and hold the presenting part off the umbilical cord***

2) Call for help and STAT call to physician consultant; order preparation of operating room; call anesthesia; alert pediatrician

3) Do not attempt to replace cord

4) Inform woman calmly what is happening

5) ***Get woman to a knee-chest or Trendelenburg position***

6) If cord is protruding from the vagina, direct others to wrap it loosely with gauze soaked in normal saline

7) Obtain fetal heart tones

8) Prepare for emergency CS if fetus is alive

9) ***Do not remove hand from presenting part until the baby is delivered***

10) Consider administering terbutaline 0.25 mcg IV for tocolysis if appropriate

11) Alternative management for a non-engaged presenting part

a) Insert a #16 foley catheter and fill the bladder with 500 cc of normal saline or sterile water.

b) Clamp the catheter while your hand is in the vagina against the presenting part.

c) Continuous fetal monitor is necessary.

d) If bradycardia recurs, reinsert your hand to assess if the cord is compressed.

e) Bladder is to be emptied prior to CS

5. Meconium-stained amniotic fluid (MSAF)

a. Defined as presence of fetal stool in the amniotic fluid.

1) MSAF with normal FHR in term fetus is probably not related to fetal distress, and is more likely as gestation progresses.

2) With abnormal FHR and fetal acidosis, meconium aspiration syndrome (MAS) caused by fetal gasping is more likely.

3) MAS may result in persistent fetal circulation, with long term poor sequelae such as cerebral palsy and seizures.

b. Classification of MSAF: **mild, moderate, or thick; classification is subjective.**

1) Mild has no particulate and is green tinged

2) Moderate is green and may have particulate

3) Thick is like "pea soup".

4) Thick may present as no fluid with rupture of membranes (meconium is behind the presenting part and too thick to drain past it); consider no fluid with an amniotomy as thick meconium.

c. Management of labor with meconium stained amniotic fluid

1) Consult according to practice agreements

2) Note classification of MSAF

3) Continuous fetal monitoring is usually recommended

4) Observe for maternal infection

5) If there are severe variable decelerations, consider amnioinfusion (not proven to prevent MAS, but may relieve variables)

6) Suction oropharynx and nasopharynx on the perineum

7) Notify pediatrics for attendance at birth. Routine endotracheal intubation at birth in vigorous term meconium-stained babies has not been shown to be superior to routine resuscitation including pharyngeal suction. It may be associated with an increased risk of developing meconium aspiration syndrome. (The Cochrane Library, 1999)

a) In a baby depressed at birth, visualize cords and suction further if needed

b) Collect a cord blood sample for blood gases.

6. Deep transverse arrest

a. *Associated with platypelloid and android pelvis*

b. Internal rotation inhibited

c. Signs and symptoms

1) Diagnosed in second stage

2) Sagittal suture in transverse diameter of the mother's pelvis

3) Hypotonic uterus in second stage

4) Extensive molding of the fetal head
5) Large amount of caput succedaneum

d. Management
1) Position changes
2) Coach for effective pushing efforts if needed (at peak and with urge to prevent exhaustion; keep hydrated)
3) Improve contractions
4) Collaborate with physician

7. Cephalopelvic disproportion (CPD)

a. Pelvis is not large enough to accommodate the fetus. It is a relative situation, based on the size or position of the particular fetus (e.g. pelvis may accommodate a 7# fetus, but not a 9# one; it may accommodate a fetus with a well flexed head in an occiput anterior presentation, but not a deflexed head in an occiput posterior position)

b. Possible etiologies
1) Macrosomia
2) Woman's body type (narrow hips; short, square stature; small, broad hands and feet)
3) History of pelvic fracture
4) Spinal or orthopedic deformity
5) Dysfunctional labor
6) Malpresentation; malposition
7) Fetal tumor or deformity (e.g., conjoined twins)

c. Pathological retraction ring
1) May see development of a pathological retraction ring (Bandl retraction ring) in labor. There is a disproportion between the fetal head and pelvis which is so pronounced that there is no engagement and descent.
2) The lower uterine segment becomes increasingly stretched and thinned.
3) A transverse or oblique ridge extending across the uterus somewhere between the symphysis and the umbilicus is noted.
4) ***May lead to uterine rupture; immediate delivery is indicated***

d. Management
1) Position changes
2) Amniotomy
3) Rest and hydration if there is maternal exhaustion
4) Oxytocin if uterine contractions are not adequate (consider intrauterine pressure catheter)
5) Ambulation

6) Enema
7) Improve flexion of fetal head
8) Epidural for maternal exhaustion
9) Consultation and collaboration with MD

8. Uterine rupture

a. Classification

1) Complete: all layers of the uterus are interrupted. Morbidity and mortality are highest.
2) Dehiscence, or incomplete: uterine muscles are separated by the visceral peritoneum is intact

b. Risk factors

1) Previous cesarean delivery is currently the risk factor in the overwhelming majority of uterine ruptures (>90%)
   a) Classical incisions (in the contractile portion of the uterus, i.e., fundus) are prone to rupture prior to labor
   b) Lower uterine incisions, i.e., low cervical transverse cesarean incisions are much less likely to rupture, but if they do it is likely to be during labor (<1%)
2) Other uterine surgery or trauma such as curettage, perforation or myomectomy
3) Oxytocin use, particularly in multipara (uncommon no according to Williams OB 22nd);
4) Congenital uterine anomaly
5) Abnormal presentation
6) Grand multiparity
7) Intrauterine manipulation; midforcep deliveries
8) Prostaglandin use, particularly with a previous cesarean section
9) Labor dystocia, shoulder dystocia
10) External trauma, e.g., automobile accident or domestic violence; external version
11) Uterine overdistention
12) Difficult manual removal of placenta, placenta increta or percreta
13) Spontaneous rupture without risk factors is extremely rare.

b. Signs and symptoms

1) ***<u>Sudden fetal bradycardia, late decelerations, undetectable FHT</u>***
2) ***Sharp, shooting pain in lower abdomen at height of a severe contraction***
3) ***Woman feels that something has "torn" inside followed by cessation of contractions and relief of pain; note that with epidural or narcotic analgesics, there may not be much pain***

4) ***Loss of fetal station***
5) Varied vaginal bleeding -- slight to hemorrhage; bloody urine
6) Referred pain, possibly to the chest or shoulder
7) Abdominal palpation of fetal parts
8) Possible violent fetal movements that stop; loss of FHTs
9) Contracted (firm) uterus felt beside fetus
10) Woman goes into shock
11) Abnormal postpartum bleeding, including hematuria, may be a sign of uterine rupture that was not identified during labor (as infant was born)

c. **Management of uterine rupture**

1) Call physician STAT if suspected
2) Initiate an IV for electrolyte solutions and another IV for blood (16 gauge; use normal saline to keep open until blood arrives)
3) STAT blood transfusion
4) Oxygen
5) Prepare for STAT abdominal surgery, including hysterectomy
6) Maternal mortality is rare, but fetal survival is unlikely if the rupture is complete

9. **Uterine inversion**

a. Incidence is approximately 1 per 25,000 births

b. Risk factors include

1) Fundal pressure; cord traction with attached placenta, relaxed uterus, fundal implantation; short cord
2) More common in primiparas
3) Uterine atony, spontaneous (e.g., with overdistention) or drug induced (e.g., magnesium sulfate)
4) Abnormal placentation (accrete, increta, percreta)
5) History of uterine inversion

c. **Signs and symptoms**

1) **The placenta appears at introitus attached to mass**
2) **Shock**
3) **Bradycardia associated with vagal response**
4) **Hemorrhage**

d. Management

1) This is an emergency situation and the midwife should call for obstetrical and anesthesia consultation.

2) **Try to replace the fundus into the uterus, even if the placenta is still attached. Maintain internal pressure if successful. If unable to replace the uterine fundus, at least push it into the vagina.**
3) Manage to prevent or treat shock, including two large bore intravenous lines, oxygen, type and cross match blood.
4) Uterine relaxation with tocolytics or anesthesia if needed for fundal replacement
5) NO OXYTOCICS until the uterus is replaced.
6) Observe for recurrence of prolapse
7) Laparotomy or even hysterectomy may be needed.

10. Maternal mortality safe motherhood

a. In the United States
   1) Every day one woman dies from pregnant related causes (primarily preventable)
   2) Since 1982, there has been minimal improvement in the maternal mortality rate
   3) Black women are three times more likely than white women to die of pregnancy related causes

According to CDC, there has been no progress made toward achieving the Healthy People 2000 goal of 3.3 maternal deaths per 100,000 live births set in 1987. During the same time period, infant mortality has declined steadily, probably due to advances in survival of low birth weight infants and preterm babies and decrease in some etiologies for postneonatal mortality such as sudden infant death syndrome.

b. Maternal mortality definition
   1) Deaths that occur during pregnancy or within 42 days of the end of a pregnancy;
   2) AND cause of death listed as complication of pregnancy, childbirth or puerperium
   3) CDC uses term maternal mortality rate or numbers per 100,000 live births

c. Difficulty in currently assessing the incidence; probably underestimated

d. Causes
   1) Has been said that hemorrhage, preeclampsia, infection and ectopic pregnancy account for 59% of maternal deaths—and in many areas homicide is now a major component

e. Actions
   1) 25 states have reinitiated maternal mortality review committees
   2) Healthy People 2010 goal is still 3.3 maternal deaths/100,000
   3) Probably will not be met
   4) The American College of Nurse-Midwives has a Safe Motherhood Initiative (SMI-USA)
   5) Other partners include ACOG, MANA, MOD, National Black Women's Caucus

Safe Motherhood: The goals/vision

Women and men are equal partners in all aspects of society
Every girl and boy arrives at maturity with full physical, emotional and spiritual health
Women and men assume responsibility for making motherhood safe and for parenting
Women trust their bodies and view birth as a normal, positive, growth-producing experience for the family
Women are educated and empowered to make informed decisions for choices during childbearing, including choice of birth attendant and site of birth
Motherhood takes place within a physical environment and social system that promotes well-being for all women
Women receive appropriate care based on need, and there is no discrimination based on ability to pay, place of residence, culture, religion or ethnic background
The use of technology, drugs and interventions in childbearing is based on research and fully informed consent and is individualized to the health needs of each woman
Safe motherhood in the United States is a woman-centered effort within the community that requires the support and efforts of many people and in which midwifery care is an integral component
The United States will use its intellectual and material resources fairly and have the political will to ensure that safe motherhood becomes a reality to all women

From ACNM, 1998

11. Intrapartum care of women with HIV

Factors that increase perinatal infection

Increased viral load
Drug naïve
Rupture of membranes more than 4 hours
Chorioamnionitis
Scalp sampling, scalp electrode, IUPC
Less than 37 weeks or 2500 gm

Stein et al. 2000

Current recommendations are for cesarean delivery if HIV+

12. Hypertension in pregnancy (5 types)

- Gestational hypertension (Formerly PIH or transient hypertension)
- Preeclampsia
- Eclampsia
- Preeclampsia superimposed on chronic hypertension
- Chronic hypertension

a. Gestational hypertension

1) BP $\geq$ 140/90
2) No proteinuria
3) Returns to normal within 12 weeks postpartum
4) Retrospective diagnosis
5) Risk of hypertension later in life rises

b. Preeclampsia

1) ***Minimum criteria***

(a) BP greater ≥ 140/90 after 20 weeks

(b) Proteinuria ≥ +1 on dipstick or ≥ 300 mg in 24 hours

2) ***Increased certainty***

(a) BP ≥ 160/110

(b) Proteinuria ≥ + 2 on dipstick or 2.0g/24 hours

(c) Serum creatinine > 1.2 mg/dL

(d) Platelet count < $100,000/mm^3$

(e) Increased LDH, ALT, AST (liver enzymes)

(f) Headache or visual disturbances and/or epigastric pain

c. Eclampsia

1) Seizures that can not be attributed to other causes

d. Superimposed preeclampsia on chronic hypertension

1) New onset proteinuria in hypertensive women but no proteinuria before 20 weeks

2) OR a sudden increase in proteinuria or BP or platelets less than $100,000mm^3$

e. Chronic hypertension

1) BP ≥ 140/90 before pregnancy or before 20 weeks gestation

2) OR hypertension first diagnosed after 20 weeks but persists after 12 weeks postpartum

f. Hospital management of hypertension: (comanagement)

1) Consider when hypertension is persistent or worsening, or in the presence of proteinuria

2) Weigh on admission and every day

3) BP sitting every 4 hours

4) Plasma creatinine, hematocrit, platelets, and serum liver enzymes periodically

5) Fetal testing for amniotic fluid volume, fetal size, nonstress test periodically (e.g., every other day)

6) Reduced activity

7) No fluid or nutritional restrictions

8) For severe preeclampsia characterized by headache, visual disturbances, epigastric pain, and/or oliguria, prescribe anticonvulsant therapy (i.e. magnesium sulfate -- $MgSO_4$) and antihypertensives, and anticipate delivery

g. $MgSO_4$ treatment

1) 4-6 g IV loading dose; 2 grams per hour in 100 mL IV fluid
2) Measure serum $MgSO_4$ at 4-6 hr and adjust infusion
3) Therapeutic plasma levels are between 4-7 mEq/L
4) ***Signs of toxicity include loss of patellar reflexes and decreased respiratory rate***
    a) Antidote is: Calcium gluconate 1 g IV and discontinue MgSo4 when symptoms present or serum level is greater than 10mEq per L

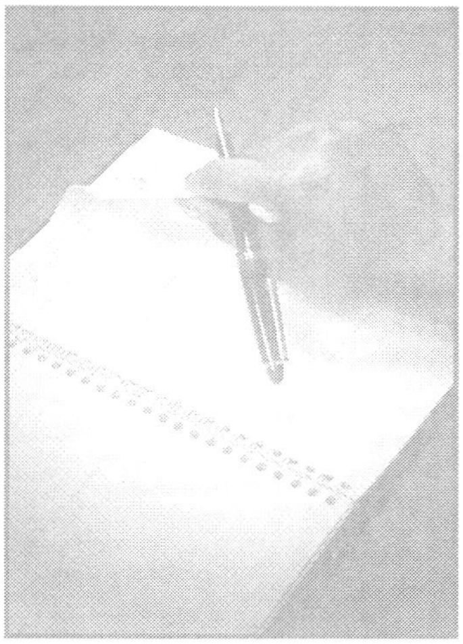

Chapter IV

Postpartum Care

IV. Postpartum (5%-10%)

IV. Postpartum (5%-10%)

A. Physiology/Pathophysiology

1. Postpartum
2. Lactation

B. Postpartum physical assessment

1. Breasts
2. Uterine involution
3. Perineum
4. Lochia
5. Urinary bladder
6. Extremities
7. Vital signs

C. Management of the normal postpartum period

1. Breast care
2. Physical adaptation/recovery (includes diastasis recti, uterine involution, exercise, nutrition)
3. Family planning/resumption of sexuality
4. Psychosocial adaptation/parental-infant relationship
5. Postpartum Rh immune globulin/immunizations

D. Six week postpartum examination

E. Laboratory tests (order/obtain/interpret)

F. **Assessment and management of deviations from normal in the postpartum period; consultation, co-management or referral, as indicated**.

1. Late (delayed) postpartum hemorrhage
2. Postpartum vulvar hematoma
3. Thromboembolic disease
4. Pulmonary embolism
5. Superficial thrombophlebitis
6. Postpartum eclampsia
7. Postpartum depression
8. Infection

IV. Postpartum (5%-10%)

A. Physiology/pathophysiology

1. Postpartum (PP)

a. Endocrine changes:

Postpartum changes occur secondary to removal of placenta (with its hormones) and to changes in prolactin secretion, initiating return of systems to the nonpregnant state. Placental hormones disappear based on their half-life. The first half-life involves removal of a substance from the blood and is relatively short. The second half-life involves removal of substances from the extravascular compartments and is lengthier. ***Most substances reach nonpregnant levels by 6 weeks postpartum.***

b. Prolactin

1) Secreted by anterior pituitary
2) During pregnancy, effects of increasing prolactin levels are suppressed by estrogen
3) Immediately after delivery, prolactin increases and peaks at 3 hours postpartum
4) Secretion of prolactin is stimulated by suckling and prolactin stimulates alveolar cells to produce milk
5) Levels fall in nonlactating women and return to nonpregnant range by 7-14 days

c. Oxytocin

1) Produced in hypothalamus; stored and secreted by posterior pituitary
2) Causes myoepithelial cells to contract, leading to milk ejection
3) Causes contraction and postpartum involution of uterus
4) Release is inhibited by stresses, such as fear, anxiety, embarrassment
5) Release is enhanced or stimulated by relaxation, orgasm, hearing a baby cry, or breast stimulation

d. Estrogen

1) Disappears rapidly postpartum with the removal of placenta
2) Plasma estradiol reaches levels that are <2% of pregnancy levels by 24 hours
3) The drop in levels at delivery aids in initiation of lactation
4) At 1-3 days, levels are similar to those found during the follicular phase
5) Levels fall further to day 7 postpartum, then rise to follicular phase levels over several weeks

e. Progesterone

1) Levels similar to luteal phase reached by 24-48 hours
2) Levels equal to follicular phase by 3-7 days
3) The drop in levels at delivery aids initiation of lactation

f. Pituitary-ovarian-hypothalamic axis

1) The pituitary-hypothalamic axis and production of FSH & LH are suppressed during pregnancy
2) Ovarian production of estrogen & progesterone is low in first 2 weeks postpartum in both lactating and nonlactating women. Then, estrogen and progesterone slowly increase and pituitary function is resumed at 4-6 weeks.

g. **Return of ovulation and menstruation**

1) Resumption of ovulation is associated with a rise in plasma progesterone
2) Initial menses following delivery is anovulatory in 75% of women

2. Lactation

HORMONAL INFLUENCES ON THE BREAST & LACTATION

HORMONE	SITE OF ORIGIN	INFLUENCE IN NONPREGNANT AND/OR PREGNANT STATE	INFLUENCE IN POSTPARTUM STATE
prolactin (prl)	anterior pituitary	prl increases but estrogen suppresses effect; alveoli & glandular proliferation	stimulates alveolar cells to produce milk; initiates lactation with suckling; inverse relationship between catecholamines & prl
prolactin inhibiting factor (pif)	hypo-thalamus	suppresses prl	suppresses release of prl; phenothiazides & reserpine decrease catecholamines, which in turn decrease pif (increasing prl)
oxytocin	posterior pituitary	sensitivity of myoepithelial cells to oxytocin increases during pregnancy	"milk ejection" reflex (let down)
estrogen	ovary & placenta	stimulates proliferation of glandular tissue & ducts; stimulates alveolar growth	blood levels decrease & initiation of lactation associated
progesterone	ovary & placenta	stimulates proliferation of lobular formation; inhibits milk production	blood levels decrease & initiation of lactation associated
adrenocorti-cotropic hormone (acth)	anterior pituitary	stimulates adrenals to release corticosteroids; stimulates mammary growth of alveoli & ducts	high level is believed necessary for maintaining lactation (milk synthesis and release)
human placental lactogen (hpl)	placenta	stimulates adrenals to release corticosteroids; stimulates mammary growth of alveoli	not applicable
thyroxine	thyroid	no direct effect on lactation	important in maintaining lactation by control of metabolism; direct effect on mammary glands
thyroid releasing hormone (trl)	hypo-thalamus	no effect	stimulates release of prl; can be used to maintain lactation
growth hormone	anterior pituitary	promotes mammogenesis & alveolar growth; stimulates ductal growth	may act with prl in initiation of lactation; may act with thyroxine to potentiate milk yield; most important in maintaining lactation

B. Postpartum physical assessment

1. Breasts

a. Engorgement occurs between 2nd and 4th postpartum days; breasts become hard and tense.

b. ***Engorgement resolves in 24-48 hours***

c. Prolactin levels return to normal by 3rd-5th week in nonbreastfeeding women

d. Breastfeeding women will have glandular hypertrophy as long as they are breastfeeding.

e. Stimulation of suckling will evert nipples and permanently increase their mobility

f. Hyperpigmentation may be permanent

g. Palliative treatment of engorgement includes warm packs, frequent breastfeeding, and manual expression if needed.

1) Cabbage leaves, red or green. Keep in refrigerator, bruise vein down the middle with a knife and tuck the leaf around the breast and leave it there until wilted from body heat. Cochrane Library has found contradictory information on therapeutic use of cabbage leaves and breastfeeding women, but has found strong association between its use and longer breastfeeding rates.

2) Analgesics as needed

2. Uterine involution

a. Involves 3 processes: contractions, autolysis, and placental site regeneration

b. ***Immediately after delivery, uterus is 2/3 between pubis and umbilicus***

c. Within hours it returns to 19-20 week size, then begins descent into pelvis; expect the fundus to descend about a fingerbreadth a day after the first postpartum day

d. Halves weight in first postpartum week by decreasing size of cells

e. ***By two weeks postpartum, uterus has reached 12 week size***

f. ***By 4th to 6th week postpartum, uterus has returned to nonpregnant size***

g. Endometrium regenerates in about 3 weeks; placental site takes up to 6 weeks

h. Involution is more rapid in breastfeeding mother

3. Perineum

a. Edematous and bruised at delivery; returns to prepregnant appearance by 2 weeks with exception of gaping at introitus

b. Episiotomy or laceration should be healed by 2 weeks; may remain tender to palpation

c. Suture may be visible at 6 week exam

d. Hemorrhoids usually resolve within a few weeks, but skin tags may remain

e. Vaginal rugae may reappear by the third week and the vagina shrinks but rarely returns to pregravid size. In a lactating mother, the vagina is atrophic due to estrogen deficiency; return of rugae may be delayed.

f. Examination requires good visualization including observing for edema, inflammation, hematomas, suppuration, wound dehiscence, stitches, ecchymosis

g. Encourage good perineal hygiene

REEDA Scale

Points	Redness	Edema	Ecchymosis	Discharge	Approximation
0	None	None	None	None	Closed
1	Within 0.25 cm of incision bilaterally	Perineal, less than 1 cm from incision	Less than 1 cm from incision	Serum	Skin separation of 3 mm or less
2	Within 0.5 cm of incision bilaterally	Perinatal and / or vulvar, 1-2 cm from incision	Between 1 and 2 cm from incision	Serosanguinous	Skin and sub-cutaneous fat separation
3	Beyond 0.5 cm of incision bilaterally	Perineal and / or vulvar greater than 2 cm from incision	Greater than 2 cm from incision	Bloody, purulent	Skin, sub-cutaneous fat and fascial layer separation

From Davidson N: REEDA: Evaluating postpartum healing. J Nurse-Midwifery 19(2);6-8,1974.

h. Comfort measures for perineal pain

1) Ice packs prn (for first 24-48 hours)

2) Topical anesthetic prn

3) Witch hazel compresses (*Tucks®*)

4) Sitz baths, cold or hot

5) Analgesia

6) Rubber ring for sitting (Varney 4th ed recommends use with caution; most current sources do not list as comfort measure)

A sitz bath does not have to be warm or hot. Data show that a tepid bath with ice added by the woman provides the same degree of cleanliness and potentially greater analgesia.

4. Lochia

a. Superficial layer of uterine decidua

1) ***Rubra: lasts about 4 days;*** bright red, contains mostly blood,

2) ***Serosa: lasts about 22 days***; pink, composed of serous fluid, decidual tissue, leukocytes and erythrocytes

3) ***Alba: lasts about a week***; whitish, contains erythrocytes and decidua

b. Mean duration of lochia: 33 days, but can last up to 60 days

1) There is MUCH variation in literature regarding duration

2) Williams Ob 22nd ed reports that maternal age, parity, infant weight, and breastfeeding do not influence the duration

c. Signs of possible problem: lochia is malodorous, becomes heavier and bright red; associated with abdominal pain or fever.

d. ***Bleeding may increase temporarily with periods of increased activity***

5. Urinary bladder

a. Immediate postpartum: edematous, congested and hypotonic
b. May become overdistended, resulting in incomplete emptying
c. Encourage periodic voiding
d. Avoid catheterization if possible –base decision on amount of bladder distention, effects of uterine displacement and amount of bleeding
e. Urethra may be insensitive due to birth trauma
f. Birth related trauma usually resolves within 24 hours
g. Bladder sensation may be diminished due to anesthesia/analgesia
h. May have nonpathologic proteinuria through 2nd postpartal day
   1) Rule out UTI, preeclampsia
i. Significant diuresis from delivery to approximately 5th postpartum day
   2) Urinary output up to 3000 mL/day
j. Incontinence of urine and even stool may persist up to 6 months postpartum

6. Extremities

a. Predisposing factors for thrombembolic disease in the pregnant and postpartum woman
   1) Venous stasis from dilation of veins and compression by uterus
   2) Prolonged bed rest
   3) Lack of activity or ambulation
   4) Hypercoagulation disorders (inherited thrombophilias)
   5) Instrument-assisted and CS births
   6) Hemorrhage
   7) Sepsis
   8) Multiparity
   9) Advanced maternal age

> If a woman has difficulty walking, do not assume it must be thromboembolic disease or even foot drop from inappropriate positioning in stirrups, even though either may be possible. If she has suprapubic pain, difficulty walking and problems abducting her hips, suspect that she has a separated symphysis (**diastasis symphysis pubis**). If so, analgesics, rest and a binder tend to be the best treatment until it resolves.

b. Examination of the legs
   1) Foot flat and knees slightly bent
   2) Palpate both sides of legs for varicosities, calf tenderness and heat
   3) Inspect for edema, redness
   4) Straighten leg for Homan's sign by applying gentle pressure to keep leg straight and dorsiflex foot.
      a) +Homan's: pain in calf

7. Vital signs

a. Temperature: slight rise immediately postpartum, normal within 24 hours

b. Pulse: should remain within normal range

1) >100 may indicate infection or hemorrhage

c. Respirations: should be within realm of normal: 12-20 respirations per minute

d. Blood pressure: should remain within realm or normal: $\leq$120/80

1) Rise of 5% in both systolic and diastolic pressures may persist through the 4th postpartum day

e. For first hour after delivery, blood pressure and pulse should be taken every 15 minutes

C. Management of the normal postpartum period

1. Breast care

COMMON DISCOMFORTS ASSOCIATED WITH BREASTFEEDING

CONDITION	ETIOLOGY	PREVENTION	MANAGEMENT
SORE NIPPLES (pink, burning nipples) related to nipple stretching peaks at 3-4 days and then subsides	Differentiate between stretching feeling and true soreness Improper positioning Unrelieved negative pressure Tongue retraction behind lower gum causing biting Nipple in baby's mouth at upward angle rubbing against roof of mouth	▪ Correct position, latch on and breaking of suction ▪ Position with gums on tops of areola ▪ Mouth open wide, lower lip of infant out ▪ Frequent feeding (every 2-3 hours) ▪ Do not let infant get overly hungry ▪ Start on least sore side	▪ **Based on etiology** ▪ Air-dry nipples ▪ Correct positioning ▪ Correct breaking of suctioning ▪ Apply expressed milk/colostrum to nipples ▪ Treat thrush ▪ Least sore side first ▪ Ice for engorgement/pain relief ▪ When sore, remove infant from breast if nonnutritive sucking ▪ Acetaminophen 30 minutes before feeding if needed
CRACKED NIPPLES (blistered, scabbed, cracked due to trauma)	▪ "Chewing" motion ▪ Disorganized or dysfunctional suck ▪ Flat or inverted nipples ▪ Pathological engorgement preventing correct positioning ▪ Improper breaking of suction ▪ Breast pads with plastic or water proof liners ▪ Use of breast shields without holes ▪ Wet breast pads left on nipples ▪ Soap or shampoo on nipples ▪ Incorrect use of breast pump ▪ Allergic reaction to nipple cream ▪ Delayed healing of cracks ▪ Thrush of infant ▪ Improperly fitting bra, encouraging poor positioning	▪ Avoid nonnutritive sucking, sleeping at breast, especially first week of life ▪ Correction of flat/inverted nipples ▪ Avoidance of creams and oils ▪ Avoidance of drying agents ▪ Use cloth breast pads with frequent changing ▪ Encourage milk ejection reflex with warm compresses and massage ▪ Avoid secondary engorgement with early & frequent feedings	▪ **Based on etiology** ▪ Air-dry nipples ▪ Correct positioning ▪ Correct breaking of suctioning ▪ Apply expressed milk/colostrum to nipples ▪ Treat thrush if needed ▪ Least sore side first ▪ Ice for engorgement/pain relief ▪ When sore, remove infant from breast if nonnutritive sucking ▪ Acetaminophen 30 minutes before feeding if needed

IV. Postpartum (5%-10%)

CONDITION	ETIOLOGY	PREVENTION METHODS	MANAGEMENT
ENGORGEMENT ▪ Usually a temporary condition ▪ Physiological: Increase in milk volume at day 2 or 3 ▪ Pathological: Unrelieved physiological engorgement	▪ Increased blood flow to breast ▪ Start of milk production, for 24-48 hours ▪ Inappropriately limiting time for nursing	▪ Adequate time for feeding (20-40 minutes) ▪ Feed within first four hours of birth and then every 2-3 hours	▪ Dispel myth of limiting nursing time ▪ Use good bra ▪ Facilitate drainage of breasts ▪ Massage breast during nursing ▪ Feed every 2 hours ▪ Soften areola before beginning the feeding ▪ Good latch on ▪ Warm pack or shower before feeding ▪ Cool compresses, mild analgesic ▪ (Anecdotal) cool cabbage leaves --astringent
UNCONTROLLED LEAKAGE ▪ Normal sign of letdown ▪ Usually temporary ▪ and decreases after several weeks	▪ Overstimulation of nipple ▪ Overfull breasts ▪ Can be increased by pumping ▪ Use of breast shells instead of pads to keep dry	▪ Proper pads ▪ Avoidance of overstimulation with clothing or bra ▪ Hand expression if feedings are missed ▪ Frequent nursing	▪ Use cloth breast pads ▪ Use towels to absorb leaking milk while nursing ▪ Change pads when wet ▪ Wear patterned clothing ▪ Mechanical pressure on the nipple with fingers or arm
INSUFFICIENT MILK Let down failure Short infrequent feeds prevent letdown and release of hindmilk	▪ Infrequent feedings ▪ Limitation of feeding time ▪ Not nursing on both breasts ▪ Improper use of breast shields ▪ Engorgement ▪ Nonfunctioning milk ejection reflex ▪ Maternal stress, inadequate diet and/or fatigue ▪ Improper latch on ▪ Poor sucking response ▪ Overuse of pacifier or other soothing techniques ▪ Smoking ▪ Oral contraceptive use ▪ Formula supplementation	▪ feed every 2-3 hours ▪ feed when baby is hungry ▪ Avoid supplementation ▪ Increase comfort when feeding ▪ Condition milk ejection reflex ▪ Minimize stress ▪ Proper latch on ▪ Avoid smoking, drugs, skipping feedings ▪ Avoid overusing soothing technique ▪ Appropriate rest, nursing while napping ▪ Avoid rapid maternal weight loss	▪ Nurse every 1-3 hours in relaxing place ▪ Facilitate nursing with heat, gentle massage, good position and latch on ▪ Increased rest and dietary changes ▪ Massage base of breast when infant changes sucking from nutritive (with swallow) to nonnutritive ▪ Change breasts frequently ▪ Syntocinon spray 1-2 sprays each nostril 3-4 minutes before feeding ▪ Feed every 2 hours at night because there is increased prolactin production at night.

2. **Physical adaptation/recovery (diastasis recti, uterine involution, exercise, nutrition)**

a. **Abdominal wall relaxation**

1) Diastasis – separation of the rectus muscles
   a) Varies in severity depending on woman's muscle tone, fitness level
   b) Parity and multiple gestation also influences degree of relaxation
2) Usually measured by fingerbreadth: length, width, and depth
3) Exercises (simple curl ups) can be initiated within a day or two of delivery
4) If muscle tone is not regained, woman may experience a pendulous abdomen and back problems with subsequent pregnancies.

b. **Uterine involution**

1) Uterus descends into pelvis by 2 weeks and cannot be palpated abdominally
2) Nonpregnant size by 4-6 weeks
3) Cervix will admit 2 fingers for few days PP
4) Vaginal rugae by 3 weeks
5) Lochia for 3-8 weeks (large variation)
6) Brief (<2 hour) episode of heavier vaginal bleeding during second week PP, when placental eschar sloughs.
7) Gabbe 4th ed states tampons ok if no lacerations, day time use only

c. **Exercise**

1) Prenatal fitness level
   a) General fitness before and during pregnancy enhances PP recovery
2) Physiologically, early postpartum exercise dictated by recovery from birth (e.g., CS)
   a) Return to exercise promotes healthy emotional status
   b) Exercise will not decrease volume or quality of breast milk
   c) Consider cultural variations in assessing woman's willingness to exercise in the early postpartum period
3) Prior to initiating an exercise program that involves sustained activity
   a) Cessation of lochia
   b) Healed episiotomy
   c) CS scar closed, no discomfort
   d) Pelvic relaxation resolving
   e) Adequate milk production
4) Exercises to initiate
   a) Kegels- begin within a few hours of birth
   b) Leg stretches within first 24 hours

c) Abdominals- begin within a day or two of vaginal birth, simple curl ups

d) Walking-during first week, walk 5-10 minutes once or twice/day

(1) Increase to 20-30 minutes by end of 3rd week

e) Fatigue, pain, numbness, increased bleeding: slow down or modify activity

d. Postpartum nutrition/weight reduction

1) Pregnancy weight gain predicts PP weight retention

2) Breastfeeding women may return to prepregnancy weight sooner (data is conflicting) and have lower risk of obesity later in life

a) Advise against rapid weight loss (≥4 lb/month)

3) Parameters

a) Average 12 pound loss at delivery

b) Further loss during first 6 weeks, but many do not return to prepregnancy weight until 6 months PP

4) Advise eating reasonable amounts of variety of healthy foods each day

5) Encourage regular exercise

6) Avoid low calorie intake (crash dieting) especially when breastfeeding

7) Consider cultural variations – certain foods may be prohibited during PP period

3. Family planning/resumption of sexuality

a. Physiologic aspects

1) Bleeding, episiotomies & lacerations may resolve as early as 2-4 weeks

2) Low estrogen during first three months (longer in breastfeeding women) is associated with fewer vaginal rugae, less lubrication, and possibly a sexual response that is less rapid and intense

b. Changes in libido

1) Body changes and body image changes

2) Role conflict

3) Fatigue

4) Breast discomfort or leakage

5) There is little consensus on whether libido increases or decreases

c. Breastfeeding and sexuality

1) Breastfeeding may enhance or decrease sexuality

2) Sexual feelings about breastfeeding can inhibit breastfeeding; some women may have an erotic response to nursing

3) Decreased vaginal lubrication due to hypoestrogenic state

4) May experience letdown with orgasm, sex play

d. **Ask about resumption of sexual activity at PP visits**
   1) Woman and/or partner may be hesitant to ask questions without "permission"
   2) Many cultures proscribe sexual intercourse until bleeding has subsided, or for a specific period of time; some even include the period of lactation
e. **Family planning: Postpartum contraception** (for full discussion various contraceptive methods, see Chapter VI)
   1) **Breastfeeding woman**
      a) ***Combination methods with estrogen have been associated with decreased milk volume and early discontinuation of breastfeeding.***
      b) Progestin only methods may boost milk production
      c) Hormonal methods in postpartum period are controversial if breastfeeding
      d) Controversy
         (1) ***ACOG recommends delaying combined contraceptives until at least six weeks PP, and then only if lactation is well established***
         (2) The World Health Organization (WHO) recommends delaying the initiation of combined contraceptives until six months PP.
      e) Symptothermal method may be difficult during lactation
      f) Barrier, spermicidal methods ideal
      g) IUD is appropriate if no contraindications
   2) ***No combination oral contraceptives the first 21 days PP for any women due to risk of thromboembolic disease; progestin only methods for nonlactating women (e.g., DepoProvera) may be initiated immediately***
   3) Fit diaphragm no earlier than 6 weeks PP
   4) ***Spermicides and condoms may be used in immediate PP period; condoms offer additional protection against endometritis from introduction of bacteria before complete healing of the placental site***
   5) IUD
      a) Copper IUD may be inserted immediately following vaginal delivery (within 15 minutes of placental delivery, and follow with oxytocic); expulsion rate is slightly higher, but lower for immediate insertion than for insertion delayed during the first PP week. If insertion is not within the first PP week, delay until 6-8 weeks PP.
      b) Progestin-containing IUDs are not recommended for the lactating woman until after 6 weeks postpartum.

6) **Lactational Amenorrhea Method (LAM)**

   a) Breastfeed full-time without the use of supplements: 93 percent do not ovulate for three months PP; 88 to 89 percent for up to six months.

   b) If supplemental feedings are used or woman menstruates, or if baby is sleeping through the night, ovulation is more likely and back-up contraception is highly recommended.

   c) Milk expression is not sufficient to prevent ovulation; frequent suckling is needed

7) Withdrawal is suggested as a potential postpartum contraceptive by in Contraceptive Technology 18th ed., with a higher risk of failure than male condom; similar risk of failure as spermicide use.

8) **Sterilization – Tubal ligation**

   a) Should be considered irreversible

   b) May be done within 24 hours of vaginal delivery, during CS, or several weeks PP

   c) Discuss possibility of regret with woman; higher rates of regret if tubal ligation within 1 year of birth in women <30 years old.

4. Psychosocial adaptation/parental-infant relationship

a. Developmental tasks of fourth trimester

   1) Reconcile conflicting conceptions of role
   2) Accept and adjust to pressures of parenthood
   3) Learn to care for infant with competence and confidence
   4) Establish/maintain healthful family routines
   5) Provide for child's development
   6) Provide a nurturing marital relationship
   7) Adjust to the practical realities of life
   8) Maintain personal autonomy
   9) Explore and develop a sense of family

b. Fourth trimester critical issues

   1) Unprepared for parenthood role
   2) Abruptness of role change
   3) Cultural/familial pressure of role
   4) Permanency of role

c. Reva Rubin observations on postpartum

   1) Woman varies in state of readiness to learn based on various stages
   2) Taking in—relatively passive
   3) **Taking hold—assuming tasks of caring for infant and self**

d. Other aspects of maternal/parental/baby relationships
   1) Difficult to study because of multiple factors
   2) Multiple instruments used to assess relationships and environment with various levels of reliability and validity (e.g. NCAST, HOMES, Broussard)
   3) Some terms often used:
      a) *En Face*—caregiver to infant with faces both on same plane
      b) Detachment—infant yawning, crying, breaking eye contact, often because tired
      c) Engrossment—engaging in close contact such as eye to eye or *en face*
      d) ***Brazelton test assesses infant's abilities on wide scale of activities, not exactly a test of relationships but often used to illustrate to new parents what their children can do***

5. Postpartum Rh immune globulin/immunizations

a. Review of Rh status
   1) Rh is an antigen on the red blood cell of approximately 85% of the Caucasian population and 93% of the African American population
   2) Has been found on fetal cells as early as 6 weeks after conception
   3) People with the factor (antigen) are Rh positive
   4) Those without the factor are Rh negative

b. Antibody screen (indirect Coombs in some older texts)
   1) Used to identify women with antibodies dangerous to fetal well being
   2) 2% of hemolytic disease in newborns is result of rare red blood cell antigens
   3) ***An Rh negative woman with a positive Rh antibody screen should be referred***
   4) A repeat antibody screen should be done for Rh negative women at 26-28 weeks and within 72 hours PP, prior to administration of Anti D serum (*RhoGAM*).

c. Postpartum
   1) 75% of gravidas have some fetal-maternal transplacental exchange of blood during pregnancy or at delivery (most often the latter)
   2) Risk factors for acquiring fetal blood in maternal circulation
      a) Birth
      b) Chorionic villus sampling (CVS)
      c) Spontaneous, therapeutic or elective abortion
      d) Amniocentesis
      e) Hypertension in pregnancy
      f) External version
      g) Hemorrhage from placenta previa or abruption

h) Cesarean Section

i) Manual removal of placenta

3) **Anti D serum, Rh Immune Globulin (RhIG) (*RhoGAM*) suppresses maternal production of antibodies against the Rh factor on fetal blood cells in the Rh negative mother**

   a) ***Presence of Rh antibodies in the mother's blood may cause hemolytic disease of the newborn in future pregnancies if the fetus is Rh positive***

   b) Anti D serum is given at 28-30 weeks antenatally and within 72 hours PP. Also given following invasive antepartum procedures (CVS, amniocentesis), abortion, external version, and antepartum hemorrhage.

   c) These women should receive Rh Immune Globulin (RhIG) during antepartum period or following the procedures listed in b) above:

      (1) Rh negative AND

      (2) Negative maternal antibody screen (indirect Coombs)

   d) ***Women who qualified for antenatal RhIG should receive another dose within 72 hours PP if the infant is Rh positive:***

      (1) Infant may have weakly positive direct Coombs test (antibody screen on cord blood) if mother received antenatal RhIG

      (2) RhIG is injected intramuscularly

   e) ***RhIG protects for up to 12 weeks***; theoretically if undelivered 12 weeks after antenatal dose, it should be repeated (but usually is not)

   f) Note that the standard dose is 300 micrograms, which protects up to 30 mL fetal blood

      (1) Larger doses may be needed; ***Kleihauer-Betke test will be used to determine the amount of fetal blood in the mother's system.***

      (2) For abortion before 12 weeks gestation, 50 micrograms is adequate; after 12 weeks, full 300 microgram dose is given.

4) **Rubella vaccine**

   a) Given in the postpartum period to rubella non-immune women

   b) 0.5 ml subcutaneous

   c) May check rubella titer to confirm immunity prior to subsequent pregnancies

      (1) Less than 1:8 usually is considered negative

      (2) Some labs report "immune", "non immune", or "equivocal"

   d) Contraindicated if woman allergic to neomycin.

   e) ***Woman should refrain from pregnancy for 1 month after rubella vaccine***

f) ***Breastfeeding is not contraindicated and she will NOT transmit rubella to other children***

g) OK to give rubella immunization if mother is also receiving RhIG.

D. "Six week" postpartum examination

1. May be performed between weeks 4-8
2. Some sites/providers do 2 week visits, particularly if indicated by factors such as extensive perineal repair, fetal loss, history of depression, or other risk factor for physical or emotional problems.
3. Postpartum complete history and anticipatory guidance
    a. Review pregnancy and birth experience
    b. Discuss problems
    c. Assess for depression
    d. Provide emotional support
    e. Answer questions
    f. Assess health risks
    g. Determine resumption of sexual intercourse/dyspareunia/contraception used?
    h. Provide contraceptive options/prescriptions/instructions
    i. Consider referrals
4. Complete chart review
    a. Antepartum, intrapartum, postpartum records
    b. Lab tests
5. Postpartum physical examination to assess if woman's reproductive tract has returned or is returning to non-pregnant condition. Complete physical is recommended, with particular attention to:
    a. Blood pressure
    b. Thyroid
    c. Breasts
        1) Masses, signs of nipple trauma if breastfeeding
        2) Exam may be difficult if breast full of milk-consider rescheduling
        3) Discuss importance of self breast exam
    d. Abdomen: diastasis recti, scar if CS, masses, tenderness, CVAT
    e. Extremities: edema, varicosities, Homan's sign
    f. Pelvic
        1) External: inspect and palpate perineum, labia, anus
        2) Speculum: cervix, vaginal secretions; Pap, gonorrhea and chlamydia cultures if indicated

3) Bimanual: tenderness of perineum, cervix, uterus; size, shape, position of cervix and uterus; adnexa; pelvic and perineal support (instruct in Kegel exercises)

4) Rectovaginal: hemorrhoids, evaluate sphincter, rectovaginal septum

E. Laboratory tests (order/obtain/interpret)

1. Lab tests may vary by site-specific guidelines and may include

   a. Urinalysis: dipstick for glucose, protein, nitrites

   b. Hematocrit or Hemoglobin – compare antepartum and postpartum values as indicated

   c. Pap smear; may need followup for abnormal pap during pregnancy

   d. Gonorrhea and/or chlamydia tests

   e. Thyroid stimulating hormone if indicated

   f. 75 g oral glucose tolerance test if she had gestational diabetes

F. Assessment and management of deviations from normal in the postpartum period; indications for consultation, co-management or referral

1. Late (delayed) hemorrhage

   a. ***Early postpartum hemorrhage: Blood loss greater than 500 cc with a vaginal birth in the first 24 hours postpartum; or a 10% change in Hematocrit between admission and the postpartum period***. Expected blood loss of cesarean is approximately 1000 cc and 1500 cc with cesarean and hysterectomy.

   b. ***Late postpartum hemorrhage (PPH): Blood loss greater than 500 cc more than 24 hours post delivery*** (quantity is not specified in most sources)

   1) Etiology:

      a) ***Usually sub-involution*** i.e., involution is not occurring as it should. May be caused by retained products of conception. This type of hemorrhage most frequently occurs in the second week PP (when the placental eschar sloughs).

      b) Infection

      c) vonWillebrand's factor increases during pregnancy, so women with this disease are protected until pregnancy changes begin to resolve. They may hemorrhage 2-5 days PP.

   c. Signs and symptoms of PP hemorrhage

   1) Persistent lochia

   2) Failure of uterus to decrease in size

   3) Painless fresh bleeding

   4) Coagulopathy

   5) Uterine inversion

6) Infection

7) Retained products of conception

d. Management of PP hemorrhage

1) Prevention - early ambulation and breastfeeding; ensure complete removal of placenta

2) Treatment of PP hemorrhage

a) Methylergonovine (Methergine) .2 mg PO q 4h X 6 doses

b) If indicated by heavy bleeding, treat as immediate PP hemorrhage, i.e., consider need for IV fluids, IV oxytocin, IM prostaglandins

c) Consult if not controlled by methylergonovine; curettage, though not the first line of treatment, may be needed if bleeding persists or medical management does not control it.

d) Antibiotics as indicated

2. Postpartum vulvar hematoma

a. Result of an injury to a blood vessel without noticeable trauma to the superficial tissue

1) Incidence - 1/800 to 1/1000

2) Predisposing factors

a) Traumatic delivery

b) Lower genital tract trauma

c) Large babies

d) Precipitous deliveries

b. Signs and symptoms of vulvar hematoma

1) Unilateral bulging

2) Bluish red discoloration

3) Pain

4) Difficulty voiding

5) Rapid development

6) Signs and symptoms of shock

7) Severe perineal or rectal pain unrelieved by usual measures

> **Midwifery Message**
> Codeine often is an excellent analgesic postpartally. It is not an antipyretic such as NSAIDs or acetaminophen and thus, will not mask an infection.

c. Prevention of vulvar hematoma

1) Check for hemostasis with repair

2) Proper suturing

3) Care in handling tissues

d. Management and treatment of vulvar hematoma

1) Ice packs (also for prevention)

2) Monitor size and approximate blood loss

3) Sitz bath

4) Analgesia for small vulvar hematomas

5) *Monitor signs and symptoms of shock in presence of firm uterus*

e. Consult for

1) Evacuation of hematoma

2) Ligate vessels

3) Suturing dead space

3. Thromboembolic disease

a. Incidence 1% with vaginal deliveries
2% with C/S deliveries

b. Predisposing Factors

1) Venous stasis

2) Immobility

3) Vascular anoxia

4) Endothelial damage

5) Increased clotting factors of pregnancy

c. **Risk factors for thromboembolic disease:**

1) Wound infection

2) Obesity

3) Previous history

4) Heart disease

5) CS

6) Varicosities

7) Inherited thrombophilias such as Factor V Leiden, Activated protein C etc.

d. Signs and symptoms

1) *Fever and tachycardia*

2) *Abrupt onset; severe leg pain*

3) *Edema of ankle*

4) *Positive Homan's sign*

5) *Pain with calf pressure*

e. Treatment of thromboembolic disease

1) Anticoagulant therapy (e.g. coumarin) AAP considers coumarin compatible with breastfeeding

2) Heparin is generally preferred in pregnancy since it has a large molecular weight and low placental transfer

3) Consult; probably refer for management

4. **Pulmonary embolism**
   a. ***Precursor may be deep vein thrombosis***
      1) **Presentation**
         a) ***Sharp chest pain***
         b) ***Shortness of breath***
         c) ***Air hunger***
         d) ***Respiratory rales***
         e) ***Hemoptysis***
         f) ***(vi)Apprehension/anxiety***
   b. Management: **REFER** for medical treatment
5. **Superficial thrombophlebitis**
   a. ***Location - Saphenous vein***
   b. Predisposing factor: Pre-existing varicosities
   c. Onset 3rd to 4th postpartum day
   d. Signs and symptoms
      1) Tenderness
      2) Warmth and redness over site
      3) Low grade fever
      4) Elevation of pulse
   e. **Treatment of superficial thrombophlebitis**
      1) Heat
      2) Limb elevation
      3) Bedrest
      4) Analgesia usually is first line of treatment, sometimes anticoagulants, but not always needed
      5) Support hose
   f. **Prevention of superficial thrombophlebitis**
      1) Maintain good hydration
      2) Early ambulation
      3) Avoid pressure of stirrups
      4) Minimize blood loss
      5) Avoid combination oral contraceptives until 2-4 weeks postpartum
      6) Elastic support hose
   g. Consult for management

6. Postpartum eclampsia

a. Incidence - Rare due to aggressive antepartal management
   Predisposing factor: preeclampsia

b. Differential diagnosis

   1) Cerebrovascular accident
   2) Pulmonary emboli
   3) Cerebral tumor
   4) Meningitis, encephalitis
   5) Metabolic disease
   6) Seizure disorder/epilepsy

c. Management and prevention

   1) ***Magnesium sulfate therapy for at least 24 hours postpartum with preeclampsia***
   2) Management will be in collaboration with MD (referred for medical management if eclamptic)

7. Postpartum depression

a. Incidence - 10% - 20%

b. Predisposing factors

   1) Lack of support systems
   2) Marital problems
   3) Current family crisis
   4) High risk birth
   5) Lack of empathetic mothering in own life
   6) Past history of depression or other mental condition

> PP "blues" usually peaks between days 3 and 5, resolving by day 10.
> PP depression begins between 2 and 30 weeks postpartum. It lasts up to a year.

c. Signs and symptoms

   1) Differentiate from postpartum "blues"

      a) Transient emotional lability during first week postpartum
      b) More than half of women experience
      c) Insomnia, weepiness, depression, anxiety, poor concentration, irritability
      d) Symptoms are mild
      e) Manage with reassurance and support; monitor for development of severe psychiatric disorders.

   2) Prenatal depression may be a precursor of postpartum depression

      a) Lack of acceptance of pregnancy
      b) Excessive mood swings
      c) Emotional withdrawal/failure to prepare for infant
      d) Preoccupation with appearance/numerous physical complaints

3) **Postpartum depression**
   a) Excessive fatigue, sleep disturbance etc.; similar to other major and minor depression disorders
      (1) Symptoms present for most of each day for at least 2 weeks
      (2) Begins within 4 weeks to 3 months of delivery

d. Risk factors: antenatal depression, young maternal age, unmarried, cigarette smoking, illegal drug use during pregnancy, hyperemesis gravidarum, frequent use of emergency services and absenteeism during pregnancy, previous affective disorder; **previous postpartum depression**.

e. Management
   1) Refer to support groups
   2) Check thyroid function as hypothyroidism can be masked as PP depression.
   3) Use team approach
   4) Support and develop positive behavior
   5) Family-centered maternity care
   6) Consult or refer for psychiatric care. Anticipate treatment with antidepressant drugs, probably a SSRI for at least 6 months.
   7) ***If the mother is detached from reality, has any thoughts of suicide or infanticide, or any other signs of psychosis, consider the situation an emergency*** and she needs to be hospitalized.

8. Infection

Puerperal morbidity is defined by the Joint Committee on Maternal Welfare as a ***"temperature of 100.4 degrees F.*** (38.0 degrees C.), the temperature to occur on any two of the first ten days postpartum exclusive of the first 24 hours and to be taken by mouth by a standard technique at least 4 times daily." Not only genital infections but also due to UTI, upper respiratory tract infection and mastitis.

a. Endometritis

1) Symptomatology for endometritis
   a) ***Fever, chills, malaise, anorexia***
   b) ***Foul smelling discharge*** (due to anaerobes); odorless scant lochia with β-hemolytic streptococcus
   c) Nausea and vomiting
   d) Abdominal/distention
   e) Uterine tenderness
   f) Decreased bowel sounds
   g) Signs: Leukocytosis (WBC 15,000-30,000)

2) **Risk factors for endometritis:**
   a) CS, especially if woman labored
   b) Instrumental delivery, manual delivery of placenta
   c) ROM greater than 24 hours (mode of delivery more important), especially preterm premature rupture of membranes
   d) Chorioamnionitis
   e) Vaginal exams - the number of vaginal exams is of greater relative importance in puerperal infection than use of internal monitors
   f) Pathogenic colonization of vagina
   g) Anemia, poor nutrition and hygiene
3) **Management**
   a) Blood cultures - organisms present in blood cultures originate from the endometrial source of infection
   b) CBC with differential
   c) UA, culture and sensitivity
   d) Endocervical cultures
   e) Parenteral antimicrobials: penicillin, aminoglycoside.
   f) Rest, good nutrition
   g) Consult; co-management or referral
4) **Complications**
   a) Pelvic cellulitis (extension of infection to surrounding areas and development of abscess
   b) Septic pelvic thrombophlebitis

b. **Infection of episiotomy/perineal laceration**
   1) Incidence 0.09% - 0.3%
   2) Signs and symptoms
      a) Localized pain
      b) Dysuria
      c) Low grade fever 101 or less
      d) Pulse greater than 100
      e) Edema
      f) Repaired edges red & inflamed
      g) Oozing pus
      h) Wound separation

3) Treatment of **episiotomy/perineal laceration infection**
    a) Antimicrobials
    b) Sitz baths
    c) Cochrane library has found secondary closure superior than healing by secondary intention
    d) Consult; co-management or referral depending on treatment chosen

c. **Puerperal mastitis**

1) Inflammation of the breast parenchyma
2) Common pathogens; *Staphylococcus aureus* (40% of cases), *Streptococci,* usually from infant's respiratory tract. Organisms enter breast through fissure or abrasion.
3) Incidence – 2-33% breastfeeding women (Williams 22nd ed)
4) ***Commonly presents weeks 3-4 PP.*** Seldom occurs before end of first week PP Usually unilateral; engorgement may precede.
5) ***Presentation: chills, followed by fever (100.4-104) and tachycardia. Breast is hard, red, and painful. Sick!***
6) **Start antimicrobial therapy within 48 hours** with constitutional symptoms,. (Some recommend culture first). Use penicillinase-resistant penicillin or cephalosporin that covers *S. aureus*.
    a) Dicloxacillin, cephalexin, cephradine, cefaclor for 10-14 days is recommended
        - Erythromycin if allergic to penicillin
    b) Continue breastfeeding – reduces chance of abscess
        - Pump if breast is too engorged for latch on
        - Start nursing on uninvolved breast to encourage let down
7) **Breast abscess**
    a) 10% with mastitis develop abscess
    b) Suspect if fever persists after starting antibiotic or palpable mass develops
    c) Breast ultrasound is indicated if abscess is suspected by fluctuant mass
    d) Needle aspiration may cure; traditional treatment is surgical drainage
    e) Refer for medical management

8) **Prevention of puerperal mastitis**:

   a) Meticulous hand washing

   b) Early, frequent breastfeeding with appropriate technique

   c) Supportive, nonrestrictive bra

   d) Observe baby for skin, cord infection

   e) If breast lump is detected:

      - Empty breasts frequently
      - Moist heat, massage before and during feeding
      - Begin feeding on affected breast
      - Change feeding positions – point baby's nose toward affected area
      - Pump before nursing if engorged
      - Rest, fluids, analgesic, good nutrition (vitamin C), etc
      - Eliminate cow milk from mother's diet if repeated infections

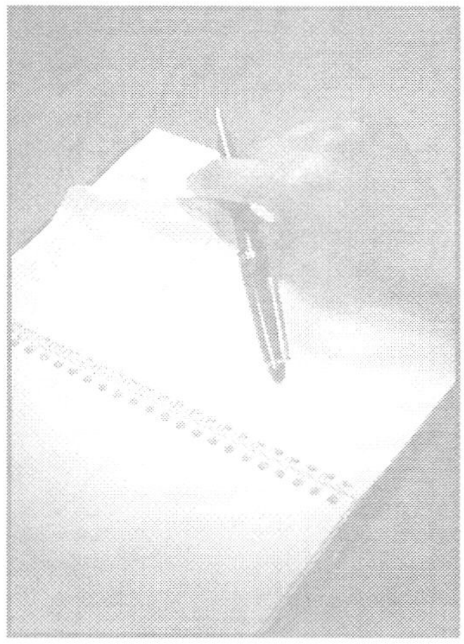

Chapter V

Neonatal Care

V. Neonatal Care (5%-10%)

A. **Physiology/Pathophysiology of the newborn**

B. **Assessment and management of transition to extrauterine life**

1. **Assignment of the Apgar score**
2. **Support of normal transition**
   a. Suction
   b. Stimulation
   c. Temperature maintenance
3. **Intervention**
   a. CPR of the newborn
   b. Medications used in resuscitation
   c. Transfer/transport

C. **Newborn assessment**

1. Physical examination
2. Newborn reflexes
3. Gestational age assessment

D. **Infant nutrition**

1. Support and instruction for breastfeeding
2. Support and instruction for bottle-feeding

E. **Newborn care and interventions**

1. Eye prophylaxis
2. Administration of medications (e.g. vitamin K, immunizations)
3. Circumcision counseling
4. Education of family for infant care

F. **Laboratory tests (order/obtain/interpret)**

1. Routine assessments and interventions (e.g. PKU)
2. Those indicated by status of newborn (e.g. bilirubin)

G. **Assessment and management of deviations from normal in the newborn period: indications for** consultation, co-management or referral

a. Neonatal jaundice
b. Hypothermia
c. Hyperthermia
d. Respiratory disorders
e. Hypoglycemia
f. Congenital heart defects
g. Neonatal bacterial sepsis
h. Congenital anomalies

i. Drug exposure

j. Congenital infections

k. Stillbirth, miscarriage or loss of perfect child

A. **Physiology/Pathophysiology of the newborn**

1. **Respiratory system**

a. **Fetal respiration**

1) **Gas exchange occurs in the placenta**
2) Partial pressure of oxygen (Po_2) of fetal blood is less than maternal blood and fetal hemoglobin (hgb F) has greater affinity for oxygen than adult hgb A, so oxygen diffuses easily from mother to fetus
3) Pco_2 and CO_2 content of fetal blood are higher than mother's, so CO_2 diffuses readily from fetus to mother for elimination
4) Fetal respirations (movement of chest and abdomen) permit neuromuscular maturation

b. **Changes at birth**

1) **Chest compression creates negative pressure**, which sucks air into lungs as the chest recoils after birth
2) **Decrease in blood oxygenation with cessation of placental blood flow stimulates respiration.**
   a) Surfactant reduces surface tension in pulmonary alveoli to allow expansion
   b) Pulmonary capillaries fill with blood
3) Drop in temperature and peripheral tactile stimuli transmit impulses to respiratory center
4) Amniotic fluid drains from the respiratory tract or is absorbed.

c. **Normal umbilical cord acid-base values**

	Vein	**Artery**
pH	7.32	7.26
Po_2	38.9	17.7
Pco_2	37.1	40
Base deficit	6.8	6.7

2. **Circulatory system**

a. **Fetal circulation**

1) **Umbilical vein carries oxygenated blood** from placenta to fetus
2) Ductus venosus shunts blood directly to inferior vena cava
3) Blood from inferior vena cava passes directly through foramen ovale into the left atrium and left ventricle to be ejected into the ascending aorta; most left ventricular output goes to fetal head
4) Blood from superior vena cava goes to right ventricle, then to pulmonary trunk

5) The ductus arteriosus arises from the pulmonary artery and shunts most blood to the descending aorta, to fetal body and placenta via umbilical arteries.
   a) High pulmonary resistance in fetal lungs forces blood through ductus arteriosus. Decreased systemic resistance.

b. Changes at birth

1) **Pulmonary capillary resistance falls** with expansion of lungs, and pulmonary blood flow increases
   a) Most blood from right ventricle enters lungs via pulmonary artery
2) **Systemic vascular resistance increases** (blood pressure rises) with cessation of placental flow, causing pressure changes in heart
   a) **Increased pressure in left heart** (along with decreased resistance in lungs) **closes the ductus arteriosus** in a few hours and the foramen ovale immediately.
3) Refinement of circulation continues for the first 1-2 months of life.

3. Gastrointestinal function

a. Fetus can absorb glucose, amino acids and other nutrients

b. ***Meconium is produced in late pregnancy***

1) ***Hypoxia increases intestinal peristalsis and relaxes the anal sphincter, causing passage into amniotic fluid***
2) Meconium passage also occurs with increasing frequency as fetus reaches and passes term and may represent maturity, not hypoxia.
3) Rarely seen before 36 weeks; 25% pass meconium between 36-42 weeks.

c. Liver function is deficient, as the placenta performs these functions prior to birth.

1) Reduced production of fibrinogen and other coagulation factors
2) ***Vitamin K storage is deficient*** because formation depends on bacteria in the intestine; ***predisposes infant to hemorrhage in first few days after birth***
3) ***Gluconeogenesis*** (formation of glucose from amino acids) and glucose storage are immature; decreased levels of carbohydrate-regulating hormones (cortisol, epinephrine, glucagon); these factors present risk of hypoglycemia if neonate is stressed.
4) ***Conjugation of bilirubin for excretion is limited***, predisposing baby to hyperbilirubinemia and jaundice.
5) Metabolism of drugs is deficient, e.g., sulfonamides.

d. **Digestive enzymes are present, but gastric contents are not acidic.** This may delay the growth of bacteria necessary for vitamin K synthesis in the gut.

1) Newborn is able to absorb simple solutions and breast milk

2) Cow's milk cannot be digested well until days 2-3, after excess gastric mucus is eliminated

e. **Peristalsis of large intestines increases after birth, and 1-6 stools are produced.**

1) ***Absence of stool within 48 hours of birth is abnormal, and may indicate intestinal obstruction or imperforate anus.***

4. **Renal function**

a. In fetal period, placenta is main regulator of fluid and electrolytes

b. Fetus begins to produce urine at 9-12 gestational weeks, and urine becomes the major component of amniotic fluid.

1) The amount of amniotic fluid is a function of fetal renal status

c. At birth, renal blood flow increases, but not proportionate to adult

d. At least 24 hours is needed for the glomerular filtration rate to adapt to extrauterine environment

e. Newborn has limited ability to excrete salt; increased renal excretion of glucose and amino acids due to immaturity of tubules. Decreased ability to concentrate, dilute, and acidify urine.

f. 93% normal infants void in first 24 hours of life; 99% within 48 hours.

5. Central nervous system

a. Fetal movement begins very early in gestation, during the first few weeks.

b. Brain development occurs early with major development between 12 and 18 weeks gestation and continues through the first year.

c. Sleep-wake patterns evolve; by term the fetus is awake about 30% of the time.

d. Term fetus has high endorphin levels, perhaps contributing to apnea and limiting pain during the birth experience.

e. See section on newborn reflexes for further information.

B. Assessment and management of transition to extrauterine life

1. Assignment of the Apgar score

> **TIP**
> 5 minute, not 1 minute, Apgar score is predictor of survival in infancy

a. Apgar scoring has been used since 1952; it is scored at 1 minute and 5 minutes

b. According to American Academy of Pediatrics and the American College of Obstetricians and Gynecologists:

1) The Apgar Score is useful in assessing the condition of the infant at birth

2) Apgar score alone should not be used as evidence that neurologic damage was caused by hypoxia or from inappropriate intrapartum treatment.

3) Apgar can be used to assess the efficacy of resuscitation efforts.

4) An infant who has had "asphyxia" proximate to delivery that is severe enough to result in acute neurologic injury should demonstrate all of the following:

a) Profound metabolic or mixed acidemia (ph <7.00) on an umbilical arterial blood sample and

b) Apgar score of 0 to 3 for longer than 5 minutes and

c) Neurologic manifestation, e.g., seizure, coma, or hypotonia, and evidence of multiorgan dysfunction

Traditional	Mnemonic of APGAR	0	1	2
Muscle Tone	Activity	Flaccid	Some flexion extremities	Well flexed
Heart Rate	Pulse	Absent	Below 100 bpm	Above 100 bpm
Reflex Irritability	Grimace	No response	Grimace	Cry, Sneeze, cough, pulls away
Skin Color	Appearance	Blue-gray, overall pallor	Normal, except for acrocyanosis	Completely pink
Respiration	Respiration	Absent	Slow, irregular, weak cry	Good, crying

c. Key Points: What the Apgar is NOT

1) Predictor of neurological development; it has been used (misused) for this, but is not an intention of the score

2) Determination of whether or not to resuscitate—remember you initiate prompt resuscitation efforts, do not wait for 1 minute

3) Determination of perinatal asphyxia; neither can it predict cerebral palsy—most infants with the condition do not have poor Apgar scores

2. Support of normal transition

a. Suction

1) Not generally required with vigorous infant

2) If needed, gentle use of bulb syringe or suction catheter

3) Aggressive pharyngeal suction can cause laryngeal spasm, vagal bradycardia, and delay the onset of spontaneous breathing

4) If no meconium, limit mechanical suction to a depth of 5 cm from lips and duration of 5 seconds

b. Stimulation

1) Drying with towel

2) Flicking the bottoms of the feet

3) Gently rubbing the back

4) If unsuccessful in initiating spontaneous respirations, proceed to assisted ventilation

5) DO NOT shake, slap, or hold upside down.

c. **Temperature maintenance**

1) Deliver in a warm, draft-free area if possible

2) Mechanisms of heat loss

a) Convection

- Depends upon air speed and air temperature

b) Conduction

- Heat exchange by conduction is relatively small
- Conduction depends on the thermal conductivity of a substance in contact with the body

c) Radiation

- Radiant heat loss is slightly more complex since it is dependent on the surface area and geometry, the surface temperature of the newborn's body, and the temperature of the surface area on which the baby is placed

d) Evaporation

- Evaporative loss depends upon air speed and the absolute humidity of the air
- If a baby is clothed (e.g. hat) or nursed in a regular warm air incubator of moderate humidity, evaporative heat loss is only a small fraction of the total heat lost

3) Ways to decrease heat loss

a) Skin-to-skin contact with mother (front-to-front)

b) Rapidly dry the skin and hair

c) Remove wet linen after delivery

d) Wrap in prewarmed blankets

e) Place under a radiant warmer

f) Cap

3. Intervention

a. **CPR of the newborn**: Follow the ABC's

Airway

Breathing

Resuscitation

1) Airway

a) Position face upward with the head in a neutral position (i.e. no neck flexion or hyperextension)

b) Vigorous respiratory efforts without breath sounds indicate airway obstruction

c) Reposition

d) Gently suction mouth first and then nostrils. Newborns are obligate nose breathers, but the first few breaths may be gasps and cries; even nose breathing will aspirate substances in the mouth.

2) Breathing
   a) For shallow or slow respiratory effort without meconium, stimulate gently and administer oxygen.
   b) If heart rate is <100 beats/minute or decreasing, start positive pressure ventilation with bag and mask resuscitation.
   c) If no response, prepare to intubate and call for help
   d) Signs of adequate ventilation include symmetric rise of the chest along with increasing heart rate, improving color, and resumption of spontaneous breathing efforts.
      - If the chest rises asymmetrically after intubation, the tube may be a main stem bronchus.
      - If the chest does not rise at all the tube may be in the esophagus (stomach would rise).
      - If placement is correct and chest excursion is asymmetrical or absent suspect pneumothorax, diaphragmatic hernia, pulmonary hypoplasia, etc.
3) Circulation
   a) Evaluate by heart rate and color
   b) Monitor heart rate at chest with stethoscope or palpation of base of the cord.
      - If ≥100 beats/minute, continue to observe
      - If < 100 beats/minute and decreasing, start or continue positive pressure ventilation (bag and mask) (i.e. respiratory resuscitation)
      - If heart rate < 60 beats/minute, start chest compressions
   c) Medications are initiated when the heart remains below 60 bpm after 30 seconds of coordinated chest compressions and PPV.
4) Positive pressure ventilation
   a) Ensure mask fits snugly around both mouth and nose
   b) Ventilation rate should be approximately 30-40 breaths/minute
   c) Observe that chest wall rises with inflation (vs. stomach)
5) **Chest compressions**
   a) Place two fingers over lower third of sternum OR use two thumbs with the hands around the chest (latter is current recommendation for infants)
   b) Compression depth of 1/3 to ½ the depth of the chest: ¾-1 inch (1.5-2.5cm)

c) Rate of 2 compressions/second – 100 per minute

d) Ratio of ventilation to chest compression is 1:3

6) **Meconium**

a) ***No need to intubate with light stained fluid and a vigorous baby***

b) With particulate meconium, DeLee suction on the perineum as the head is delivered.

c) If baby is not vigorous, intubate and aspirate meconium from the trachea by applying suction directly to the tracheal tube while withdrawing and removing the tube OR through a wide-bore suction catheter passed down a tracheal tube. Do not try to stimulate prior to intubation as the baby could aspirate meconium.

d) Ventilate the baby when as much meconium as possible has been removed.

7) Severe congenital anomaly: resuscitate baby until informed decisions about further management can be made.

b. Medications used in resuscitation

MEDICATIONS USED IN NEWBORN RESUSCITATION			
DRUG	DOSAGE	STRENGTH	ROUTE
Naloxone Hydrochloride-*Narcan* (reverse opiate depression)	0.1 mg/kg	0.4 mg/ml OR 1.0 mg/ml	IV, ET, or IM
Epinephrine (stimulant)	0.1—0.3 ml/kg	1:10,000 = 0.1—0.3 mg/kg	IV, ET Rapidly
Sodium Bicarbonate (correct acidic milieu)	1-2 mEq/kg	0.5 mEq/ml (4.2%)	Slow IV push after adequate ventilation & perfusion established
Volume Expanders (Crystalloid = normal saline, Ringer's lactate) (Colloid = blood, 4-5% albumin, plasma substitute) (treat blood loss)	10 ml/kg		Slow IV push (over 5-10 minutes)

Adapted from American Heart Association , *Neonatal Resuscitation Textbook* (4th ed), 2000.

c. Transfer/transport

1) Candidates

a) Resuscitation

b) Congenital anomalies

c) Any condition needing further evaluation (e.g. hypothermia, hypoglycemia, lethargy)

2) Information to provide to receiving facility
    a) Bring the chart and all pertinent information needed for giving a detailed report of baby's status and history.
3) While waiting for transport, maintain charting, prepare copies of charts to transfer with infant, continue stabilization efforts, and attend to parents
4) Stabilization efforts:
    a) Maintenance of thermoregulation
    b) Maintenance of oxygenation and ventilation
    c) Monitoring oxygen (oxygen saturation in 95-97% range if equipment available for this)
    d) Newborn assessment (if feasible)
    e) Gestational age assessment (if feasible)

C. Newborn assessment

1. Physical examination – may vary order of exam depending on newborn state. Possible findings are listed.

a. Ensure adequate lighting and temperature

b. Newborn state
    1) Sleep (deep or light)
    2) Transitional (drowsiness)
    3) Awake (quiet alert, active alert)
    4) Crying
    5) If ill, may be lethargic, stuporous, comatose

c. Posture
    1) Flexion, symmetrical
    2) Extension, asymmetrical
    3) Decerebrate

d. Tone
    1) Obtuse popliteal angle
    2) Limp

e. Movement
    1) All extremities, random, symmetrical
    2) Jitteriness, tremors, seizures

f. Gross anomalies
    1) Malformations, deformities, or disruptions

g. Measurements
    1) Weight, length, head circumference, chest circumference

h. Skin

1) Texture

a) Soft & moist is normal

b) Dry, peeling areas in post-mature infant

c) Vernix caseosa (more extensive in premature infants)

d) Lanugo (more extensive in premature infants)

e) Nails (longer in mature infants)

f) Tags, defects, or sinus formations may indicate underlying cyst or mass, especially if preauricular, along sternocleidomastoid, or midline from nose, over head and down back to coccyx.

2) Color: pallor, cyanosis, jaundice, plethora

a) Acrocyanosis or peripheral mottling common

b) ~50% of infants develop physiologic jaundice. Early onset is more likely to be problematic. The lower and more peripheral the jaundice, the higher the bilirubin level. Clinically apparent jaundice occurs when bilirubin > 6 mg/dl.

c) Melanin not fully apparent at birth: skin color is more apparent in nail beds and on scrotum or vulva

d) Common "spots"

- ***Milia*** -- yellow or white keratin-filled papules (~1 mm). Disappear within days to weeks
- ***Erythema toxicum*** -- red macular rash on face, upper trunk, upper extremities. Tiny central vesicle develops. Appears within 48 hours and disappears by 4-5 days of life
- ***Mottling (cutis mamorata)*** -- splotchy macular patches forming a network. Associated with cooling. Tends to disappear with warming.
- ***Café au lait*** -- light brown patches. Large (>3 cm) and/or > 6 patches may indicate neurofibromatosis
- ***Mongolian spots*** -- blue-black macular lesion, usually on back and buttocks. Seen frequently in blacks and Asians. Fades within a couple of years
- ***Hemangioma telangiectasia*** -- on forehead, lids, lips, and nape of neck. Of capillary origin, "strawberry" marks fade over time
- ***Nevus flammeus (salmon patch)*** -- light red, macular blotch on nose, eyelids, or nape of neck; "stork bites" fade within a year. Mainly seen in Caucasians.

- ***Port wine stain*** -- Flat, intensely red or purple, large. Seen mainly on face, arms, or legs. Requires cosmetic repair. Stain on eyelid (ophthalmic branch of trigeminal nerve) suggests Sturge-Weber syndrome.
- ***NOTE: Vesicles are always a concern, as they may indicate herpes***
- ***Meconium***-staining of cord, vernix or nails

i. Vital signs & statistics (term newborn)

1) Temperature 95.9°-99.5° F (36.5°-37.5° C)
2) Heart rate: 110-140 beats per minute
3) Respirations: 30-60 per minute
4) Length: 18-23 inches (46-57.5 cm)
5) Head Circumference: 13.2-14.8 inches (33-37 cm)
6) Chest Circumference: ¾-1 inch (2-2.5 cm) < head circumference

j. Head and neck

1) ***Caput succedaneum crosses suture lines*** (more common)
2) ***Cephalhematoma limited by suture lines***
3) Molding common in vaginal birth
4) Note if suture lines are overriding or widely separated; also note presence and condition of fontanels (tense, bulging, sunken)
5) Eyes
   a) Pupils equal, reactive, responsive to light and accommodation
   b) Congenital cataracts (seen with TORCH infections)
   c) Lid ptosis—trauma or palsy
   d) Mongolian slant or crease at inner canthus with trisomy 21
6) Ears
   a) Pinna flat, curved, degree of recoil, cartilage
   b) Low-set ears common with other anomalies, especially renal and hearing loss
7) Nose
   a) Flaring (respiratory distress)
   b) Choanal atresia: obstructed nares-infant is blue when sleeping; pink when crying
8) Mouth
   a) Check for intact palate or cleft lip/palate
   b) Epstein pearls on gums or neonatal teeth are innocuous
   c) Large tongue may indicate hypothyroidism or trisomy 21

9) Neck
   a) ~90° rotation
   b) Dimples in neck or near ears: possible cysts
   c) Webbing (possible Turner syndrome)

k. Chest

1) Lungs
   a) Respiration rate & rhythm
   b) Retractions, grunting
   c) Breath sounds
2) Heart
   a) Rate & rhythm
   b) Murmurs (systolic <24 hr. of age is normal)
3) Observations
   a) Asymmetry
   b) Accessory nipples (normal)
   c) Breast nodule size (for gestational age)
   d) Nipple discharge (normal)
   e) Crepitus over clavicle (abnormal, rule out fracture)

l. Abdomen

1) Shape -- round, scaphoid, distended
2) Diastasis recti
3) Umbilical cord
   a) Number of vessels: should be 3 (2 arteries and one vein). 2 vessel cord indicates possible anomaly.
   b) Omphalocele
4) Hernia
5) Gastroschisis: abdominal wall defect
6) Masses
7) Liver: smooth edge or enlarged
8) Spleen: nonpalpable, palpable, enlarged
9) Kidneys: palpable, enlarged
10) Bowel sounds

m. Perineum

1) Ambiguous genitalia: Most authorities suggest that any surgical repair reflect the biological sex as determined by chromosome analysis.
    - If ambiguous genitalia is due to congenital adrenal hyperplasia, there may be a medical emergency.
2) Male
    a) Testes: undescended, upper part of scrotum, descended; rugated
    b) Penis: phimosis (normal), hypospadias
3) Female
    a) Clitoris: enlarged, hooded
    b) Vagina: white or pinkish discharge, imperforate
    c) Labia: minora & majora equal, minora covered

n. Extremities

1) Lower
    a) Femoral pulses
    b) Hip abduction (Ortolani's click with hip dysplasia)
    c) Persistent extension
    d) Tibial bowing
    e) Constriction bands
    f) Joint range of motion
    g) Syndactyly, polydactyly
    h) Sole creases: anterior, anterior 2/3, entire
2) Upper
    a) Joint range of motion
    b) Constriction bands
    c) Hand webbing
    d) Cortical thumb; overlapping fingers; short, incurved little finger
    e) Syndactyly, polydactyly

o. Back

1) Spine shape
2) Dimples, open or closed neural tube defects, hair
3) Imperforate anus
4) Gluteal folds symmetric or asymmetric

p. Brazelton's neonatal behavioral assessment scale (NBAS)

1) The NBAS was developed in 1973 by Dr. T. Berry Brazelton and colleagues.

2) The scale includes 28 behavioral and 18 reflex items to assess the baby's capabilities across different developmental areas and describes how the baby integrates these areas as she deals with her new environment.

2. Newborn reflexes

a. Suck

1) A finger or nipple placed in baby's mouth elicits rhythmical sucking.
2) Depressed sucking may be due to medication administered during labor and birth.

b. Rooting

1) Turns head to suck
2) When cheek is stroked at the corner of the mouth, head turns toward touch and baby makes sucking motions.
3) If this reflex doesn't vanish in 3-4 months, there may be a CNS problem

c. Moro (startle)

1) Baby is held horizontally, then swiftly lowered a few inches; or the head may be lowered a few inches; or a loud sudden noise makes baby's arms fling out and then come together as hands open then clutch.
2) Absence or weakness of this reflex suggests a severely disturbed CNS.

d. Palmar grasp

1) By pressing just one of baby's palms, fingers should grasp the object.
2) Absence or weakness of this reflex could reflect an injured spinal chord or depressed CNS

e. Plantar grasp

1) Pressing thumbs against the balls of baby's feet will make toes flex.
2) Absence of this reflex may indicate damage to the spinal chord

f. Placing and stepping

1) Holding baby upright with feet touching a solid surface and moving him forward should elicit stepping movements.
2) After 3-4 months, this reflex should vanish. If it reappears, there may be an injury of the upper spinal cord.

g. Babinski

1) Baby's foot is stroked from heel toward the toes. The big toe should lift up, while the others fan out.
2) Absence of reflex may suggest immaturity of the CNS, defective spinal chord, or other problems. Reflex may be seen up to age one, then reaction will be reversed with the toes curling downward.

h. Babkin

1) When both palms are pressed, eyes will close, mouth will open and head will turn to one side.
2) Absence of this reflex or if it reappears after vanishing around 3-4 months, may signify a malfunctioning CNS.

i. Doll's Eyes

1) While manually turning baby's head, eyes will stay fixed instead of moving with the head.
2) While normally vanishing around one month of age, if it reappears later, there may be damage to the CNS.

j. Galant (trunk incurvation reflex)

1) While stroking back to one side, spine and trunk arch toward that side.
2) Absence may indicate spinal injury or depression of the CNS.

k. Perez

1) Firmly stroking spine from tail to head elicits cry out and head rises.
2) If this reflex does not vanish in 4-6 months, CNS may be severely depressed

l. Withdrawal

1) A pin prick to the sole of baby's foot will make the knee and foot flex.
2) Absence of this reflex could indicate a damaged sciatic nerve.

3. **Gestational age assessment**: Dubowitz-Ballard assessment criteria -- estimation of gestational age

a. Neuromuscular maturity

1) Posture

a) Degree of extremity flexion
b) Greater flexion➔maturity

2) Square window

a) Flexion of hand to forearm
b) Greater flexion (0 degrees)➔maturity

3) Arm recoil

a) Recoil of arm after full extension
b) Full recoil➔maturity

4) Popliteal angle

a) Angle of knee, with thigh on chest
b) Lesser angle (90 degrees)➔maturity

5) ***Scarf sign***
   a) Put hand on opposite shoulder
   b) Lesser travel of elbow across midline→maturity
6) ***Heel to ear***
   a) Non-forceful movement of heel toward ear
   b) Greater distance between heel and ear→increased maturity

b. Physical maturity
1) Skin
2) Lanugo
3) Plantar surface
4) Breast
5) Eye/ear
6) Genitalia

c. Scoring: Each item is scored in each of the sections. The two section scores are added and the total is compared to a rating scale to determine the gestational age.

D. Infant nutrition

1. Support and instruction for breastfeeding

a. Recommend and encourage breastfeeding for all pregnant and postpartum mothers except (in developed countries) those who are HIV positive
   1) Other contraindications to breastfeeding include strong maternal preference, substance abuse, HTLV-1 infection, and certain maternal medications.

b. Breast milk
1) Composition: 10% solids for energy [e.g. lactose, protein (casein and non-casein) and fat]; 90% water
2) Influenced by stage of lactation
   a) Maturity of milk varies greatly from woman to woman
   b) Colostrum; transitional milk; mature milk (10 days)
3) Human milk does not supply vitamin K (synthesized in infant gut when it becomes colonized); vitamin D (supplementation or sun exposure); fluoride (unless mother drinks fluoridated water); vitamin B_{12} if the mother is vegan.

c. Benefits
1) Protection against infection
2) Protection from allergy
3) A lower incidence of Sudden Infant Death Syndrome (SIDS)
4) A lower risk of childhood diabetes, cancer, and ear infection
5) A better response to vaccinations and a faster ability to fight disease

6) Better psychomotor, emotional, and social development

7) An association with higher intelligence

d. Factors related to success

1) Breastfeeding immediately after birth results in greater continuation

2) *Women who had analgesia/anesthesia for birth need support for successful breastfeeding initiation and continuation*

3) Let-down is activated by the infant suck which stimulates release of oxytocin from the posterior pituitary

e. Engorgement

1) Some is normal

2) Increased by feeding delays and supplementation

3) Prevention

a) Nurse early and often

b) Hand express

c) Cool & warm compresses

d) Chilled whole cabbage leaves with veins crushed (anecdotal evidence)

e) Feed on demand

f) Use both breasts at each feeding

g) Milk "comes in" day 3-4; accelerated by early frequent feeds

f. Cracked/sore nipples: usually due to malposition; prevent by insuring areola is in the newborn's mouth; could be caused by yeast when everything else has been eliminated

g. Positioning instructions

1) Recommend "en face" position, baby's belly to mother's belly

2) C-hold of breast

3) Infant grasps surrounding areola, not just the nipple

h. Nipple care

1) Proper positioning and latch-on

2) Breast shells to protect nipples between feedings

3) No soaps

4) No drying with hairdryers or nipple preparation with terry washcloths

i. Assessment of sucking

1) Regular audible swallowing heard

2) No clicking or smacking noises

j. Breast milk storage

1) Wash hands thoroughly before pumping

2) Freezer vs. refrigerator
    a) Freeze if stored longer than five days; ideal is 2 days
    b) Store as far away from the freezer door as possible
    c) If stored in refrigerator freezer, milk should be used within six months
    d) Milk stored in deep freezer should be used within 12 months
    e) Fresh milk may be stored in the refrigerator from 5-7 days at 39 F
    f) Defrosted milk should be used within 24 hours
    g) Place frozen milk in the refrigerator the night before
    h) Milk should be thawed under running warm water or placed in a pan of warm water, not hot; the latter destroys immunological properties of breast milk; it should be used immediately
    i) Shake while thawing to mix creamy portion
    j) Never refreeze

> **Milk protein: woman vs. cow**
> **W**oman: **W**hey (mostly)
> **C**ow: **C**asein (mostly)

3) Type of container
    a) A clean container must be used and labeled with the date and time of earliest milk expressed
    b) Hard plastic or glass for sick or premature infants
    c) Ziplocs for healthy babies
    d) Some immunological properties may be lost but this is not a problem for healthy term infants
    e) Vitamin C and IgA are lost when milk is heated too quickly or when it is too hot
    f) Fat content is altered with refrigeration and freezing
    g) Loss can be minimized with shaking

2. Support and instruction for bottle-feeding

a. Information regarding supplies needed

1) Glass, plastic, or disposable refillable bottle
2) Keep opened cans of liquid formula covered and refrigerated
3) Discard unused formula within 24 hours
4) Nipples should be firm enough for infant to suck vigorously
5) Soft nipples allow milk to go in so fast that sucking needs may not be satisfied
6) Bottle caps to cover the nipples are recommended during transportation to maintain cleanliness

b. Information regarding formula preparation

1) If using pre-sterilized formula:

a) Wash top of can with warm, soapy water and rinse

b) Open and pour into clean bottle

c) Put on nipples, being careful not to handle nipple projection

d) Place bottle caps over nipples and refrigerate

e) To prepare a single bottle from powder or concentrate, combine clean water with formula in bottle, cap the bottle, and shake to mix.

2) If commercial formula is not to be used

a) 15 oz water, 1 Tablespoon sugar, 10 oz evaporated milk

b) Produces 25 oz formula, 20 cal/oz

c) Supplement with multivitamin with iron

c. Information regarding feeding techniques

1) Warming is optional

2) If warming, use care with microwave as milk in center is hotter than near side

3) Shake bottle well after microwaving to mix cool and warm portions

4) If warming in a pan of hot water on stove, do not allow pan to boil dry (bottle will burst)

5) Check temperature of formula by allowing a drop or two to fall on your inside wrist

6) Do not warm disposable bottles with plastic liners on the stove—tend to melt and leak during feeding

7) Once bottle has been used, discard any remaining contents

8) Ensure adequate time (at least 30 minutes) and a comfortable chair for feeding

9) Hold baby with head slightly elevated; bottle should not be propped.

10) Ensure nipple is filled and baby is sucking milk, not air.

11) A baby who develops colic may do better with an angled or disposable liner bottle

12) Burp infant regularly and after every feeding.

13) Baby will take about 1-2 oz every 2-3 hr for the first 2 weeks

d. Supplementation

1) Iron

a) In formula fed newborns, begin at 3 months

b) Side effect may be constipation

2) Fluoride

a) Indicated at 6 months when using ready to use formula

b) Unfluoridated water to prepare formula and when breastfeeding

e. **Honey and corn syrup**: Do not use before 1 year of age due to risk for *Clostridium botulinum*

f. **Solids can be added at 4-6 months**

1) Add new food one week at a time; start with cereal, followed by fruits and vegetables
2) Cues for self-feeding usual at 6-8 months
3) Never put the baby to bed with a bottle. Causes ear infections.
4) Add crackers/cereal first
5) Cow's milk can be added after 1 year
    a) Before that time may cause iron-deficiency anemia due to GI blood loss

E. **Newborn care and interventions**

1. **Eye prophylaxis**

a. ***Prevention of neonatal gonococcal and chlamydial infection (ophthalmia neonatorum)***

b. Recommend routine administration of one of following to all newborns within the first hour of life

1) **Erythromycin 0.5%** ophthalmic ointment in each eye is effective for gonorrhea and chlamydia
2) **1% silver nitrate** drops in each eye (associated with high incidence of chemical conjunctivitis). *Silver nitrate* d*oes not protect against chlamydia.*

c. These agents are equally effective in prevention of gonococcal infection

d. Prophylaxis for *Chlamydia trachomatis* requires erythromycin

2. **Administration of medications (e.g. vitamin K, immunizations)**

a. **Vitamin K** is required for conversion of processor proteins into proteins with procoagulant and anticoagulant activity

1) Vitamin K is synthesized in the gut by bacteria; newborn is not colonized for several days following birth, so he is deficient
2) Administration of vitamin K to a healthy term infant prevents decrease in prothrombin activity and prolonged clotting time in the first days of life
3) The premature infant responds to vitamin K less predictably
4) Recommended: vitamin K (K-1 phytonadione) 0.5-1.0 mg intramuscularly to newborn soon after birth
5) Oral vitamin K is used in many countries but is not yet recommended in U.S.
6) Prevention of hemorrhagic disease of newborn (HDNB)
    a) Self limited, hemorrhagic disease usually evident 2-3rd day of life
    b) Rarely occurs later
    c) GI tract most common site of bleeding
    d) Cause is vitamin K deficiency and consequent deficiency of factor II, VII, IX, X

e) More common in breast fed babies not provided preventive vitamin K

f) Vitamin K not well transported across placenta

g) Response to treatment is rapid

h) Diagnosis by neonatal bleeding, prolonged PT, PTT

i) Treat disease with intravenous or intramuscular vitamin K

j) Serious hemorrhage treatment may include transfusion

b. **Cord care**

1) Recommended cord care has included topical antistaphylococcus agents and antistreptococcal agents

2) Drug classification: Antiseptics

a) Triple dye

b) Silvadene

c) Hexachlorophene

d) Bacitracin

e) Isopropyl alcohol

f) Iodophor

3) Conclusions of Cochrane review

a) Simply keeping the cord clean appears to be as effective and safe as using antibiotics or antiseptics

c. **Narcotic antagonist**: Naloxone

1) Indicated when mother has had an opioid within 4 hours of delivery

2) Do not give if mother is a known opioid abuser

3) Opioid antagonist with the greatest affinity for mu receptor

4) Dosage is 0.1mg/kg

d. **Hepatitis B immunization** #1 is given at birth (see Chapter I, Primary Care)

1) Hepatitis B immune globulin if mother is HBsAg+

e. Other vitamin/mineral supplements

1) *Vitamin D supplementation for breastfed infants (especially African American) unless exposed to sun at least 30 minutes diapered or 2 hours fully clothed per week.*

2) Fluoride for breastfed infants unless mother's water is fluoridated

3) Vitamin B_{12} for breastfed infants if mother is vegan

3. Circumcision counseling

a. Circumcision is the surgical removal of foreskin of penis.

b. Indication: parental choice – not medically necessary according to AAP.

c. Complications of circumcision

1) 1 in 200 to 1 in 500
2) Infection
3) Bleeding
4) Urethrocutaneous fistulas
5) Meatal stenosis
6) Amputation of distal glans
7) Removal of excessive foreskin
8) Scarring of the penile shaft
9) Anesthesia complications
10) Skin tags and bridges
11) Curvature of penis
12) Possible psychological ramifications

d. Benefits of newborn circumcision

1) Decreased incidence of UTI (1:100 uncircumcised, 1:1000 circumcised)
2) Prevention of penile cancer (rate is tripled in uncircumcised males, but incidence is very low, 9 per million)
3) Prevention of phimosis (unable to retract foreskin) and paraphimosis (unable to replace foreskin once retracted)
4) Avoidance of potential need for circumcision later in life when procedure is more risky and more expensive

e. Risk of balanitis (inflammation and sclerosis of the foreskin around the meatus; foreskin also does not retract) is the same for circumcised and uncircumcised.

f. Risk of sexually transmitted infections is lower in circumcised males, but unsafe behavior is a more important risk factor.

g. AAP recommends analgesia for all circumcisions

1) EMLA cream
2) Dorsal penile block
3) Subcutaneous ring block

h. Care of newly circumcised penis

1) Careful hand washing
2) Vaseline gauze dressing for 24 hr
3) Glans is red for 24 hours, then edematous
4) Serosanguinous drainage
5) Healing begins in 2 days; complete at 7 days
6) Sponge bath until healed; no soap or alcohol

i. Care of uncircumcised penis

1) Wash external structures only
2) Needs no special care
3) Foreskin should not be forcibly retracted
4) Foreskin usually retractable by puberty when child can retract it himself
5) If irritation occurs, A&D ointment can be applied

4. Education of family for infant care

a. Infant care & parenting instructions

1) Promote breastfeeding if not contraindicated
2) If bottle-feeding, hold baby during feeds, do not prop bottles
3) Stroking baby's lip with nipple helps grasp
4) Hold bottle so that milk stays in the neck to prevent swallowing of air
5) Average amount to feed during week one is 30-60 mL every 2-3 hours
6) During first weeks, waken baby to feed at least every 4 hours
7) Supplemental food sources not necessary until 4-6 months. Newborns are not able to transfer food to back of tongue for swallowing until then.

b. Diaper rash

1) Reaction to ammonia in urine
2) Clean with mild soap and warm water
3) Leave open to air whenever possible
4) Frequent diaper changes
5) Zinc oxide cream as a barrier for prevention
6) Usually not involving folds of skin or confluent

c. Candida albicans rash

1) Involves skin folds; confluent and often around anus
2) Nystatin, miconazole or clotrimazole
3) Consultation needed if skin is peeling or if vesicles or exudate are present

d. Weight loss

1) Weight loss of 5-10% is normal first week

e. Weight gain

1) Bottle-fed: 1 oz per day and 1 in. per month
2) Breastfed: slightly less than 1oz per day
3) Should regain birth weight by 2 weeks
4) Birth weight doubles by 6 months; by one year birth weight triples

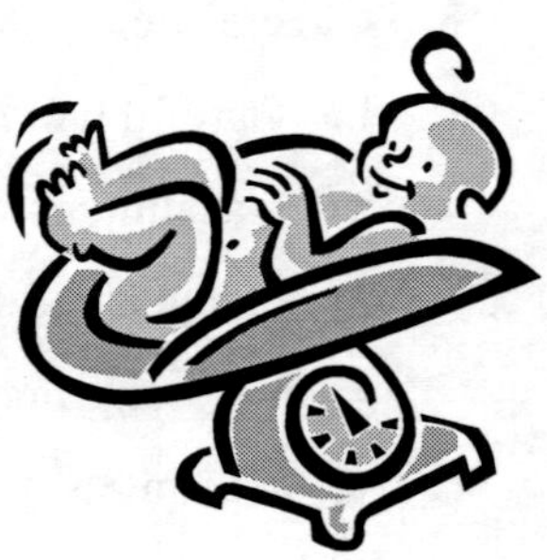

f. Voiding and elimination

1) 6-8 wet diapers a day
2) 2-5 bowel movements a day, more with breastfed babies

g. Sleeping

1) Baby sleeps 2-3 hours at a time.
2) During the first week he/she will sleep about 16 hours/day.
3) Put the baby on his/her side or back for sleeping; switch sides after feeding so fluid/mucus will not collect in one lung.

h. Crying

1) Babies can cry for about 2 hours total out of every 24 hours (day).
2) Crying will usually increase until 6-7 weeks of age and then will slow down.
3) Fussy periods are usually in the evening.

i. Cord care

1) Keep the cord above the diaper. It will turn black and dry within a couple of days. The clamp will be taken off at the first visit, if not before discharge from health care facility.
2) The cord will fall off in about a week.

j. Bathing

1) Don't immerse in water until after cord falls off. Until then, sponge baths.
2) Be certain the room is warm (about 75°).
3) Bathe before a feeding so the baby does not spit up during the bath or have a bowel movement.
4) Get everything you will need for the bath and after together before starting.
5) Never leave the baby.
6) The water should feel warm to mother's elbow or wrist. Use a mild soap on the body & hair—no soap on the face.
7) Start with the cleanest area (face) & move to the dirtiest area (diaper area).
8) Rinse the soap off well. Wipe eyes from the inside to the outside.
9) For boys: Do not push the foreskin of the penis back at this time.
10) For girls: Wash the vulva from the front to the back.
11) Wash the hair at the end of the bath.
12) Dry immediately & put a hat on.
13) Powders and lotions are not needed.
14) Dress the baby quickly after the bath.

k. Car seat

1) The best location is in the back seat, away from any air bags.
2) Car seat and infant should face back of the car.
3) Put rolled up blankets or diapers on either side of his/her head.
4) Buckle the baby in properly, passing the strap through the legs.

l. Signs of wellness

1) Eats as if hungry
2) Spits up no more than a slight amount after feeding
3) Bowel movements are loose, but not runny or watery
4) Sleeps 2-3 hours at a time and seems content overall
5) Normal temperature
6) Breathes faster than an adult, but is not stressed with breathing
7) Skin is not blue or yellow

m. Signs to call the midwife/pediatric health care provider

1) Not eating
2) Vomits (more than "spitting up")-large, "projectile"
3) No wet or dirty diapers in a day
4) Runny, watery stools
5) Lethargic, difficult to wake up at all
6) Prolonged crying
7) High pitched/shrill cry
8) Very low or high temperature (<97° or >100.4° F axillary)
9) Oozing, redness or foul odor around the cord

F. Laboratory tests (order/obtain/interpret)

1. Routine assessments and interventions (e.g. PKU)

a. Metabolic screening labs

1) State regulations

a) No federal guidelines
b) Practitioners must be aware of regulations in their state
c) Wide variation among states in what disorders are screened and mandatory versus voluntary screening

2) All states screen

a) Phenylketonuria (**PKU**), Hypothyroidism (**TSH**)
b) Both are conditions that lead to preventable mental retardation
c) Initial screening done at 48-72 hours of age
d) Formula fed can be screened as early as 24 hours

e) Should be repeated at between 2 and 4 weeks

f) State law mandated

3) Other metabolic diseases screened for in one or more states

a) Biotinidase deficiency

b) Congenital adrenal hyperplasia

c) Cystic fibrosis

d) Galactosemia

e) Homocystinuria

f) Branched chained ketoaciduria (maple syrup urine disease)

g) Sickle cell disease

h) Tyrosinemia

i) For discussion of expert recommendations for expanded newborn screening, see http://www.mchb.hrsa.gov/screening

b. Newborn hearing screening

1) The screening of newborns and infants involves use of non-invasive, objective physiologic measures that include otoacoustic emissions and/or auditory brainstem response. Both procedures can be done painlessly while the infant is resting quietly.

2) Prevalence of congenital hearing loss is 1.5 to 6/1000 live births

3) Early identification important so interventions can be initiated that will affect speech and language development

4) Screening neonates based on risk factors misses 50% of hearing impaired newborns

5) Universal hearing screening is recommended and is mandated by law in many states

2. Those indicated by status of newborn (e.g. bilirubin)

a. **Blood glucose screening**

1) ***Normal range: 40-130 mg/dL***

2) Indications for screening

a) Large (LGA) or small (SGA) for gestational age

b) Infant of gestational diabetic or insulin dependent mother

c) Prematurity

d) Apgar <5 at 5 minutes,

e) Perinatal asphyxia

f) Multiple gestation

g) Symptoms of hypoglycemia
(1) Poor feeding
(2) Plethora
(3) Hypotonia or hypertonia
(4) Changes in level of consciousness
(5) Excessive tremors
(6) Hypothermia

3) *Continue to monitor those infants with low blood glucose before feedings until levels are $\geq$ 40 mg/dL for 12 hours*

b. **Hematocrit/hemoglobin/WBC**

1) Fetal hemoglobin
a) Higher affinity for oxygen than adult Hgb
b) Present in newborn with adult Hgb up to 1 year

2) *Normal range is hct 45-65%; Hb 15-22g/dL; WBC ~18,000*

3) Indications for screening for anemia or polycythemia
a) Perinatal asphyxia
b) Respiratory distress
c) Pallor
d) Plethora
e) Multiple gestation
f) Infant of diabetic mother
g) SGA
h) Maternal antepartum or intrapartum hemorrhage

c. **Blood type and Coomb's test** or direct antiglobulin test (DAT)

1) DAT: detects presence of antibody in infant's blood
Indications for screening; quantified from <+1 to +4

2) Indications

a) Mother is Rh negative
b) Mother is O+ (to rule out ABO incompatibility)
c) Maternal blood type is unknown

3) All infants with a positive DAT should have a cord bilirubin drawn

d. **Bilirubin**

1) ***Normal ranges***

a) Direct bilirubin <1.8md/dL

b) Total bilirubin

- Birth <2mg/dL
- 0-1 days <6mg/dL
- 1-2 days <8mg/dL
- 3-5 days <12mg/dL

2) ****Major concern is when total bilirubin level rising rapidly*** (>.5mg/dL per hour)

3) ***Indications for screening***

a) **Any baby with jaundice under 24 hours of age**

b) Full term infant with apparent clinical jaundice greater than expected for age

c) Full term healthy infant with clinical jaundice persisting for more than a week

e. **Drug screening**: Urinary and meconium drug screening if there is maternal history of drug abuse or baby has symptoms of withdrawal

G. Assessment and management of deviations from normal in the newborn period: indications for consultation, co-management or referral

a. Neonatal jaundice

1) General information

a) Infants are born with relative polycythemia

b) Majority of hemoglobin in newborn's red blood cells is fetal hemoglobin

c) These factors contribute to the fetus's ability to be well oxygenated in the reduced oxygen environment in utero

d) Fetal red blood cells have a short life span

e) As the cells are hemolyzed, bilirubin is released

f) After birth, the neonatal liver often is unable to manage the amount of bilirubin that is released into the blood stream

g) The newborn generates three times more bilirubin per kilogram of body weight than the adult

h) **There are four types of jaundice**

(1) **Physiologic:** usually peaks on day three to four

(2) **Pathologic:** jaundice in the first 24 hours after birth; rising faster that 5 mg/dL per day; a high direct bilirubin level

(3) **Breast milk:** late onset (> 6 days)

(4) **Breastfeeding-associated or "starvation" jaundice**: by day 3-4

2) **Physiology**

   a) Hemoglobin released from lysed red blood cells is broken down to heme and globin. Heme is converted in the reticuloentothelial cells to bilirubin (fat soluble). Most of this bilirubin is bound to albumin in the blood stream and transported to the liver where it is conjugated (attached) to glucoronide -- this process is facilitated by urdine diphosphoglucuronosyl transferase (UDPGT) -- formerly named glucoronyl transferase.
   b) UDPGT is not abundant in the immature neonatal liver, leading to jaundice.
   c) Once the bilirubin is conjugated, it is water soluble and can be cleared from the bloodstream via the bile ducts and deposited in the gut.
   d) The bilirubin is then excreted in the stool.
   e) If the infant is not stooling regularly, water soluble bilirubin can be converted back to fat soluble bilirubin and reabsorbed into the blood stream.
   f) This fat soluble bilirubin is deposited in tissues causing the jaundice color.
   g) Bilirubin can be deposited in brain tissue, causing condition known as kernicterus.
   h) While kernicterus can lead to brain damage, there is no evidence that kernicterus occurs as a result of physiologic hyperbilirubinemia.

3) **Laboratory diagnosis**

   a) When a total bilirubin level is ordered, total amount of serum bilirubin, the direct bilirubin, and the indirect bilirubin level
   b) The direct reflects the amount of conjugated bilirubin in circulation, the indirect is the unbound and unconjugated bilirubin. (Unbound bili is found when the amount of bilirubin exceeds the albumin binding site capacity.) The indirect bilirubin level is the value of interest in physiologic hyperbilirubinemia.

4) **Physiologic jaundice**

   a) Physiologic jaundice accounts for >81% of jaundiced newborns
   b) By the second day of life the process is well underway
   c) Physiologic jaundice peaks between 72- 96 hours after birth
   d) It is completely dissipated by 10 to 14 days
   e) Physiologic jaundice occurs in all mammal newborns

5) **Pathologic jaundice**

   a) Occurs within 24 hours or after one week
   b) Total bili serum levels rise faster than 0.5 mg/dL/hour; a direct bilirubin > 1.5 - 2 mg/dL.

c) Increased RBC hemolysis is associated with the following symptoms and/or causes:

(1) ABO incompatibility is more common than Rh incompatibility but is usually considerably milder than Rh disease

(2) Rh incompatibility (erythroblastosis fetalis) is infrequently seen because of the widespread use of anti-Rh gamma globulin or *RhoGAM*.

(a) ABO incompatibility is somewhat protective if it occurs simultaneously

(3) Polycythemia

(4) Cephalhematoma

(5) Petechiae

(6) Ecchymosis

(7) Delayed clamping of the cord. If the newborn is held below the level of the placenta as much as 40 to 60% increase in blood volume is transferred from the placenta to the newborn. The infant acquires about 25% additional blood volume within 15 seconds after birth and at the end of one minute 50% more.

(8) Liver disorders such as hepatitis

(9) Bile duct obstruction such as biliary atresia

(10) Infections

(11) Metabolic disorders such as galactosemia, hypothyroidism

(12) Decreased albumin sites (e.g. preterm, hypoglycemia, acidosis, hypoxia)

(13) Medications (e.g. oxytocin, aspirin, sulfas)

6) Breast milk jaundice

a) Occurs in only one to two percent of all term newborns

b) Cause is uncertain

c) Begins 5 to 7 days after lactogenesis

d) May be superimposed on normal physiologic jaundice

e) Peaks at 7 to 10 days

f) Persists for several weeks

g) No reported cases of kernicterus

h) 70 % chance siblings will be affected

7) Breastfeeding associated jaundice

a) Generally iatrogenic/schedule or management induced

b) Aggravated by glucose water (and formula) supplementation

c) Breastfeeding management will decrease bilirubin levels

d) Breastmilk contains lactalbumin and albumin is necessary for bilirubin to bind with for excretion

e) ***Need early, frequent feedings on demand (and unlimited)***

f) Non-separation of mother and infant

g) Be aware of events in labor (analgesia, anesthesia, hypoxia and precipitous birth) which may affect infant behavior; set in place mechanisms to assist the newborn when a more difficult transition is anticipated. (e.g. sleeping baby)

8) When is treatment necessary?

a) Phototherapy should be considered for an infant between 48 and 72 hours of age when the total bili is $\geq$15 and in a term infant older than 72 hours if the bili is $\geq$17. Most pediatricians will begin phototherapy in a term newborn, older than 72 hours, whose bilirubin level is $\geq$ 20.

b) **When there is evidence of hemolysis or baby is sick**

(1) Interrupting breastfeeding probably of little use

(2) Phototherapy (may use 'double banks' of lights if bilirubin is rapidly rising)

(3) Exchange transfusion may be necessary

9) Jaundice first appears in the face, then on torso, extremities, and last in hands and feet. It disappears in reverse order. If the soles of the feet or palms of the hands show pink/white on pressure and release then this zone is clear of jaundice.

b. Hypothermia

1) ***Rectal temperature < 36.5 °C (96.5 °F)***

2) Etiology

a) Evaporative heat loss

b) Increased surface area/body mass ratio

c) Decreased subcutaneous tissue

d) Sepsis

3) Risk situations

a) Prematurity and SGA infants

b) Air conditioned rooms

c) Inadequate or delayed drying and warming after birth

4) Neonatal response

a) Nonshivering thermogenesis

b) Hypoxemia

c) Metabolic acidosis

d) Depletion of oxygen stores

e) Reduction of blood glucose levels

f) Increased oxygen consumption

5) Treatment

a) If temperature is <96.5° F (36.5°C) axillary, take rectally

b) Double wrap infant in warm blankets and cover head with hat

c) Check blood glucose level. If <40 mg/dL, follow care for hypoglycemia

d) Repeat assessment in 1 hr. If still <96.5° F (36.5°C), place under radiant warmer (unclothed), and consult with pediatric provider

e) ***NOTE: Insure that skin probe is attached to upper abdomen (not over bone) when infant is placed under a radiant warmer***

c. Hyperthermia

1) *Rectal temperature >99.5 ° F (37.5 °C)*

2) Etiology

a) Impaired ability to sweat in response to environmental temperatures

b) Sepsis

c) Maternal fever at birth

d) Over bundling or over warming

3) Risk situations

a) Maternal fever

b) Prolonged resuscitation under the warmer

c) Improper probe placement when under warmer

4) Neonatal response

a) Hypernatremia

b) Dehydration

c) Increased metabolic demand

d) Apnea

5) Treatment

a) Unwrap infant and recheck temperature in 1 hour. If still elevated, consult with pediatrician

b) If under warmer, check probe placement, and adjust warmer if needed

d. Respiratory disorders

1) Causes of respiratory distress

a) Sepsis

b) Hematologic (polycythemia)

c) Cardiac (cyanotic and noncyanotic heart disease

d) Shock

e) Metabolic (acidosis, hypoglycemia)

f) Respiratory

2) **Transient tachypnea of the newborn*: Wet Lung***

a) Diagnosis of exclusion, more common in Cesarean and precipitous births

b) Caused by delayed clearance of lung fluid

c) Clinical presentation of tachypnea, minimal respiratory distress

d) Radiographs reveal fluid in fissures, pleural effusion, streaky parenchymal changes

e) **Management**

(1) Short-term oxygen supplementation. Self limited illness that resolves spontaneously in 24-48 hours

3) **Respiratory distress syndrome (RDS)**

a) Most common in preterm infants related to surfactant deficiency

b) Higher incidence with maternal diabetes, acute asphyxia, second twin, meconium aspiration, lower gestational age, white male infants

c) Primary prevention

(1) Identify mothers at risk for PTL; administration of prenatal betamethethasone (multiple doses of prenatal steriods might be deleterious)

d) Clinical presentation of tachypnea, grunting, retractions, cyanosis, flaring

e) Radiographs of ground glass reticulogranular appearance, air bronchograms

f) Management

(1) Prompt resuscitation at delivery; rule out infection; mechanical ventilatory support, exogenous surfactant

4) **Spontaneous pneumothorax**

a) 1-2% of live births

b) Symptomatic in 1 of 1500 live births

c) Clinical presentation of tachypnea, minimal retractions, grunting, nasal flaring, cyanosis; May notice diminished air entry on affected side, shifting of cardiac impulse, muffled heart tones

d) **Management**

(1) Supportive, spontaneous resolution is common; if not resolving, consider pneumoncentesis or chest tube

5) **Meconium aspiration syndrome**

a) Caused by the presence of thick meconium in the distal airways, causing a valve-like mechanism that obstructs air movement

b) Incidence rare <37 weeks, since meconium is rare before that gestational age

c) Can occur in a stressed neonate in utero or at time of delivery

d) Deep fetal gasping causes the aspiration of the meconium-mixed amniotic fluid

e) **Prevention of meconium aspiration**

(1) Suction oral and nasopharynx after birth of head and again after body; if thick or particulate meconium present, infant should receive endotracheal suctioning

f) Radiographs of thick infiltrates, air entrapment, pneumothorax

g) Treatment is complex, requiring multi-system support

6) **Apnea**

a) Types

(1) Central

(a) No respiratory effort for 15 seconds because of arrest of respiratory drive

(b) May have secondary bradycardia

(c) May be secondary to CNS disorder

(2) Obstructive

(a) Cessation of gas exchange in the lungs because of obstruction of air flow

(b) May be infectious, due to poor tone or coordination of pharyngeal muscles, or structural

b) Causes

- Prematurity
- Hypoxia
- Anatomic abnormalities (choanal atresia, palate malformations)
- Maternal drugs
- Infections
- Metabolic imbalances
- Temperature instability
- Seizures
- Hematologic
- Cardiovascular
- Genetic
- CNS disorders
- GI reflux
- Swallowing difficulties

c) Diagnosis

(1) History

- Difficult delivery
- Chorioamnionitis
- Drug abuse
- Drugs administered to the mother
- Resuscitation of the infant needed at birth
- Low Apgar score
- Umbilical pH levels
- Gestational age

(2) Physical exam

- Temperature
- Presence of dysmorphic features or malformations
- Skin color
- Perfusion
- Blood pressure
- Irritability or lethargy
- Tone and activity
- Anterior fontanel
- Milk in nasal or nasopharyngeal passages
- Heart murmur
- Petechiae
- Hepatosplenomegaly
- Gestational age

d) Laboratory studies (if cause unknown)

(1) Glucose

(2) Electrolyte levels

(3) CBC & differential

(4) Blood gases

(5) Sepsis workup

(6) Other studies as indicated

(a) Chest x-ray

(b) Spinal tap

(c) Ultrasound of head

(d) Electroencephalogram

(e) CT scan of head

e) Treatment

(1) Address underlying cause

(2) Ventilatory support

(3) Apnea monitor

(4) Teach parents CPR

e. **Hypoglycemia**

1) Incidence: common, 2-10 per 1000 live births
2) ***Serum glucose <40mg/dL at term*** (other sources say <35 to 45), <30mg/dL premature
3) ***Risk factors***
   a) SGA
   b) Postdate infants
   c) Infants with a history of asphyxia
   d) Hypothermia
   e) Sepsis
   f) Prematurity
   g) Hypermetabolism
   h) Maternal diabetes
   i) Maternal ingestion of oral hypoglycemics or beta-agonists
4) ***Clinical presentation***
   a) Pale
   b) Cool
   c) Irritable
   d) Jittery
   e) Poor feeding
   f) Apnea
   g) Seizures
   h) Lethargy
   i) Emesis
   j) Hypotonia
   k) Temperature instability
   l) Asymptomatic
5) Evaluate: high risk infants without symptoms at 2 hours of age; repeat screening may be warranted before feedings for 12-24 hours; infants with symptoms

f. **Congenital heart defects**

1) Incidence is 1% all live births
2) Major cause of death in first year of life
3) Etiology unknown in 90% of cases
4) Some possible causes: maternal rubella, alcohol use during pregnancy, maternal age > 40, Type 1 diabetes, heredity, chromosomal abnormalities

5) Types

- Defects with increased pulmonary blood flow (acyanotic)
  a) Left to right shunting of blood
  b) Area of high pressure shunting to area of low pressure
  c) Increases pulmonary blood flow -- overloads right side of heart and pulmonary artery
  d) Symptoms of congestive heart failure: hepatomegaly, dyspnea, tachypnea, intercostal retractions, poor growth
  e) Frequent respiratory infections from pooling of blood in the lungs
  f) Pulmonary hypertension
  g) Examples
     (1) **Patent ductus arteriosus**
     (2) **Atrial septal defect**
     (3) **Ventricular septal defect (VSD)**
     (4) **Coarctation of aorta**
     (5) **Hypoplastic left heart**
- Defects with decreased pulmonary blood flow (cyanotic)
  a) Usually a vascular or valvular malformation
  b) ASD or VSD also present
  c) High right-sided pressure
  d) Saturations are decreased because deoxygenated blood shunts from right to left and into the systemic circulation
  e) Symptoms of hypoxemia
  f) Examples
     (1) **Tetralogy of Fallot** (VSD, overriding aorta, right ventricular outflow obstruction, hypertrophy of right ventricle)
     (2) **Transposition of the great vessels**
     (3) **Pulmonary stenosis**
- Mixed defects

6) **Congestive heart failure (CHF)**: Inability of the heart to pump an adequate amount of blood to the systemic circulation to meet the body's metabolic demand

a) ***CHF is due to***

- Volume overload (left to right shunts)
- Pressure overload (obstructions)
- Decreased contractility of the heart muscle (electrolyte imbalances, asphyxia, ischemia)
- Increased cardiac output demands (sepsis)

b) ***Pathophysiology***

- Right or left side is impaired, the other side attempts to compensate
- Compensates by: hypertrophy and dilation of cardiac muscle
- Over time, hypertrophy impairs oxygenation to the heart muscle and muscles overstretch. The force of the contraction decreases, leading to heart failure
- Sympathetic nervous system causes peripheral vasoconstriction and increases the force and rate of myocardial contraction resulting in tachycardia
- Peripheral vasoconstriction causes decreased renal perfusion, activating the renin-angiotensin-aldosterone system; this causes the body to retain salt and water=fluid overload
- Vasoconstriction leads to decreased coronary perfusion

7) *Diagnosis*

a) Clinical symptoms

b) Chest X ray - cardiomegaly

c) EKG- hypertrophy of ventricles

8) Medical treatment

a) Improve contractility

b) Inotropes (e.g. digoxin)

c) Decrease afterload (e.g. control fluid intake, diuretics)

d) Decrease cardiac demands and decrease oxygen consumption (treat infections, sedation)

e) Improve tissue oxygenation (administer oxygen)

g. Neonatal bacterial sepsis

Neonatal bacterial sepsis is associated with 10% to 40% mortality and significant morbidity, especially neurologic sequelae of meningitis. Infants <1 month old are immunologically deficient and are predisposed to serious infections.

1) Predisposing factors

- Premature rupture of membranes (>24 hours)
- Premature labor
- Maternal fever
- UTI
- Foul lochia
- Chorioamnionitis
- IV catheters (in infant)
- Intrapartum asphyxia
- Intrauterine monitoring (pressure catheter or scalp electrode)
- Maternal colonization

2) Organisms

a) ***Early infection (0 to 4 days of age).***

- Group B streptococcus and *Escherichia coli* 60% to 70% of infections.
- *Listeria* (rare in United States)
- *Klebsiella*
- *Enterococcus*
- *Staphylococcus aureus* (uncommon)
- *Streptococcus pneumoniae*
- Group A streptococci.

b) ***Late infection (>5 days of age)***

- *Staph. Aureus*
- *Group* B streptococcus
- *E. coli*
- *Klebsiella, Pseudomonas, Serratia, Staph. epidermidis, Haemophilus influenzae.*

3) Signs and symptoms of neonatal bacterial sepsis (require consultation)

- Presentation may be subtle; thus any febrile neonate must have a septic work-up. Fever may be absent; so watch for symptoms below.
- Irritability, vomiting, poor feeding, poor temperature control, lethargy, apneic spells
- Respiratory distress, poor perfusion, abdominal distension, jaundice, bleeding, petechiae, or seizures
- Bulging fontanel is a very late sign of neonatal meningitis.

4) **Work-up**
   a) Lumbar puncture for cell count, protein, glucose, and culture.
   b) UA, CBC (remember neutropenia or thrombocytopenia are also suggestive of infection) and repeat in 5 hours
   c) Chest X ray, C-reactive protein.
   d) Cultures of blood, urine, and any other site as indicated.
   e) Latex agglutination test for pneumococcus, *E. coli, H. influenzae,* group B streptococcus, and meningococcus in blood, urine, and CSF is done even though the usefulness is questionable. Negative latex agglutination tests do not rule out infection, but positive results may help guide therapy.
5) **Associated lab findings:** Hypocalcemia, hypoglycemia, hyponatremia, and disseminated intravascular coagulation
6) **Management**
   a) Consult with pediatric health care provider
   b) Should be tailored to age of onset, clinical setting, and initial findings.
   c) DO NOT DELAY antibiotic therapy. Begin empiric therapy after cultures are obtained or before cultures if delay is anticipated.
   d) Empiric early (0 to 4 days old): Ampicillin 50 mg/kg/day (100 mg/kg/day in meningitis) divided 12 hours IV and gentamicin 5 mg/kg/day divided 12 hours IV.
   e) Empiric late (>5 days old). Depends on cause (for example, methicillin-resistant *Staph. aureus* outbreak requires vancomycin): ampicillin 100 to 200 mg/kg/day divided Q8h plus (ceftriaxone 100 mg/kg/day IV Q12h or cefotaxime 150 mg/kg/day IV Q8h), or ampicillin-gentamicin as above usually adequate.
   f) **Repeat cultures in 24 to 48 hours**. In meningitis, repeat LP every day until clear.
   g) There are isolates of Streptococcus pneumoniae that are resistant to penicillin and cephalosporins. ***Depending on the institution, vancomycin plus rifampin should be added to the above regimens until sensitivities are known.***
   h) Other hemodynamic, respiratory, hematologic, metabolic, and nutritional support and surveillance are critical. Shock may require volume expansion
7) **Conjunctivitis**
   a) Ophthalmia neonatorum (ON)
   b) Incidence 2%
   c) Prophylaxis

(1) Erythromycin 0.5% ointment

(2) Tetracycline 1% ointment

(3) Silver nitrate 1% drops (produces chemical related conjunctivitis)

(4) Prophylaxis is highly effective against GC but less so for Chlamydia

d) Differential diagnosis regarding type of ON includes chemical, Chlamydia, bacterial (GC, Staphylococcus aureus, staphylococcus epidermidis, streptococcus pneumoniae, Haemophilus), herpes simplex

e) Treatment for N. gonorrhea-ceftriaxone; Chlamydia-erythromycin syrup; HSV-Trifluridine 1%

f) Consult

8) Thrush

a) Oral candidiasis that peaks at 14 days of life.

b) Clinically, white plaques on erythematous base over oral mucosa, tongue

c) Treatment is nystatin suspension 100,000 to 200,000 U PO QID for 7 days; Mycostatin cream to maternal areola and nipple if breastfed

h. Congenital anomalies

1) Leading cause of infant mortality is birth defects (CDC 2005)

2) Overall rate ~3%, but rates of specific defects varies greatly

3) Causes for most (75%) are unknown; multifactorial

4) Some related to exposures in pregnancy

Cause Of Human Malformation	Percent
Genetic (single gene)	20%
Chromosome Anomalies	5%
Environmental Factors	10%
Irradiation	<1%
Infections (Rubella, CMV, Toxoplasmosis, Syphilis)	2-3%
Maternal Disorders (DM, PKU, Virilizing Tumors)	1-2%
Drugs and Chemicals	4-5%
Multifactorial/Unknown	65%

Originally from Wilson

5) 55 % of Infants with birth defects have two or more malformations

6) Highest structural defect is cardiac (1/200), whereas limb defects are uncommon (1/1750)

7) Cleft lip and cleft palate

a) Incidence 1 in 700-800 births

b) Cleft varies from involvement of soft palate only, to complete cleft of soft and hard palates, alveolar process of maxilla, and lip

c) Mildest form – bifid uvula

d) Isolated cleft lip primarily a cosmetic problem

e) Can interfere with feeding and speech development

f) Early treatment – special cleft palate nipples or dental appliances that occlude the cleft so suckling can occur

g) Ultimate treatment is surgical closure

h) Consult - refer

8) Congenital dislocation of the hip

a) More common in female than male and breech presentation

b) Secondary to laxity of ligaments or in-utero position

c) Can be unilateral or bilateral

d) If unilateral, involved leg is shorter; may be **asymmetric skin creases** in thigh

e) ***Major sign of dislocation is inability to completely abduct the thigh when hip and knee are flexed***

f) Abduction and external rotation of femur may produce audible or palpable "clunk" as femoral head reenters the acetabulum (Ortolani's sign)

g) ***Early treatment critical***

(1) Splints, slings, harnesses, or large padded diapers that hold the affected hips abducted and externally rotated

(2) Consult - refer

9) Talipes equinovarus

a) ***Most common of clubfoot deformities***

b) Foot is plantar flexed, inverted, and markedly adducted

c) Deformities from in utero positioning can mimic clubfoot, but can be passively corrected

d) Orthopedic are with repeated cast applications to normalize the foot's position

e) Severe cases may require surgery

f) Consult - refer

10) Reduction deformities or congenital amputations

a) Often etiology unclear

b) Teratogenic agents (e.g., thalidomide) and amniotic bands are two known causes

c) Treatment highly individualized and consists mainly of prosthetic devices

d) Consult - refer

11) Esophageal atresia

a) ***Fistula from near the carina of the trachea to the lower esophageal segment***

b) Characteristic signs are ***excessive secretions, coughing and cyanosis after attempts at feeding, and aspiration pneumonia***

c) Soon leads to abdominal distention because as infant cries, air from trachea is forced through fistula into the lower esophagus and stomach
d) Diagnosis suggested by inability to pass nasogastric tube into stomach
e) Treatment is surgical correction
f) Oral feedings withheld
g) Continuous suction prevents aspiration of saliva
h) Refer

12) Diaphragmatic hernia

a) ***Protrusion of abdominal contents into the thorax through a defect in the diaphragm***
b) On left side in 90% of cases
c) If hernia is large, the lung on affected side is hypoplastic
d) Respiratory distress immediate in severe cases
e) In less severe cases, mild respiratory difficulty develops a few hours or days later as abdominal contents progressively herniate
f) Diagnosis by x-ray
g) Treatment by MD
   (1) Immediate intubation and ventilation (bag and mask may worsen compromise)
   (2) Surgery

13) Pyloric stenosis

a) ***Obstruction of the pyloric lumen due to pyloric muscular hypertrophy***
b) ***Forceful projectile vomiting of feedings without bile usually begins late in first month***
c) May cause almost complete gastric outlet obstruction
d) Rare at birth, develops over initial 4-6 weeks of life
d) Most common in first born boys
e) ***Diagnosis made by palpation of discrete, 2-3 cm firm moveable pyloric olive like mass deep in right side of epigastrium or by identification by abdominal ultrasound***
f) Treatment – longitudinal pyloromyotomy
g) Consult - refer

> 3 **P**'s **of P**yloric stenosis
>
> **P**alpable mass
> **P**eristalsis visible
> **P**rojectile vomiting (2-4 weeks after birth)

14) **Gastroschisis**

a) ***Protrusion of abdominal viscera through an abdominal wall defect, usually to right of umbilicus***
b) ***No membrane covering bowel***, which is markedly edematous and erythematous
c) Long standing inflammation of bowel due to direct exposure to amniotic fluid
d) No increased incidence of other anomalies
e) Surgery indicated when infant stabilized; may take several procedures to completely reduce the bowel
f) Often takes several weeks before GI function recovers
g) Consult-refer

15) **Reflux**

a) ***Regurgitation secondary to gastroesophageal reflux is normal in majority of infants***
b) Complicated reflux is accompanied by failure to thrive, esophagitis, cardiorespiratory symptoms
c) Diagnosis : Upper GI series to rule out partial obstruction
d) Treatment of complicated reflux by referral MD
   (1) Prone position
   (2) Small frequent feedings
   (3) Pharmacologic therapy for complicated reflux
   (4) Continuous nasogastric feedings may alleviate the complications of reflux
   (5) Surgery may be indicated

16) **Chromosome abnormalities**

a) Down syndrome: chromosome disorder usually resulting in mental retardation, characteristic facies and many other typical features, including microcephaly and short stature
   (1) Incidence 1/800; marked variability depending on maternal age
      Mothers <20 years old – 1/2000
      Mothers >40 years old – 1/40
   (2) Only 20% of infants with Down syndrome are born to mothers $\geq$35 y/o
   (3) May result from trisomy 21, translocation, or mosaicism
      - **Trisomy 21**: Extra whole chromosome 21 (95% of cases is maternally derived)

> Remember most babies with trisomy 21 are born to women under 35 years of age. More mothers are of that age group and they are less likely to be screened.

- **Translocation**: Have 46 chromosomes but actually have genetic material of 47 chromosomes; the additional chromosome 21 has been translocated or attached to another chromosome
- **Mosaicism**: Occurs when two different cell types are present in a person. Results from an error in chromosomal separation during cell division. Relative proportion of trisomy 21 cells highly variable. Prognosis for intelligence presumably depends on the proportion of trisomy 21 cells in the brain

(4) Signs and symptoms of chromosome abnormalities

- Newborns tend to be placid, rarely cry, demonstrate muscular hypotonia
- Extra skin around the neck is common
- Physical and mental development are retarded
- Mean intelligence quotient is about 50
- Microcephaly, flattened occiput, short stature
- Outer sides of eyes are slanted upward, and epicanthal folds at inner corner of eye usually present
- Brushfield's spots (white spots resembling grains of salt in iris)
- Bridge of nose flattened
- Mouth is often held open because of large protruding tongue
- Ears small and rounded
- Hands short and broad and often have single palmar crease
- Clinodactyly (incurving) 5th finger
- Congenital heart disease affects 40% of Down newborns
- Increased incidence of other congenital anomalies

(5) Prognosis for chromosome abnormalities

- Life expectancy decreased due to heart disease and susceptibility to leukemia
- Aging process accelerated with death often occurring in 5th or 6th decade

b) **Trisomy 18**: chromosome disorder resulting from an extra chromosome 18, producing many developmental abnormalities, including severe mental retardation; incidence 1/6000

c) **Trisomy 13**: Chromosome disorder resulting from an extra chromosome 13, producing many developmental abnormalities, including severe mental retardation and forebrain abnormalities

d) **Turner syndrome**

- ***Sex chromosome abnormality in which there is complete or partial absence of one of the two sex chromosomes, producing a phenotypic female***
- Incidence 1/4000 live female births
- 50% have 45,X karyotype
- Many are mosaics
- Typically short stature, webbing neck, low hairline on back of neck, ptosis, broad chest with widely spaced nipples, multiple pigmented nevi
- Cardiac and renal anomalies common
- Mental deficiency rare
- Gonadal dysgenesis with failure to go through puberty, develop breast tissue or begin menses occurs in 90% of affected person
- Hormonal therapy will bring on puberty

e) **Triple X syndrome**

- Sex chromosome abnormality in which there are three X chromosomes, resulting in a phenotypic female
- 1/1000 apparently normal females have 47, XXX

f) **Klinefelter syndrome**

- Sex chromosome abnormality in which there are two or more X chromosomes and one Y, resulting in a phenotypic male; 47, XXY
- 1/800 live male births
- Affected persons tend to be tall, with long arms and legs, facial hair growth light
- Often have small firm testes, and 1/3 will develop gynecomastia
- Predisposition for learning difficulties
- Probably all are sterile

i. **Drug exposure**

1) **Toxic substance screening** to detect heroin, cocaine, marijuana, and barbiturates

NEONATAL EFFECTS OF SELECTED DRUGS OF ABUSE

Pregnancy Complications	Neonatal Complications	Problems in Child Health or Development
	Alcohol	
Spontaneous Abortion Poor Weight Gain Anemia Hepatitis	Withdrawal Low birth weight Restlessness Poor suck Facial malformation Microcephaly Organ defects (muscle, bones, genitals)	Mental retardation Developmental delay Learning disabilities CNS defects Heart disease Hearing problems Fetal alcohol syndrome Fetal alcohol effects
	Cigarettes	
Spontaneous abortion Preterm Preeclampsia Placental abruption Placental previa Slow fetal growth Difficulty conceiving	Low birth weight Increased risk of SIDS Increased neonatal mortality	Slow growth Learning disabilities Behavioral problems Respiratory disease during first five years

Pregnancy Complications	Neonatal Complications	Problems in Child Health or Development
Cocaine		
Prematurity Hypertension Tachycardia Placental abruption Precipitous birth Poor nutrition Poor weight gain Slow fetal growth Polypharmacy effects	Withdrawal Cerebral vascular accident Irritability Disturbed sleep Restlessness Hyperreflexia Poor Feeding Microcephaly	Mental retardation Learning disabilities Behavior problems CNS defects Incoordination
Opiates (Heroin, Methadone)		
Prematurity Hypertension	Withdrawal Irritability High pitched cry Fever Tremulousness Disturbed sleep Poor feeding Vomiting Diarrhea Increased risk for SIDS Major seizures	Developmental delay Learning disabilities Hyperactivity Visual problems Hearing problems
Marijuana		
Possible increased risk of spontaneous abortion (controversial)	Fetal exposure to THC (possible fetal effects)	Some evidence of increased birth defects in animal models
PCP (Phencycladine)		
Injuries secondary to use	Jittery and tense Vomiting Diarrhea Poor reflex Nystagmus	Possible poor attention span Possible birth defects
LSD		
Possible chromosomal damage	Possible chromosomal abnormalities	Some evidence of increased birth defects in animal models

j. Congenital infections

1) Maternal diagnostic screening

   a) Screen early for antibody to rubella, syphilis, hepatitis B

   b) Offer HIV testing to all pregnant women

   c) Viral cultures as indicated for HSV, CMV, rubella, enterovirus

   d) Serologic test as indicated for HSV, CMV, HIV

2) ***Congenital infections should be suspected in those infants who are premature or have growth restriction, failure to thrive, hepatomegaly, lethargy, thrombocytopenia, anemia, rashes, or seizures***

3) Laboratory studies

a) TORCHS

- **T**oxoplasmosis
- **O**ther infections
- **R**ubella
- **C**ytomegalovirus (CMV)
- **H**erpes simplex (HSV)
- **S**yphilis titers on baby and mother

b) IgM antibodies-IgM does not cross the placenta and therefore indicates reaction of the infant to infection

c) Viral cultures (HSV, rubella, CMV, enterovirus)

d) Culture of cerebral spinal fluid in HSV

e) Tzanck test of vesicles for suspected HSV infant and mother; more often culture or PCR techniques for active lesions

f) Urine cytology and culture for CMV

g) Darkfield exam of lesions or umbilical cord scraping for syphilis

h) Placenta to pathology lab for culture and microscopy

i) General lab screening including liver function tests, electrolytes, glucose, CBC, and clotting studies

4) Toxoplasmosis

a) Caused by Toxoplasma gondii

b) Fetus infected by transplacental passage during maternal parasitemia

c) Infection occurs through ingestion of sporulated oocysts in cat feces or poorly cooked meats

d) 50% of infants born to mothers who seroconvert during pregnancy will become infected

e) Risk of congenital abnormalities low after 20 weeks gestation

f) Diagnosis

(1) Isolation of organism from placenta

(2) ELISA to detect specific IgG, IgM

g) **Clinical findings of toxoplasmosis**

- 10% symptomatic
- Maculopapular rash, generalized lymphadenopathy, hepatosplenomegaly, thrombocytopenia, microcephaly, cerebral calcifications, seizures, motor abnormalities, chorioretinitis, pneumonia

h) If left untreated develop mental retardation, seizures, spasticity

i) **Prevention and treatment**

- Avoid changing cat litter and eating undercooked meat during pregnancy
- If documented prenatal infection noted, consider treatment with pyrimethamine and sulfadiazine
- Treat infant with pyrimethamine and sulfadiazine for 1 year
- Corticosteroids for ocular disease and CNS infection
- Pediatric infectious disease consult

5) **Cytomegalovirus (CMV)**

a) ***Most common congenital infection with 95% asymptomatic***

b) Vertical transmission may be acquired transplacentally or at birth

c) Diagnosis: Virus isolated from urine, pharynx, WBC, CSF, human milk, cervical secretions; IgM titers

d) ***Clinical findings***

- ***Sensorineural deafness***
- ***Mental retardation***
- ***Cytomegalic inclusion disease with jaundice, hepatosplenomegaly***
- ***Petechial - purpuric rash***
- ***Microcephaly***
- ***Cerebral calcifications***

e) Treatment: Ganciclovir (efficacy limited); pediatric infectious disease/neurology consult

6) **Herpes simplex (HSV)**

a) Most type 2 transmission occurs at birth through direct contact

b) Probably 20% or more of women have had HSV-2 and carry virus

c) Many women are asymptomatic shedders at time of delivery which accounts for most neonatal infections

d) ***Clinical findings***

- Average incubation 6 days up to 20 days
- ***Disseminated disease may mimic fulminate sepsis with seizures, jaundice, hepatitis, encephalitis, DIC, pneumonia***
- Untreated 90% mortality
- Local mucocutaneous disease may be mild; conjunctivitis, keratitis, or chorioretinitis can result in vision loss

e) Prevention and treatment

- Suspicious lesions during pregnancy should be cultured
- Active disease or prodromal symptoms at onset of labor mandates CS
- If vaginal delivery occurs over active lesions or rupture of membranes greater than 4 hours, begin Acyclovir
- ***Infected mother and infant should be kept in contact isolation***

7) Rubella

a) Teratogenicity greatest in first trimester, less in second, none in third

b) ***Clinical findings: Retinopathy, cataracts, patent ductus arteriosus, pulmonary artery stenosis, deafness, thrombocytopenia with "blueberry muffin" skin lesions***

c) Treatment is supportive only; prevention by immunizing children and susceptible nonpregnant women of childbearing age

8) Syphilis

a) High probability that infected mother will transmit disease

b) Treponemes cross placenta in all trimesters

c) Clinical findings

- 50% asymptomatic
- Can be benign to fatal
- SGA***, jaundice, recurring rashes, anemia, hepatosplenomegaly, "snuffles" (serous rhinitis), meningitis, condylomata lata, osteochondritis***

d) Diagnostic studies: VDRL, RPR, FTA-ABS, CSF analysis, darkfield microscopy of vesicular fluids or condylomata lata

e) **Treatment**

- **Procaine penicillin G**
- **Follow-up titers (VDRL) at monthly intervals**
- **VDRL titer should revert to negative at 6 months post treatment**

k. Stillbirth, miscarriage or loss of perfect child

Grief is a normal and natural reaction to any type of loss. For the parents of a child with a congenital anomaly or genetic disorder, they may grieve the loss of the dreams they had envisioned for the child. For individuals diagnosed with an adult onset genetic disorder, they may grieve the loss of their health and vitality, or the loss of future dreams. Grief is an adaptive process that has several components. Harrington defines grief "not as a state or set of symptoms, but a succession of clinical pictures which blend into and replace each other." Several researchers, including Elisabeth Kubler Ross, George L. Engel, John Bowlby and C. Murray Parkes, have described the stages of grief in various ways.

1) **The four dimensions of the mourning process outlined by Bowlby and Parkes are**
    a) Shock and numbness
    b) Yearning and searching
    c) Disorientation and disorganization
    d) Resolution and reorganization

> Remember mother & fathers may grieve differently.

The four dimensions do not follow a set order and a person may experience feelings from several stages at one time.

One of the major interventions of the midwife for a family with a perinatal loss is to help them meet their needs. Photographs of a stillbirth can particularly be helpful in the bereavement process. Also families should be referred to self help groups such as Compassionate Friends or Resolve to Share.

NOTES

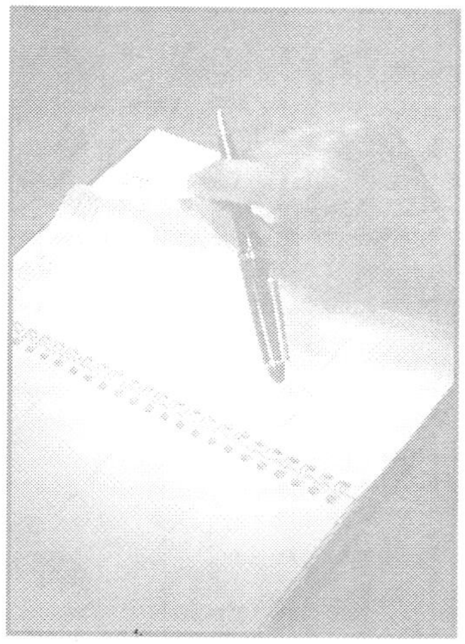

Chapter VI

Family Planning/ Gynecology

A. Physiology/Pathophysiology

1. Menstruation, interconceptional period
2. Peri-and postmenopausal period

B. **Family planning**

1. Collection of a database for the provision of contraceptive options
    a. Screening for contraindications
    b. Teaching and counseling concerning available methods
2. **Provision of contraceptive methods and devices**
    a. Natural family planning
    b. Barrier methods (e.g. condoms, diaphragm, cervical cap)
    c. Oral contraceptives
    d. Injectable contraceptives
    e. Intrauterine devices
    f. Subdermal implants
    g. Sterilization counseling
    h. Emergency contraception
3. **Fertility promotion**
    a. Preconceptional counseling
    b. Initial assessment and diagnostic procedures/referral for infertility

C. **Well-woman/perimenopausal care**

1. Laboratory tests and procedures (order/obtain/interpret)
    a. **Screening (e.g. Pap smear)**
    b. Diagnostic (e.g. wet mount, colposcopy)
    c. Ultrasound
2. Assessment and management of specific concerns
    a. **Vaginitis**
    b. Signs/symptoms of menopause
    c. Hormone replacement therapy (includes alternative therapies)
    d. Sexuality
    e. Sexual abuse/sexual assault

D. Assessment and management of deviations from normal; indications for consultation, co-management or referral

1. Amenorrhea
2. Dysmenorrhea
3. Dysfunctional uterine bleeding
4. Uterine fibroids

5. Polycystic ovary syndrome
6. Breast problems, breast cancer
7. Adnexal masses
8. Vulvar variations
9. Pelvic relaxation
10. Urinary incontinence
11. Endometriosis
12. Sexually transmitted diseases
13. Ovarian cancer
14. Cervical cancer
15. Adenomyosis

A. Physiology/Pathophysiology

1. Menstruation, interconceptional period

a. Regulation of menstrual cycle

1) Feedback loops are primarily positive in follicular phase and negative in luteal phase (but not exclusively)

2) Neuroendocrine control

a) Hypothalamus

b) Tonic and cyclic centers for gonadotropic releasing hormone (GnRH)

3) Pituitary: follicle stimulating hormone (FSH) and luteinizing hormone (LH)

4) Ovary: Estrogen (estradiol, estrone)

a) Corpus luteum: Progesterone

5) *Preovulatory*

a) Hypothalamus →GnRH→FSH and LH →follicular development

b) FSH and LH stimulate follicle maturation and ovulation

c) Production rate depends upon time in the menstrual cycle

d) Blood levels

	Estradiol	Estrone
Early Follicular	63	52
Late Follicular	235	170

6) *Ovulatory*

a) Estrogen levels increase

b) Eventually stimulate hypothalamus→FSH and LH surge →follicular development

c) Estrogen surge approximately 12 hours before LH surge

7) *Postovulatory*

a) Corpus luteum→through progesterone and estrogen inhibit pituitary (and pituitary gonadotropins) but FSH and LH continue to stimulate corpus luteum

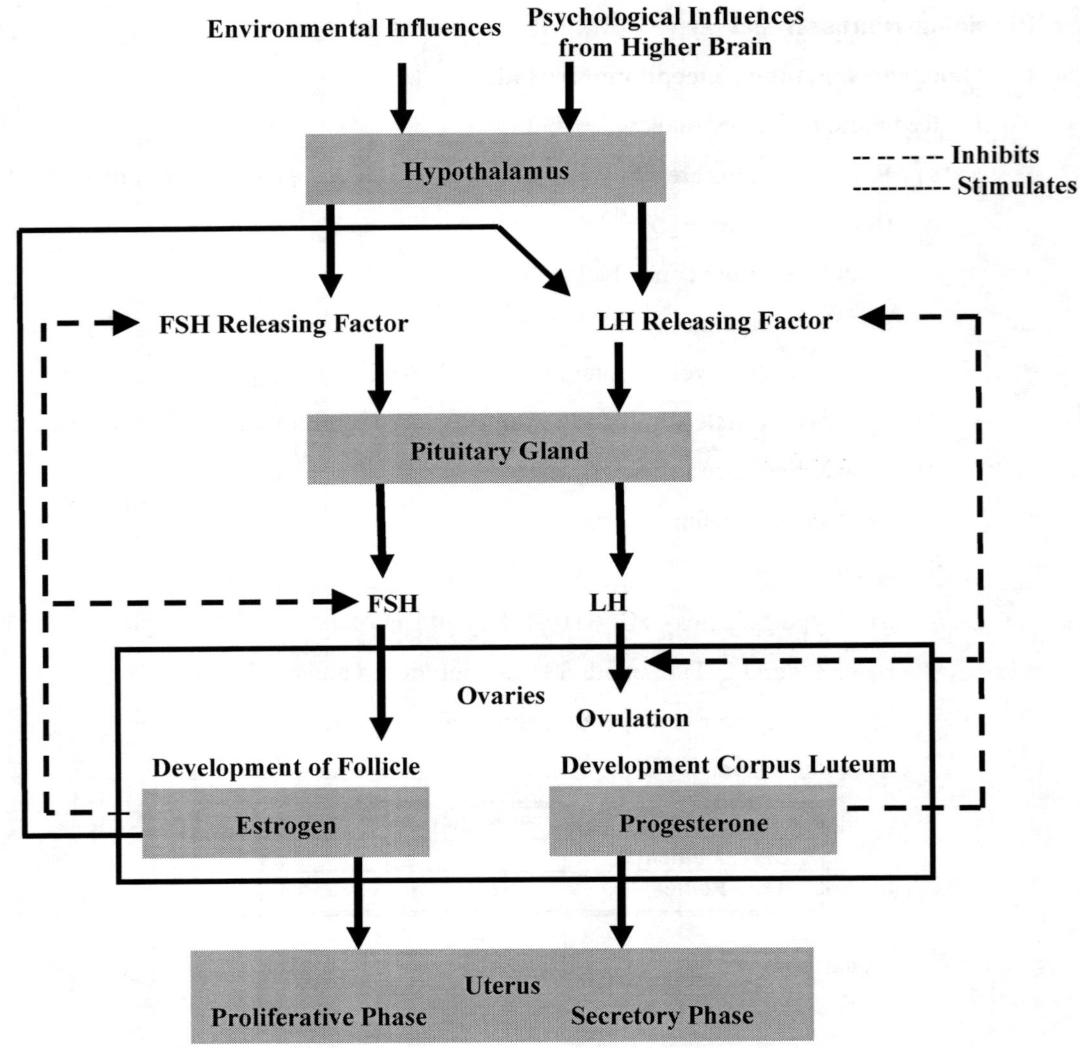

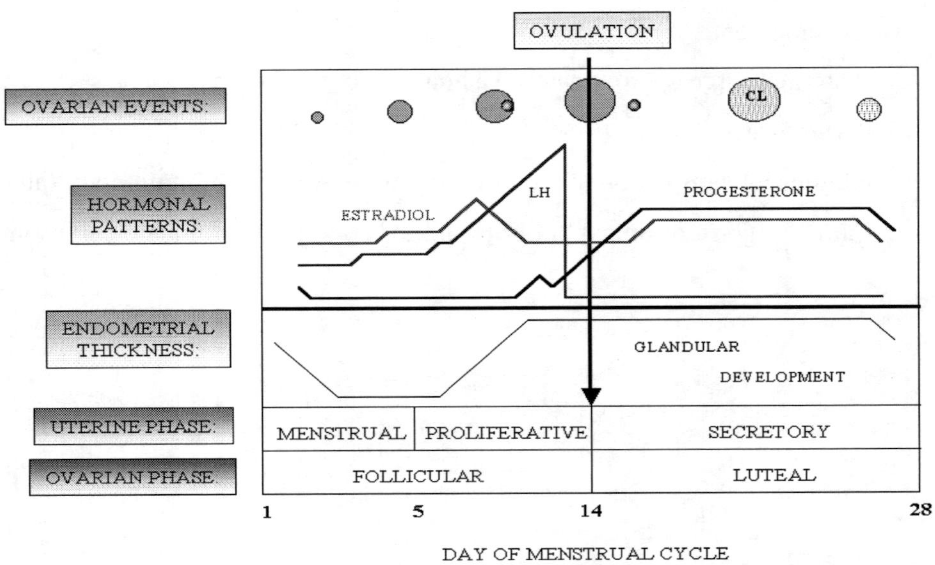

Women's Health Nursing Toward Evidence Based Practice; Breslin, Eileen T., Lucas, Vickie A.

Menstruation is the physiological phenomena of the uterus shedding its lining, approximately at monthly intervals from menarche to menopause.

- Traditionally, the first day of menstrual flow is the first day of the menstrual cycle.
- The normal phases of the menstrual cycle are defined by the endometrial and ovarian patterns of change.

The endometrium undergoes 3 distinct phases during the menstrual cycle.

- The 1st phase is the menstrual phase and corresponds with the 1st 5 days of the cycle.
- 2nd is the proliferative phase (days 6-14)
- 3rd is the secretory phase (days 15-28 or the last 14 days of the cycle)

The ovaries have 2 corresponding phases.

- **The follicular** phase starts on day 1 of the menstrual cycle and continues until ovulation or day 14 in a 28 day cycle.
  - Follicular phase is not as consistent in length as the luteal phase.
- **The luteal phase** (day 15 or post ovulation through day 28 or the last day of the cycle) follows the follicular phase and corresponds with the secretory phase of the endometrium.
  - The time interval in the LUTEAL Phase is 14 days (+/-2) and is based on the life of the corpus luteum.

KEY POINTS ON MENSTRUAL PHYSIOLOGY

(adapted from Hatcher RA, Zieman M et al. *A Pocket Guide to Managing Contraception.* Tiger, Georgia: Bridging the Gap Foundation, 2004.)

- Each woman is born with 1-2 million follicles, most of which undergo atresia before puberty.
  - About 10-20 follicles each month are recruited by rising FSH levels.
  - Recruitment occurs during the late luteal phase of the preceding cycle.
  - Of those 10-20 follicles, usually only one dominant follicle ovulates.
  - The number of follicles stimulated each month depends on the number of follicles left in the residual pool.
- FSH levels are low before ovulation as a result of negative feedback of estradiol (E2) and inhibin B.
  - The dominant follicle "escapes" the effects of falling FSH levels before ovulation because it has more granulosa cells, more FSH receptors on its granulosa cells, and increased blood flow.
  - Cut off from adequate FSH stimulation, the other nondominant follicles undergo atresia.
- When E2 production is sustained at sufficient levels (about 200 pg/mL) for more than 50 hours, negative feedback of E2 on LH reverses to positive feedback.
  - The ***LH surge*** occurs
  - About 12 hours later an oocyte is extruded (ovulation).

- About 50,000 granulosa cells form the ***corpus luteum.***
  - Some granulosa cells continue to produce E2 and inhibins but many join the outer layers of theca cells to produce progesterone (P).
  - Inhibin selectively suppresses FSH, not LH. The highest levels of inhibin are during the mid-luteal phase (primarily inhibin A), causing FSH levels to be the lowest in the mid-luteal phase.
  - At the end of the cycle (10-14 days after ovulation) if the corpus luteum is not rescued by HCG produced by the implanted trophoblast (i.e. pregnancy), the corpus luteum will undergo programmed atresia. ***Falling E2, P, and inhibin levels induce the release of FSH to initiate another cycle.***
- ***Atrophy of the corpus luteum on or about day 25 of a typical 28 day cycle initiates menses (and the next cycle)***
  - This atrophy is initiated by a decline in LH release from the anterior pituitary gland and results in a fall in serum estrogen and progesterone levels.
  - Without hormonal support, the endometrium sloughs. This drop in hormone levels is also detected by the hypothalamus and pituitary, and FSH levels increase to stimulate follicles for the next cycle
- ***Anovulation in women NOT on birth control pills leads to prolonged cycles, oligomenorrhea, amenorrhea or irregular bleeding.***
  - The absence of progesterone in anovulatory women *not* on pills places these women at risk for endometrial hyperplasia and cancer.
  - Return of ovulation has been demonstrated in women treated with cognitive behavioral therapy for coping with stress and hypnotherapy.
- ***The two-cell, two gonadotrophin theory***
  - At the very beginning of the cycle, the outer follicular theca cells can only be stimulated by LH and produce androgens (testosterone and androstenedione); the inner granulosa cells can only be stimulated by FSH.
  - Androgens diffuse toward the inner layer *granulosa* cells where they are converted into estradiol (E2) by FSH-stimulated aromatase
- ***The role of androgens***
  - In a developing follicle, ***low androgen levels*** serve as substrate for FSH induced aromatization and stimulate aromatase activity.
  - ***High levels of androgens*** (an "androgen-rich" environment as in some women with polycystic ovaries) lead to inhibition of aromatase activity and to follicular atresia.

2. Peri-and postmenopausal period

> Remember, the **estrogen of reproductive years is estradiol**. It is about 10 times more potent than estrone, the estrogen of perimenopause/menopause)

a. Estrogen--estrone
   1) No rhythmic production
   2) Can lead to persistent proliferative endometrium, anovulation, and unpredictable periods of unopposed estrogen
   3) Fibroids, endometrial hyperplasia

b. Progesterone
   1) Premenopausal—primarily from corpus luteum
   2) Postmenopausal--probably ovaries and adrenals, not yet well studied
   3) Essentially at same level as in early follicular phase (much lower in oophorectomized woman)

c. Androgens
   1) Relationship to estrogen changed, even if mean amount doesn't change
   2) Essentially at same level as in early follicular phase (much lower if oophorectomized woman)
   3) Some suggestion that androgen decrease may be due to aging itself, not hormonal changes
   4) No major decrease in testosterone until several years post menopause

d. Estrogen withdrawal and follicular exhaustion

> **Midwifery Message**
> Most oocytes are lost by atresia, not ovulation

   1) Unknown reasons for aging
   2) Aging is different than estrogen decrease
      a) Yolk sac has primordial germ cells which undergo mitosis
      b) Eventually become oogonia, then oocytes
         Fetal ovaries -- 7 million oocytes at 20 weeks GA
         Birth -- 2 million oocytes
         Puberty -- 200,000 oocytes
      c) Loss by ovulation (about 500) and all the rest by atresia
      d) What causes atresia?
         (1) Unknown
         (2) Increased by androgens, radiation, chemotherapy, surgical impairment of ovarian blood supply and smoking (some evidence that smoking most clinically significant factor)

3) **Approximately one decade <u>before</u> menopause, there is a gradual increase in production of LH and FSH**
   a) Usually a blood level of >50 MIU of FSH signals ovarian compromise
   b) After menopause FSH and LH are higher; (FSH 10 times and LH 3 times) for several decades
   c) Then they drop, although never back to premenopausal levels
   d) In late menopause, estradiol is low, Inhibin A is low, Inhibin B is low and FSH is high
4) Testosterone
   a) Mean concentration is minimally lower than premenopausal
   b) Therefore, increased testosterone production in ovary--especially androstenedione
      (1) Primary ovarian androgen for reproductive woman
      (2) If no follicular activity then decrease production to about 20% premenopausal
5) Adrenal cortex
   a) Estrone from peripheral aromatization of androstenedione
   b) Estrone also found in fat, muscle, liver, bone marrow, brain, fibroblasts, hair roots

e. Post menopause

1) E_2 and E_1 are low and $E_2 < E_1$
2) E_{1S} (Estrone sulfate) is a stabilizing reservoir of estrogen and drops from premenopausal of more than 1000 pg/ml to a mean of 350 pg/ml postmenopausal

f. Role of cholesterol and lipids

1) Serum lipoproteins
2) HDL (accelerate lecithin/cholesterol acetyltransferase activity; Promotes transfer from tissue to plasma to transport to liver for breakdown)
3) IDL, LDL, VLDL--without estrogen all changes for the worse

> **TIP:**
> **LDL as "Loser"** cholesterol and
> **HDL as "Hero"** cholesterol

B. Family planning

Overview of Family Planning

Family planning methods enable women and families to

- Have access to the information about reproduction
- Determine the number of children they want and when they want them;
- Help women have an equal voice in decisions that affect their lives;
- Promote personal health by planning their family and potentially availing themselves of noncontraceptive health benefits of some methods

A family planning method must be personally acceptable to the woman/couple, available and appropriate based on her health

Although there are a number of methods currently in the United States, not all are

- Appropriate for specific women
- Accessible to women, either due to lack of availability or cost
- Acceptable to all women for various reasons including personal choices

Approximate method failure rates, from lowest theoretical failure rate to highest
(Differs among sources)

Method	Lowest Expected Failure Rate (theoretical)	Failure Rate in Typical Users (actual)
Transdermal (few studies)	.01	0.6-1.0
Norplant	0.09	0.09
Combination Pill	0.1	3
Vasectomy	0.1	0.15
Estrogen/Progesterone Injection (Lunelle)	0.1-1.0	0.1-1.0
IUD (general)	0.1-0.5	0.1-2.0
Ring	0.2	0.2-2.0
Progesterone only injection (Depo-Provera)	0.3	0.3
Tubal ligation	0.4	0.4
Progesterone only pill	0.5	3
Fertility Awareness (BBT, calendar, cervical mucus)	1-9	20
Condom: Male	2	12
Withdrawal	4	19
Condom: Female	5	21
Diaphragm	6	18
Spermicides	6	21
Sponge (lowest rates in nulliparas)	6-9	18-28
Cervical Cap (lowest rates in nullipara)	9	18
Chance	85	85

1. **Collection of a database for the provision of contraceptive options**

   The following are some of the issues that a midwife should explore with a woman or family regarding contraception

   - *When (if ever) does she want to have a baby?* Reversibility
   - *Medical/Health Issues:* contraindications, health benefits.
   - *Efficacy.* "Typical" versus "perfect" usage, and individual tolerance for failure.
   - *How critical is efficacy?* Is avoidance of pregnancy critical to her health?
   - *Is she willing to consider emergency contraception or abortion for contraceptive failure?*
   - *Need for STD protection.*
   - *Cost.* Consider long term cost, and no cost of abstinence or withdrawal.

- *Side effects*. Latex allergies, nausea, mid-cycle "spotting".
- *Knowledge of all options.*
- *Method used by friends/family/popularity.*
- *Cultural implications.*
- *Long range effects.*
- *Convenience.*
- *Frequency of intercourse.* Hormonal methods or IUDs are often preferred if intercourse is frequent; if intercourse is infrequent, diaphragm or cervical caps may be appropriate.
- *Religious/Personal beliefs*. Woman and partner(s).
- *Availability*
- *Aesthetics/Personal needs.*
- *Comfort/Pleasure/Fun/Spontaneity*
- *Gender Bias*
- *General track record* of the method and the woman.

a. Screening for contraindications

This table summarizes World Health Organization (WHO) medical eligibility criteria for starting contraceptives.

WHO categories for temporary methods:

WHO 1 Can use the method. No restriction on use.

WHO 2 Can use the method. Advantages generally outweigh theoretical or proven risks. If the method is chosen, more than usual follow up may be needed.

WHO 3 Should not use the method unless clinician makes clinical judgment that the patient can safely use it. Theoretical or proven risks usually outweigh the advantages of method. Method of last choice, for which regular monitoring may be needed.

WHO 4 Should not use the method. Condition represents an unacceptable health risk if method is used.

Simplified 2-category system for clinical decisions regarding temporary methods.

WHO Category	*With Clinical Judgment*	With Limited Clinical Judgment
1	Use the method in any circumstances	Use the method
2	Generally use the method	
3	Use of the method not usually recommended unless other, more appropriate methods are not available or acceptable	Do not use the method
4	Method not to be used	

Note: Category 3 and 4 conditions are shaded to indicate the method should not be provided where clinical judgment is limited. In the United States experienced surgeons and general anesthesia are generally available.

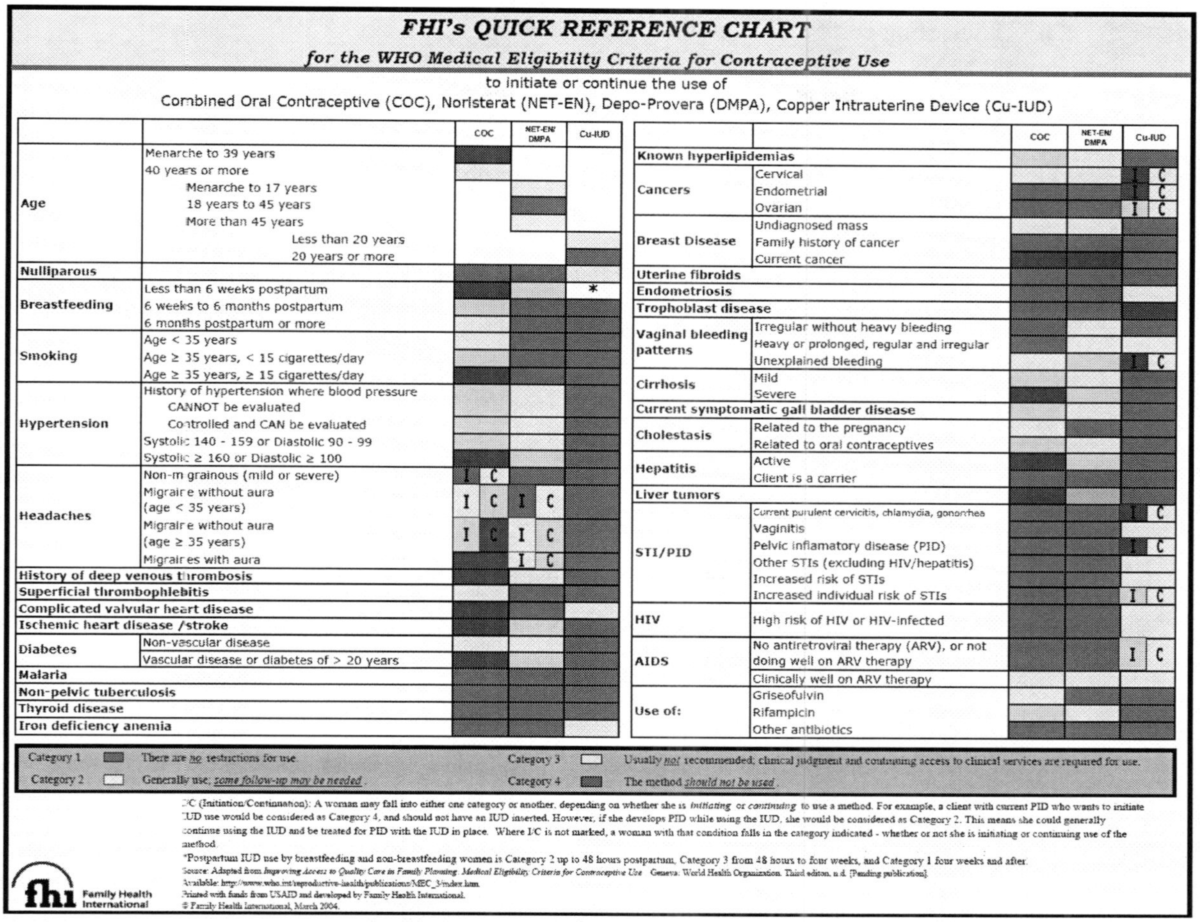

FHI's QUICK REFERENCE CHART
for the WHO Medical Eligibility Criteria for Contraceptive Use
to initiate or continue the use of
Combined Oral Contraceptive (COC), Noristerat (NET-EN), Depo-Provera (DMPA), Copper Intrauterine Device (Cu-IUD)
COC
NET-EN/ DMPA
Cu-IUD
Age
Menarche to 39 years
40 years or more
Menarche to 17 years
18 years to 45 years
More than 45 years
Less than 20 years
20 years or more
Nulliparous
Breastfeeding
Less than 6 weeks postpartum
6 weeks to 6 months postpartum
6 months postpartum or more
Smoking
Age < 35 years
Age ≥ 35 years, < 15 cigarettes/day
Age ≥ 35 years, ≥ 15 cigarettes/day
Hypertension
History of hypertension where blood pressure CANNOT be evaluated
Controlled and CAN be evaluated
Systolic 140 - 159 or Diastolic 90 - 99
Systolic ≥ 160 or Diastolic ≥ 100
Headaches
Non-migrainous (mild or severe)
Migraine without aura (age < 35 years)
Migraine without aura (age ≥ 35 years)
Migraines with aura
History of deep venous thrombosis
Superficial thrombophlebitis
Complicated valvular heart disease
Ischemic heart disease /stroke
Diabetes
Non-vascular disease
Vascular disease or diabetes of > 20 years
Malaria
Non-pelvic tuberculosis
Thyroid disease
Iron deficiency anemia
Known hyperlipidemias
Cancers
Cervical
Endometrial
Ovarian
Breast Disease
Undiagnosed mass
Family history of cancer
Current cancer
Uterine fibroids
Endometriosis
Trophoblast disease
Vaginal bleeding patterns
Irregular without heavy bleeding
Heavy or prolonged, regular and irregular
Unexplained bleeding
Cirrhosis
Mild
Severe
Current symptomatic gall bladder disease
Cholestasis
Related to the pregnancy
Related to oral contraceptives
Hepatitis
Active
Client is a carrier
Liver tumors
STI/PID
Current purulent cervicitis, chlamydia, gonorrhea
Vaginitis
Pelvic inflamatory disease (PID)
Other STIs (excluding HIV/hepatitis)
Increased risk of STIs
Increased individual risk of STIs
HIV
High risk of HIV or HIV-infected
AIDS
No antiretroviral therapy (ARV), or not doing well on ARV therapy
Clinically well on ARV therapy
Use of:
Griseofulvin
Rifampicin
Other antibiotics
Category 1 There are no restrictions for use.
Category 2 Generally use; some follow-up may be needed.
Category 3 Usually not recommended; clinical judgment and continuing access to clinical services are required for use.
Category 4 The method should not be used.
I/C (Initiation/Continuation): A woman may fall into either one category or another, depending on whether she is initiating or continuing to use a method. For example, a client with current PID who wants to initiate IUD use would be considered as Category 4, and should not have an IUD inserted. However, if she develops PID while using the IUD, she would be considered as Category 2. This means she could generally continue using the IUD and be treated for PID with the IUD in place. Where I/C is not marked, a woman with that condition falls in the category indicated - whether or not she is initiating or continuing use of the method.
*Postpartum IUD use by breastfeeding and non-breastfeeding women is Category 2 up to 48 hours postpartum, Category 3 from 48 hours to four weeks, and Category 1 four weeks and after.
Source: Adapted from Improving Access to Quality Care in Family Planning: Medical Eligibility Criteria for Contraceptive Use. Geneva: World Health Organization. Third editon, n.d. [Pending publication].
Available: http://www.who.int/reproductive-health/publications/MEC_3/index.htm.
Printed with funds from USAID and developed by Family Health International.
© Family Health International, March 2004.
fhi Family Health International

Source: http://w3.whosea.org/LinkFiles/Publications_English_MEC.pdf

b. Teaching and counseling concerning available methods

1) Counseling is an integral part of family planning. The goals of counseling are to help a woman

a) Make an informed choice among options,

b) Select a satisfactory contraceptive method for her and her partner

c) Use the method safely and effectively.

Keys to good counseling

A good counselor:

- Understands and respects the woman's rights, including the right to decide whether or not to practice family planning, the right to privacy and confidentiality and the right to refuse any type of treatment
- Earns the woman's trust
- Understands the benefits and limitations of all contraceptive methods
- Understands the cultural and emotional factors that affect a woman's (or a couple's) decision to use a particular contraceptive method
- Encourages the woman to ask questions
- Uses a nonjudgmental approach which shows the woman respect and kindness
- Presents information in an unbiased, woman-sensitive manner
- Actively listens to the woman's concerns, recognizing verbal and nonverbal communication

Adapted from Pocket Guide for Family Planning Service Providers, 1998

2) Counseling can be divided into three phases

a) Initial counseling at reception (all methods are described)

b) Method-specific counseling prior to and immediately following (the client is given instructions on how to use the method and common side effects are discussed)

c) Follow-up counseling (during the return visit, use of the method, satisfaction and any problems that may have occurred are discussed).

d) Counseling should be part of every visit/interaction.

3) Components of informed consent

a) Both information and consent

(1) Name of method and details of mechanism of action.

(2) Description of reasonably foreseeable risks or discomforts.

(3) Description of the anticipated benefits.

(4) Disclosure of appropriate alternative methods

(5) Risk of pregnancy and foreseeable risks should she be or become pregnant.

(6) Special instructions regarding food, drink, or lifestyles (e.g., COCs do not protect from HIV)

2. Provision of contraceptive methods and devices

a. Natural family planning; fertility awareness methods (FAM)

1) Typical Failure Rate: 1-15%

2) All FAMs rely on abstinence during infertile phase of the menstrual cycle

a) Infertile phase begins 24 hours following ovulation and ends several days before ovulation

b) **Fertile** days are several days preceding ovulation to 24 hours following ovulation

c) The woman identifies her fertile and infertile phases using one or several methods to determine when she ovulates

d) The most effective FAM involves using several parameters; success rate is further enhanced if the couple confines intercourse to the post ovulatory infertile period only

e) FAMs may assist women desiring conception in addition to those desiring to avoid pregnancy.

3) Calendar method (rhythm method)

a) Keep menstrual diary for 6-12 cycles

b) Assume sperm survival for 2-3 days (may be longer) and ovulation 14 days prior to menses

c) Earliest fertile day is the shortest cycle length minus 18

d) **Latest fertile day is longest cycle minus 11**

e) The woman abstains from sexual intercourse during the fertile days, e.g., if a woman's cycles are consistently 28 days, she would be abstinent from day 10 through day 17. If her cycles range from 25-30 days, she would be abstinent from day 7 through day 19.

4) **Standard days method** using color-coded beads

a) If MOST cycles are between 26 and 32 days long, the woman abstains during days 8-19; beads are white on CycleBead necklace.

b) Further information at www.cyclebeads.com

5) **Cervical mucus** ovulation detection method

a) Woman manually checks quantity and character of cervical mucus daily for several months to learn her pattern

b) Mucus types

- Post menstrual: Scant or undetectable
- Pre ovulation: Cloudy, yellow or white, sticky
- Ovulation: Clear, wet, stretchy (spinnbarkheit), slippery
- Post ovulation (fertile): Thick, cloudy, sticky
- Post ovulation (infertile): Scant or undetectable

c) Semen and vaginal secretions from intercourse may interfere with results for 24 hours (may be important in pre ovulatory period)

d) Abstinence (or contraception) begins as soon as there is noticeable mucus

e) Intercourse resumes without restriction 4 days after ovulation mucus (wet, stretchy, slippery)

6) **Basal body temperature** (BBT) method

a) BBT may drop just prior to ovulation and rises 0.4-0.8° F with ovulation

b) Fertile period is the day of first temperature drop or first elevation through 3 consecutive days of elevated temperature.

c) **Abstinence begins on first day of menses and continues through 3 consecutive days of temperature rise**

d) Woman records her temperature every morning before arising with a basal body thermometer. Prior to ovulation, the temperature is likely 97.2° - 97.4°F.

e) When the temperature remains elevated for at least three days, a woman may assume she has ovulated.

7) **Symptothermal method: *MOST EFFECTIVE Fertility Awareness Method***

a) Combines at least 2 of the FAMs – usually cervical mucus and BBT

b) Other symptoms of ovulation observed are mittelschmerz, libido changes, and changes in the cervix itself, e.g., position, texture, and dilation

(1) Just before and during ovulation the cervix is soft, moist, and open.

(2) Post ovulation, the cervix drops and is firm and closed.

8) **"TwoDay" method** is described in Hatcher, 2004
   a) New; variation of cervical mucus method
   b) Woman monitors presence or absence of cervical secretions
   c) "Secretion" is anything from the vagina except menstrual bleeding
   d) The woman asks herself 2 questions: (1) Did I note secretions today? and (2)Did I note secretions yesterday?
   e) If the answer to EITHER question is yes, she abstains if attempting to avoid pregnancy. If the answer to BOTH is no, she may consider herself infertile.

9) **Limiting intercourse to post-ovulatory periods is the most effective variation of FAMs, with a failure rate of only 1% among perfect users.**

10) **Lactational Amenorrhea Method (LAM)**
   a) Typical failure rate: 2% in first 6 months PP; Perfect use failure rate 0.5%.
   b) Breastfeeding prevents more pregnancies in the world than all other methods of birth control combined.
   c) It can be used as long as a woman nurses her baby frequently and is amenorrheic.
   d) Woman must nurse ten or more times throughout the day and introduce no other foods into her baby's diet. **Because food is usually introduced at about six months, LAM as birth control is not recommended beyond that time. Nor is it recommended when the baby begins sleeping through the night.**
   e) Menstruation will usually not occur for several months postpartum, perhaps 4 to 24 months after delivery (non-lactating women can ovulate as early as 3-8 weeks PP).
   f) Prolactin stimulates lactation and interrupts release of gonadotropins
   g) LAM may be effective for as long as three years in some. **Hatcher recommends use of LAM alone only for the first 6 months PP.**
   h) Many breastfeeding women do not ovulate until after the first period, but ***the longer LAM is used, the more likely it is that ovulation will precede the first menses.***
   i) Cervical mucus changes will herald the first ovulation; a woman should start checking daily at six weeks postpartum.

> **Midwifery Message**
> Do not ignore the fact that LAM can be an effective contraceptive method. It often is not considered in mainstream America. Approximately half of women leave the hospital not breastfeeding and among those that do, the majority supplement which significantly decreases the efficacy of the method. But it is not the fault of the method.

11) **Electronic monitors to augment natural family planning**

a) Marketed under the name *Persona;* fertile days are indicated with a red light and infertile days with a green light. If the light is yellow, the woman takes a urine test that changes the light to green or red, based on hormonal amount.

b) Clinical trials are now being conducted to obtain FDA approval, but such devices are currently not on the market in the US.

c) One advantage of this method is that charting body signs is not necessary. Disadvantages include the expense of the computer and the need to purchase urine test sticks for use eight days out of each cycle. Additionally, this method is currently only being recommended for women whose cycles are between 23 and 35 days). Other models measure and store basal temperature readings: *LadyComp* and *BioSelf*. The *LadyComp* device can be used by women with longer or irregular cycles, such as those experienced postpartally.

12) **Other– Coitus interruptus (withdrawal)**

a) Typical Failure Rate: 27% first year

b) Mechanism of action: Taking the penis out of the vagina before ejaculation, thereby preventing deposition of sperm in the female genital tract.

c) Advantages: It requires no devices, involves no chemicals, and is available in any situation at no cost, there are no health risks and no complications (except high failure rate). May be surprisingly effective for individual couples, and withdrawal is definitely **better than no contraception**.

d) Disadvantages: The man may not withdraw in enough time to prevent semen from escaping into the vagina, especially if ejaculation is premature or unpredictable. Requires high commitment, self control, communication, dedication. May interfere with quality of sexual experience. No protection against STD.

e) Offer emergency contraception.

f) With repeated orgasm, there may be sperm in pre-ejaculatory fluid.

13) **NFP method problems and complications**

a) There are no complications associated directly with the methods

b) Careful instruction is important

c) No protection from STDs

d) Provide emergency contraception if acceptable

Cervical, Cervical Mucus and BBT Changes During the Fertility Cycle

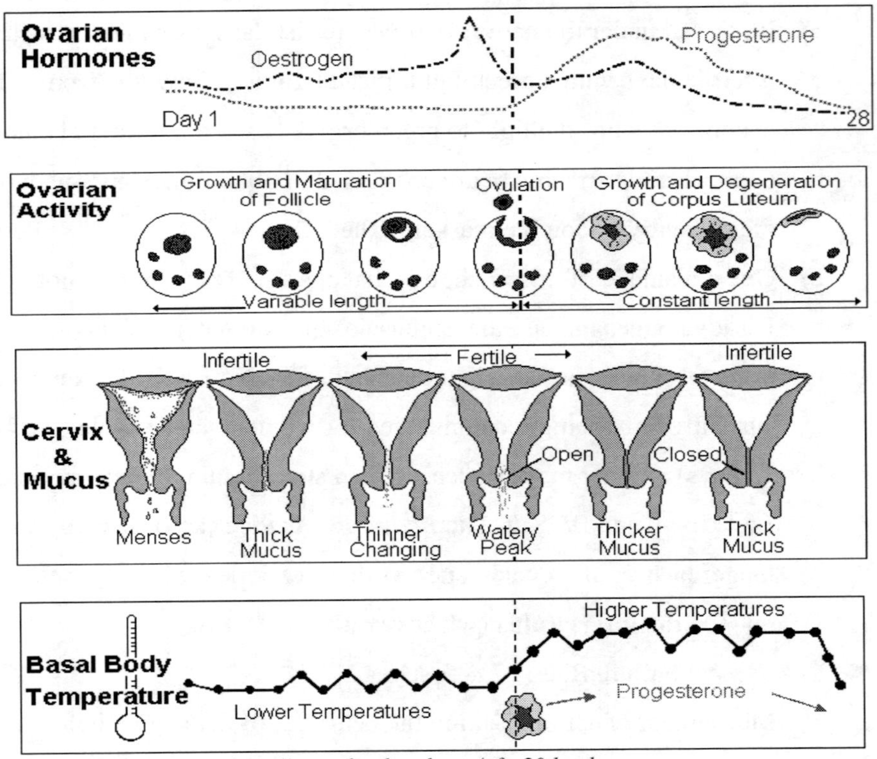

Source of illustration: *http://www.fertilityuk.org/nfps20.html*

b. Barrier methods (e.g. condoms, diaphragm)

1) Barrier methods for women

a) Diaphragm and cervical cap used with spermicide, and contraceptive sponge provide a physical barrier to semen and immobilize sperm before they enter the uterus and fertilize an egg.

b) After intercourse, diaphragm must be left in place for six hours.

c) May provide some protection from STDs (note use of spermicide without barrier increases risk of HIV transmission)

d) The reliability of these methods varies widely, even among perfect users.

e) For intercourse more than three times weekly, may be less effective. Infrequent intercourse or low fertility (e.g., older) -- more reliable.

f) Higher risk of vaginal infection, urinary tract infection, and possibly toxic shock syndrome.

g) Neither cap nor sponge should be used during menstruation.

h) Should not use with oils-based lubricants or vaginal creams

2) Diaphragm

For multiple acts of intercourse, do not remove the diaphragm to place more spermicide on it.

a) Typical Failure Rate: 16% first year

b) Soft rubber or latex cup fitted for size by provider. Spermicide is applied to the diaphragm, which is inserted into the vagina; it covers the cervix and is held securely in place behind the pubic bone and posterior vaginal wall.

c) Insert just prior to intercourse or up to 6 hours before.

d) If intercourse is repeated, contraceptive cream or jelly should be applied each time, inserted with applicator while the diaphragm is still in place. **The diaphragm should not be removed.**

e) Leave in place for >6 hours post intercourse, but no more than 24 hours.

g) Each time the diaphragm is used it should be checked for holes or tears

h) **Replace every two years**. Keep dry and clean and in a dark place.

i) Sizing should be checked after a pregnancy and after a gain or loss of more than ten pounds.

j) Many failures result from failure to actually use the diaphragm correctly.

k) The woman returns 1 week after fitting with the diaphragm in situ for the midwife to check fit.

l) Complications: increases risk for UTI; may increase risk of toxic shock syndrome; large poorly fitted diaphragm may cause erosion of tissue; allergic reaction to latex.

S&S of Toxic Shock
- Sudden onset of fever > 102
- Sunburn – like rash esp. on palms and soles of feet
- H/A
- Sore throat
- Nausea & vomiting
- Watery diarrhea

m) **Types of diaphragms**

- The **arcing spring** is most commonly used.
  Can be used by women with good pelvic tone or mild cystocele/rectocele.
- **Coil spring** is for women with average tone
- **Wide seal rims** to contain spermicide

3) Diaphragm problems and complications

a) Risk of latex or spermicide allergy as above: discontinue use.

(1) Avoid nonoxynol 9 if at risk of STD

b) Increased risk of UTI

(1) Instruct woman to void after intercourse

(2) Ensure proper fit to avoid urethral compression

4) **Cervical cap**

a) Typical failure rate in first year 16% nulliparous woman; 32% multiparous

b) The cap, held in place by suction, is partially filled with contraceptive jelly or cream and then inserted so that it covers the cervix. If intercourse is repeated, it is not necessary to reapply spermicide, but the woman should check to make certain that the cap is still in place.

c) The cervical cap is as effective as a diaphragm in nullipara; ***higher failure rates apply to multiparous women.***

d) UTIs may increase for some brands; cervical erosion may occur; toxic shock syndrome is theoretical risk if left in too long; allergic reaction may be life threatening.

e) Should be inserted >30 minutes prior to intercourse

f) Should be left in for >6 hours after final intercourse

g) May be left in place for up to 48 hours.

5) **Spermicides for use with barrier methods**

a) Failure rates zero to 50% for typical users with average approximately 21%

b) Spermicides prevent pregnancy by killing sperm.

c) Must be used every time intercourse occurs and before the penis is placed anywhere near the vagina.

d) May cause allergy and irritation; because of this, they have been associated with higher rates of STD transmission (especially among women who had very frequent intercourse). It should NOT be used as a lubricant for anal intercourse.

e) An advantage is that spermicides may be purchased without a prescription and are relatively inexpensive.

f) Spermicides increase the risk of urinary tract infections in some women.

g) Nonoxynol-9 was once thought to help prevent HIV infection, but newer studies show an ***increased risk*** because the chemical irritates the vagina, facilitating infection.

h) The more nonoxynol-9 in a gel, the more contraceptive protection

> **Myth—**
> Contrary to some popular thought, spermicides are not linked to teratogenic effects should they fail and pregnancy occur

i) Contraceptive films, (thin spermicidal squares), are placed over the cervix before intercourse. They are less messy than creams, jellies, or foams; film dissolves completely in the vagina.

j) Suppositories, small waxy spermicidal inserts, are inserted by hand or with an applicator.

6) **Spermicide problems and complications**
   a) Instruct woman carefully so there is no confusion with edible fruit jelly and contraceptive gel; instruct that cosmetics containing octoxynols and other nonoxynols (4, 10, 12, 14) are not substitutes for nonoxynol 9.
   b) Risk of allergy: discontinue use
   c) Risk of STD transmission with nonoxynol 9 is higher than without
7) **Condoms**
   a) Several types are available; most are made of latex rubber, but some are made from polyurethane or animal tissue (e.g., "natural skin").
   b) May be lubricated, ribbed, or treated with spermicide, and may be purchased without a prescription.
   c) Main advantage is that ***latex condoms can provide protection from both pregnancy and STDs***. Polyurethane condoms are not as effective in protecting against STD's.
   d) Latex condoms can only be used with water-based lubricants but polyurethane may be used with oil – based lubricants.
   e) Male condoms
      (1) Typical Failure Rate: 12%
      (2) Thin shield worn on the penis.
      (3) Traps ejaculated semen.
      (4) Must be put on while the man has an erection but before intercourse.
      (5) After ejaculation, he should withdraw immediately to prevent leakage.
      (6) To decrease the risk of breaking, store them in a cool, dry place; ***oil-based lubricants (such as Vaseline or baby oil) should not be used with latex condoms*** as they weaken the rubber.
      (7) Increased risk of urinary tract infections in women (especially if they contain spermicide). Spermicidal condoms have not been shown to be more effective than condoms without spermicide, and they can worsen the allergenic properties of the latex.
      (8) For sensitive individuals, non-spermicidal polyurethane or natural skin condoms may be preferable. ***Natural skin condoms are expensive and do not protect against STD;*** polyurethane condoms are more likely to break but can be used with oil-based lubricants.

(9) Most men report reduced sensitivity during intercourse; some men cannot maintain an erection when one is used; may affect the spontaneity of intercourse. For men with premature ejaculation, use of the condom may prolong erection.

(10)A new condom must be worn if intercourse is repeated.

(11)Don't use two condoms at once, latex rubbing may cause tearing.

8) **Condom problems and complications**

a) **Risk of latex allergy** (not female condoms or male condoms that are made from polyurethane), which is potentially life threatening. 2-3% Americans are latex allergic. Also risk of allergy to spermicide if used with condom.

(1) Discontinue use of latex products; switch to polyurethane condom

(2) Discontinue use of spermicide

(3) Avoid use of nonoxynol 9 if at risk of STD

b) **Retained condom in vagina poses risk of infection and pregnancy**

(1) Patient and/or partner should try to remove as soon as possible or

(2) Removal by clinician as soon as possible

(3) Use emergency contraception (EC) as soon as possible, within 72 hours after sexual intercourse, but can be taken up to 96 –120 hours (ideally should have on hand)

9) **Female condoms**

a) Typical Failure Rate 21%

b) Thin polyurethane sheath with two soft rings at each end. One ring, covered with the polyurethane, fits over the cervix, acting as an anchor. The larger, open ring stays outside the vagina, covering part of the perineum and labia during intercourse.

c) No prescription. (one brand is *Reality Female Condom*)

d) Will not deteriorate when used with oil-based lubricants (because it is not latex). It can be inserted up to eight hours before intercourse but should be removed immediately after. Some women find the outer ring causes discomfort during use.

e) Can have increased effectiveness in protecting against HPV and genital herpes as the female condom covers a larger surface area.

f) Male and female condoms should not be used at the same time.

10) **Female condom problems and complications**

a) May pose increased risk of vaginal infection and UTI

b) Difficulty with insertion: offer clinician instruction

c) Condom dislodged or penis inserted outside it: insert new condom; use EC if semen spillage; evaluate for STD if indicated

11) Contraceptive Sponge (*Today*®)

a) Average Failure: 18-28%

b) Small, disposable sponge containing nonoxynol 9; available without prescription.

c) The sponge should be moistened with water (not saliva) just before inserting, then placed over the cervix. Once in place, it provides protection for twenty-four hours, no matter how often the woman has intercourse.

d) The sponge is about as effective as a diaphragm, but, like the cap, it is less effective for multiparous women.

e) In addition to toxic shock syndrome, women who use the sponge may be at higher risk of vaginal yeast infections.

f) The sponge was removed from the US market in 1995 due to manufacturing problems which were resulting in contamination of the product. It is now available again in the United States.

c. Oral contraceptives (OC or OCP)

1) Typical failure rate is 3%, theoretically more for progestin only pills (POP) than combined oral contraceptives (COC) but similar in studies

2) Mechanism of action

a) Prevents LH surge, thus preventing ovulation. (High levels of estrogen and progestin suppress GnRH, FSH, and LH secretion through negative feedback on the hypothalamus and pituitary. Note that the progestin is the active hormone, although estrogen also participates.)

> **Midwife Message**
> Estrogen is included for cycle control and progesterone for suppression of ovulation and other changes that reduce likelihood of conception

b) Suppress FSH rise early in the cycle, **preventing follicle development**.

c) **Thickens cervical mucus,** making it impenetrable to sperm.

d) Makes the **endometrium hostile** to implantation.

e) **Decreases fallopian tube motility** / function.

f) No increase in libido at mid cycle.

3) Formulations of oral contraceptives

a) A wide variety of oral contraceptive formulations exists with little research comparing one pill to another

b) The "active ingredient" in oral contraceptives is the progestin (suppresses ovulation)

c) Estrogen is added to reduce break-through bleeding and amenorrhea (cycle control, although it does contribute somewhat to contraceptive efficacy)

d) Essentially all pills use the same type of estrogen (ethinyl estradiol, EE)

e) Several progestins are marketed.

f) Progestational assays may not compare.

g) All progestins except one are derived from nortestosterone and then manipulated at different carbon chain points to have various effects (e.g. antiandrogenic). The one not derived from nortestosterone is drosperinone (found in *Yasmin*) which comes from spironolactone, a mild diuretic with antiandrogenic effects.

h) COCs with estranes (e.g. norethindrone) and levonorgestrel often are called second generation; those with desogestrel, norgestimate and gestodene are termed third generation.

i) Many pills are generically identical

4) **Prescribing guidelines**: Most are arbitrary

a) Use lowest dose reasonable. Start women on 35 mcg EE or less

b) Progestin-only pills are usually recommended for breast-feeding women or those for whom any estrogen administration is contraindicated. ***Remember, if a woman has regular predictable menses on progestin only pills, she probably is ovulating and may be at a higher risk of pregnancy***.

c) Of the remaining pills, it is very difficult to show any superiority of one pill over another. Most women will do equally well or poorly on any pill in this group.

d) Makers of pills with 20 μg of EE claim that their pills have lower side effects and are advantageous for smokers.

e) The lower theoretic androgenicity of desogestrel and norgestimate pills makes them potentially preferable, as they may have beneficial cosmetic effects and possibly less effect on blood lipids. *Ortho TriCyclen* and *Estrostep* have an FDA indication for treating acne, although that side effect is probably true for all combination oral contraceptives because of impact on sex hormone binding globulin (remember if you are treating an adolescent for acne only, not contraception, you need parental permission).

5) **Benefits and risks of oral contraceptives**

a) Cancer

(1) Decreased: ovarian cancer, endometrial cancer.

(2) Questionable or low effect on breast cancer (some studies have found increase of 17-24%, but remember since breast cancer is rare in younger women, the individual's risk remains small).

(3) Questionable effect on cervical cancer. Some studies have found oral contraceptive treatment raises the risk of cervical cancer (1.5 times); probably, women on oral contraceptives are more likely to obtain medical care (surveillance bias), be more sexually active, and smoke, all confounding influences.

b) Menstrual problems

(1) Less anemia and dysmenorrhea

6) Method of taking

a) Starting the pill

(1) May start with Sunday after menses - although the entire area of when to start and how long to use backup is lacking evidence

(a) Sunday may be easier day for woman to notice and remember

(b) Helps verify not pregnant

(c) If menses begins on Sunday, start pills on that day and use back-up for 7 days.

(2) "Quick Start" is starting a woman when she presents for care as long as she is not pregnant.

(a) The later in the cycle, the more likely breakthrough bleeding (BTB); up to 1/3 of women may have BTB first cycle anyway.

(b) Quick start has demonstrated more women start and continue COCs.

(c) Backup method on first cycle of pills for 7 days (some areas say all month; others say backup unnecessary if start pills on first day of menses instead of Sunday after period starts)

(3) **If 7 days or more since start of menses, ovulation is more likely in first pill week**.

7) Pill problems

a) Ideally take a pill each day at the same time (more important for POP than COC)

(1) One pill missed: take missed pill as soon as possible. Offer emergency contraception (EC) if missed during first week of pack (WHO does not recommend EC for one missed pill).

(2) Two pills missed: Take one pill every 12 hours until she catches up, then continue pack. May need antiemetic before second pill. Backup contraception for 7 days. Offer EC, especially if early in cycle; restart pills next day.

(3) More than 2 pills missed: Offer EC if she had intercourse, and restart COCs the next day. Use barrier for 7 days. If she declines EC, recommend discard missed pills, restart COCs and continue to end of pack. She will need to use barrier contraception until the end of the cycle, as she is not protected from pregnancy.

b) If woman uses EC, advise her to skip the missed pills in her pack and resume her COCs the day after she takes EC pills.

c) **No withdrawal bleed** (not taking *Seasonale* or continuous COCs)

(1) ***Rule out pregnancy***

(2) If she missed pills, offer EC if appropriate

(3) Reassurance

(4) Switch to higher estrogen or lower progestin activity pill if she desires monthly bleed

8) Special considerations

a) See section on contraindications

b) Screen regularly for major complications by teaching the woman using the ACHES or other method to rule out major issues

c) Remember to do a lipid profile if strong family history of hypercholesterolemia or if woman is over 35

d) Support women during first three months when BTB is most common.

e) Common side effects include BTB, amenorrhea

f) No evidence on how to switch women from one pill to another. Since you cannot change estrogen type, consider changing progestin type; **there is no data as to how to make scientific choice**

g) Most commonly continue until woman is 55 (at which time >90% are menopausal)

9) Follow up

a) Should include blood pressure since a few women develop significant hypertension on OCs

b) Usual exam timing is 3 months after pill initiation and then every year

> **Odd Observation**
> Women on COCs are more likely to get chlamydia (probably due to cervical eversion) but less likely to get PID. Recent evidence suggests that if a woman is on OCs and has cervical HPV—it may be more likely to be malignant.

10) Hormonal contraceptive problems (including oral, patch, and ring):

a) Venous thromboembolism (DVT) - Includes deep venous thrombosis, pulmonary embolism and retinal vein thrombosis

(1) Seems related to dose of estrogen - When estrogen was decreased from 50 mcg to 30 mcg for COCs in general use, VTE dropped by 2/3

(2) Also related to type of progestin: some third generation progestins (desogestrel and gestodene, and perhaps drosperinone) have been associated with increased VTE incidence when compared to second generation—but still less risky than pregnancy.

(3) Risk of DVT is associated with inherited thrombophilias, e.g., Factor V Leiden mutation, Protein S or C abnormalities.

(4) Instruct woman on danger signs (ACHES), consult if DVT is suspected

(5) Do not prescribe for women with documented risk factors

b) Myocardial infarction (MI), stroke

(1) No increased risk for young women on low dose OCPs who do not smoke, have hypertension, and do not have migraines with neurological findings

(2) Women at highest risk for MI or stroke are

(a) ***Smokers over age 35: do not prescribe COCs***; encourage and assist all smokers to quit.

(b) Hypertension, diabetes mellitus, hyperlipidemia, obesity

(c) Severe migraines or new onset headaches (stroke risk)

(3) Teach woman to report ACHES: **A**bdominal pain, **C**hest pain, **H**eadache, **E**xtremity pain, or changes in **S**ight

<u>ACHES</u>
Abdominal pain **C**hest pain **H**eadache **E**xtremity pain **S**hortness of breath

c) Hypertension

(1) 1% users develop; usually reversible with discontinuation of COC

(2) Hypertension may be stronger factor than smoking in women >35 (reason for checking BP before initiating COC—and for recheck in 3 months)

(3) Discontinue estrogen; may try progestin only pills (POPs)

(4) Recommend health promotion activities, e.g., stop smoking, maintain healthy body weight, exercise regularly, use salt in moderation, reduce stress, etc

d) Neoplasias

(1) Users of early generation high dose pills at higher risk of adenocarcinoma of cervix and hepatic adenomas (both rare)

(2) Breast cancer:

(a) Current users have higher risk of being diagnosed with cancer; reason is not known – may be detected more often because of increased breast exams or OCPs may promote growth of cancer cells already present. These breast cancers are more likely to be localized (i.e., not metastatic)

(b) Women who ever used OCPs have no higher risk

(c) Conclusions drawn are that women with strong family history of breast cancer do **not** increase the risk of breast cancer by taking OCPs.

(d) Still "unanswered questions about pills and breast cancer" (Hatcher, 2004), but the **overall conclusion is that OCPs do not cause breast cancer**.

e) Cholelithiasis/cholecystitis

(1) Higher doses were associated with risk of gallbladder disease.

(2) COCs should be used with caution in women who are known to have gallstones

(3) Sub 50 mcg preparations may pose a slight risk

f) Visual changes

(1) Retinal thrombosis may occur rarely

(2) Stop OCPs

(3) Contact lens wearers may experience dryness; use drops or switch methods

11) COC Problem management

a) **Nausea/vomiting**

(1) ***Rule out pregnancy***

(2) Change to lower dose pill or a non oral method (e.g., patch, vaginal ring)

(3) Take pills at night if morning nausea; vice versa

(4) If woman vomits within 1 hour of taking pill, take antiemetic and retake pill; use backup method for 7 days

(5) Rule out serious complication: thrombosis of intra abdominal vessels, gallstones, pancreatitis, liver adenoma, Chrohn's disease, porphyria

b) **Breakthrough spotting or bleeding**

(1) ***Rule out pregnancy, intrauterine or ectopic***

(2) Rule out cervical or endometrial cancer, infection

(3) Determine if there are any potential drug interactions

(4) Evaluate adherence to pill taking regimen

(5) Provide EC if needed

(6) Reassurance if appropriate

(7) Switch to another pill (not evidence based for any of the sub 50 mcg pills)

(8) If on continuous hormones (*Seasonale*, or no active pill breaks), consider stopping the pills for 2-3 days, restart and stop again for next spotting episode. MUST have taken pills for at least 21 days before stopping.

c) **New headaches or preexisting headaches worsen on pills**

(1) Rule out causes: hypertension, vision problems, medications, etc

(2) Evaluate headache. ***If associated with neurological symptoms, discontinue COCs and refer to MD***. May try POP in consultation with MD or non hormonal contraceptive.

(a) Neurological symptoms: scotomata, blindness, weakness, slurred speech, dizziness, abnormal cranial nerve function.

(3) If no neurological symptoms, keep diary.

(a) Headaches with menses: start new pack with onset of period (first day start), use COC continuously. If persistent headaches, switch to POP or non hormone method.

(b) Headaches not associated with menses: if symptoms severe or woman at risk for stroke, discontinue COC immediately and refer. Offer POP in consultation with MD or non hormone method. If symptoms are mild, switch to lower estrogen content and monitor closely. Discontinue if headaches do not resolve and use POP or non hormone method.

d) Hot flashes during placebo pill week

(1) Start pills on first day of bleeding (first day start) or use continuously

(2) Low dose transdermal or oral estrogen during pill free week.

e) **Depression, mood swings**

(1) Monitor closely with history of depression

(2) Decrease progesterone activity

(3) If irritability and edema, decrease estrogen activity

(4) Diet changes to avoid hypoglycemia

(5) Vitamin B6 10 mg daily

f) Weight gain

(1) Decrease progesterone effect

(2) If cyclic (fluid) decrease estrogen activity

(3) Recommend diet, exercise

g) **Mastalgia (breast tenderness)**

   (1) *Rule out breast mass, pregnancy*

   (2) Lower estrogen or progesterone component

   (3) Low dose pill

h) Note: for many of the discomforts associated with oral contraceptives, consider the effects of estrogen and progesterone excess in pregnancy and hormone deficiency in menopause; alter pill preparation accordingly.

12) Progesterone only pills (POPs)

- Start on day 1 of cycle
- If >3 hours late taking pill, use back-up for 48 hours
- If >1 pill missed, take 2 pills for 2 days and use back-up for the rest of cycle.
- Notify provider if no withdrawal bleed in 4-6 weeks.

13) POP complications

a) Allergy (rare)

b) Ectopic pregnancy

c) Diabetes mellitus type 2, especially if woman had gestational diabetes

d) May be used by women who are not good candidates for COCs (some in consultation with MD)

   (1) Personal or strong family history of venous thromboembolism

   (2) Recent postpartum

   (3) Breastfeeding (controversial)

   (4) Smokers over age 35

   (5) Women with estrogen related side effects (e.g., chloasma, migraine headaches)

   (6) Women with hypertension, coronary artery disease, cerebrovascular disease

14) **POP Problems**

a) Amenorrhea

   (1) ***Rule out pregnancy*** with first episode or with symptoms

   (2) Reassurance if appropriate

b) Irregular bleeding

   (1) Evaluate adherence

   (2) ***Rule out STD, pregnancy, cancer***

   (3) If no pathology or pregnancy, reassure

   (4) 3 day course of NSAID

c) **Heavy bleeding**

(1) ***Rule out STD, pregnancy, cancer***

(2) Evaluate for anemia

(3) 3 days high dose NSAIDs

(4) May need contraceptive doses of estrogen. ***Physiologic doses of estrogen as with estrogen replacement therapy may compromise cervical mucus barrier***. If unable to take estrogen, may need a non hormone method of contraception.

d) **Abdominal pain**

(1) ***Rule out ectopic pregnancy, ovarian torsion, PID***

(2) Refer as needed; ovarian cysts usually resolve spontaneously

Possible drug to drug interactions	
Oral Contraceptive and...	**Possible effect**
Acetaminophen	Decrease effectiveness of analgesic; may need higher dosage of analgesic
Antimicrobials	Probably no effect except increased breakthrough bleeding with common drugs like ampicillin and tetracycline; decreased pill efficacy with rifampin and would need contraceptive backup. OC labeling contains precaution about antibiotic interaction; if woman has vomiting, diarrhea, or just prefers it, suggest a back up method.
Antifungals e.g., griseofulvin	Decreased contraceptive efficacy, use backup
Theophylline	Increased theophylline effect, may need lower dosage of theophylline
Vitamin C	Increase estrogen activity of pill, can decrease temporary side effect like break through bleeding
Hepatic enzyme-inducing agents, e.g., anticonvulsants (except valproic acid); St John's wort	Prescribe high dose COC (50 μg EE); or 30-35 μg pill with reduced pill-free interval (first day start, bicycling, continuous use) due to decreased effectiveness of contraceptive.

15) **Other hormonal combination methods—not specifically mentioned in AMCB blueprint**

a) **Transdermal patch**

(1) Perfect use failure rate: Less than 1% (no typical user failure studies)

(2) FDA approval 2001. Slightly more expensive per month than OCPs.

(3) *Ortho-Evra®* (ethinyl estradiol/norelgestromin) is a patch that is effective for 7 days. One patch is used each week for three weeks and after a patch free one week interval, the cycle is restarted. Each patch contains the same amount of both estrogen and progesterone; delivers 20 μg EE and 150 μg norelgestromin daily.

(4) May be useful for women who tend to have problems with daily pill taking.

(5) The patch can be placed on abdomen, buttocks, arm or upper abdomen (not the breasts). Adherent during swimming or bathing. Similar to oral contraceptives, it is prescribed in cycles, each consisting of 3 patches.

(6) Side effects are similar also to other estrogen/progesterone methods, including bleeding. People also complain of skin irritation.

(7) Continuation rates higher than COCs and ability to use perfectly is higher for all age groups than COCs, including adolescents.

(8) The transdermal may rarely detach; new patch is applied if detaches partially or fully.

(9) **Caution women who weigh more than 198 pounds; studies have consistently reported higher risk for pregnancy**.

b) **Ring** impregnated with estrogen and progestin ***(NuvaRing***®***)***

(1) Typical user failure rate: similar to COCs

(2) It is soft, flexible, transparent ring that is easily self-administered and provides month-long contraceptive protection.

(3) **Leave ring in Vagina for 3 weeks and then remove. New ring is inserted after 7 days.** The ring is inserted into the vagina; it releases on average 0.120 mg of etonogestrel and 0.015 mg of EE per day over 3 weeks (21 days).

(4) The exact positioning within the vagina is not critical for it to work because it is not a barrier contraceptive; therefore, it cannot be incorrectly inserted within the vagina.

(5) If ring is removed or expelled for > 3 hours, use back up for 7 days after reinserting ring into vagina.

d. Injectable contraceptives

The only injectable available in the US at this time (April 2005) is depot medroxyprogesterone acetate (*DepoProvera*®). *The combined injectable, medroxyprogesterone/estradiol cypionate (Lunelle®) is currently not available in the US.*

> Remember methods that decrease bleeding may be particularly helpful for women with anemia and HIV positive status

1) Depot medroxyprogesterone acetate (*Depo Provera*, DMPA)

a) Typical user failure rate: 0.3%

b) Medroxyprogesterone acetate in oil—150 mg

c) Mechanism of action

(1) Suppresses LH surge: inhibits ovulation

(2) Decreases sperm penetration through cervical mucous

(3) Decrease tubal motility

(4) Hostile endometrium

> **Midwifery Message**
> Ask woman considering DMPA when (if ever) she wants to get pregnant. May take 7-9 months after last injection before fertility resumes

d) Candidate
   (1) Wants reversible contraceptive
   (2) Contraindications to estrogen
e) Side effects
   (1) Bone loss after prolonged use. FDA says that **prolonged use may result in the loss of bone density and that the loss is greater the longer the drug is administered**. The bone density loss **may not be completely reversible** after discontinuation of the drug. The warning states that women should use Depo-Provera Contraceptive Injection for **no longer than two years.**
      (a) In March 2005, the World Health Organization published a statement **on DPMA and bone mineral density** acknowledging that the new evidence confirms prior evidence of reduction in bone mineral density in DMPA users. Currently, WHO recommends that women who are ages 18 to 45 years can use DMPA without restriction (WHO Category "1"). For women ages less than 18 or greater than 45 years, the benefits of using DMPA generally outweigh the known or theoretical risks (WHO Category "2").
      (b) Recommend adequate dietary calcium and exercise.
   (2) Amenorrhea is common, as is break through bleeding
   (3) Weight gain is common (more than 60% of women gain an average of 5 pounds)
   (4) Breast tenderness, bloating, headaches, etc.
   (5) Possible increase in depression, anxiety, irritation, premenstrual syndrome (PMS), fatigue, mood changes; severe depression is rare
   (6) Rare but possible liver problems—do liver studies if jaundice occurs
f) Injection
   (1) Within first three days of menses, within 5 days postpartum or at 4-6 weeks postpartum
   (2) Every 3 months
   (3) If longer than 14 weeks, do a pregnancy test before administration
   (4) Compatible with breastfeeding
   (5) Inject into deep muscle (gluteal or deltoid) using 1.5 to 3 inch needle
   (6) Do not massage after injection
   (7) Anaphylaxis is possible; some recommend having patient remain in clinic for 20 minutes; at least, have patient report itching at injection site

(8) Great choice for women with seizure disorder or sickle cell anemia. Has an anti-convulsant effect and reduces the number of sickle cell crises.

g) ***Initiation of DMPA in immediate PP period for breastfeeding women is controversial***

2) **Problems and complications associated with DMPA**

a) **Progressive significant weight gain**

(1) Recommend dietary changes, exercise, support groups

b) **Severe depression**

(1) DMPA as causative agent is controversial

(2) Evaluate suicide potential and refer as indicated

(3) Recommend avoidance of alcohol

(4) Antidepressant therapy if needed

(5) Recommend psychotherapy, refer for treatment

(6) Change contraceptive method

c) **Severe allergic or vasovagal reaction, including anaphylaxis (very rare)**

(1) Have woman remain in clinic for 20 minutes following injection (controversial)

(2) Have woman report itching at injection site

(3) Benadryl to reduce pruritus and swelling

(4) Oxygen and CPR if needed

(5) Refer

(6) Change contraceptive method

3) **Problem management**

a) **Vaginal dryness, dyspareunia, atrophic vaginitis**

(1) Estrogen replacement therapy as cream, ring, tablets, patch

(2) Water soluble silicone lubricant for dyspareunia

b) **Pain** or infection at injection site

(1) NSAIDs for pain; rule out nerve damage, infection

(2) Antibiotics as indicated

c) Woman presents **early for reinjection**: give it

d) Woman presents **late (>13 weeks) for reinjection**

(1) If LMP onset ≤5 days ago, give it

(2) If LMP onset >5 days ago, and she has not had intercourse, consider pregnancy test and give DMPA

(3) If LMP onset >5 days ago and she has had intercourse, do pregnancy test

(a) If pregnancy test negative, may give DMPA with precaution that it may be false negative but DMPA will not harm fetus. ***Use backup method for 7 days.*** Repeat pregnancy test in 2 weeks. If negative, resume regular DMPA regimen (i.e., return in 11 weeks)

e) **Heavy bleeding**

(1) ***Rule out pregnancy, cervical infection, neoplasia or other pathology***

(2) Rule out anemia

(3) Treat with NSAIDs for 3 days (avoid if GI problems or asthma) or estrogen supplements, including may use estrogenic COC for 1-2 months in addition to DMPA. Physiologic estrogen may be continued indefinitely with DMPA.

f) Irregular bleeding/spotting

(1) Rule out pregnancy (unlikely), cervical lesion or infection

(2) Reassurance if appropriate

(3) May use NSAIDs and estrogen as described above

g) Amenorrhea

(1) Reassurance; pregnancy test if other symptoms or woman desires

(2) Switch to another method if woman desires menses

4) Lunelle: not available in US at present

e. Intrauterine contraceptive devices (IUCD; IUD; IUS)

***ParaGard® T380A*, Levonorgestrel intrauterine system (*Mirena LNG- IUS*)**

1) Typical user failure rate: In general 0.1-2.0

2) Mechanism of action

a) **Copper IUDs** work primarily as a spermicide by inhibiting sperm capacitation and survival. A sterile inflammatory reaction phagocytizes the sperm. They are approved for use for 10 years.

b) **Levonorgestrel-containing IUDs** (*Mirena®*) releases 20 μg/day levonorgestrel (14 μg/day after 5 years). This progestin causes cervical mucus thickening, preventing sperm migration to the fallopian tubes. Alteration of the endometrium prevents implantation of a fertilized ovum; to some extent it may also prevent ovulation. Replace after 5 years.

Note: IUDs will be considered separately because of the differences in their mechanisms of action, indications, and side effects.

3) **Copper IUD (*ParaGard*®)**

a) **Advantages**:

- Possible protection from endometrial cancer, possible protection from cervical cancer
- Rapid return to fertility
- Cost effective
- Good alternative for women who cannot use hormonal methods
- High level of user satisfaction.
- ***May be used for emergency contraception.***

b) **Disadvantages:**

- Increased menstrual blood loss (may be diminished by NSAIDs),
- Increased dysmenorrheal, spotting and cramping with and following insertion
- Strings may cause discomfort for partner during intercourse.
- Increased risk of infection in first 20 days after insertion (PID 1/1000).

c) Candidates

(1) Stable mutually monogamous relationship

(2) Desires long term contraception

(3) Nulligravida, primigravida, multigravida at low risk of STD

(4) History of past PID with monogamous uninfected partner now and successful pregnancy since PID

(5) Cannot or does not want to use hormones

(6) **Need for emergency contraception** within 5 days of unprotected intercourse; may be used within 8 days if ovulation is known to have occurred at least 3 days after intercourse.

d) Contraindications and precautions

(1) Pregnancy

(2) Current STD or STD within 3 months, or at risk (e. g., multiple partners)

(3) Uterus sounds <6 cm or >9 cm (package insert; some use 10-12 as upper limit)

(4) Undiagnosed vaginal bleeding

(5) Active cervicitis, active pelvic infection, known symptomatic Actinomycosis

(6) Recent endometritis (past 3 months)

(7) Allergy to copper; Wilson's disease

(8) Uterine structural abnormality

(9) AIDS, HIV (not evidenced based; theoretically at risk for other STDs)

(10) Known or suspected uterine or cervical cancer; unresolved abnormal Pap

(11) Severe anemia (Levonorgestrel IUD would be a good choice)

(12) Relative contraindication is nulligravid or non-monogamous.

e) Insertion timing

(1) Any time in cycle when pregnancy is ruled out; lowest expulsion rates at mid cycle

(2) Immediately after induced or spontaneous abortion if no infection

(3) Immediately after delivery of placenta or after complete involution

f) Notes

(1) **Routine antibiotic prophylaxis is not recommended**; women with high risk of bacterial endocarditis need antibiotics

(2) Check position, size and mobility of uterus prior to insertion

(3) Cleanse upper vagina, outer cervix, and cervical os and canal with antiseptic

(4) Place tenaculum to stabilize cervix and straighten uterine axis

(5) May use paracervical block: 0.5 cc lidocaine in tenaculum site

(6) Sound uterus to fundus

(7) Trim strings to 2" and document length in chart

(8) Teach woman to report PAINS: **P**elvic pain, **A**bnormal bleeding, signs of **I**nfection, **N**o period, **S**tring not palpable

PAINS

Period late
Abdominal pain, Dyspareunia
Infection exposure, STD
Not feeling well, fever, chills
String missing, shorter/longer than normal

g) Complications

(1) Excessive bleeding

(2) Cramping and pain

(3) Expulsion

(4) Perforation

(5) Unable to palpate string

(6) Risk of ectopic pregnancy (IF pregnancy occurs), spontaneous abortion (early removal reduces the risk)

(7) Upper genital tract infection; there is controversy about whether or not to remove the IUD at the time of treatment

4) Levonorgestrel Intrauterine System (*Mirena®; LNG IUS*)

a) **Advantages:**

➢ Menorrhagia improves (90% less blood loss with *LNG IUS* than without; 20% amenorrheic within a year, 60% by 5 years)

- Decreased surgery for menorrhagia; may protect against endometrial cancer, extremely effective (as effective as tubal ligation);
- May be used as progestin by women on hormone replacement therapy
- Reduces endometrial polyps in breast cancer patients taking tamoxifen (safety in breast cancer is not documented)

b) **Disadvantages:**

- Irregular spotting and bleeding for first few months
- Amenorrhea
- Expulsion rate higher in women using Mirena to control heavy menstrual bleeding
- 5-8% of pregnancies while on IUD are ectopic.
- Ovarian cysts (most resolve spontaneously)
- Headaches, acne, mastalgia during first few months.

c) **Candidates**

(1) Same as *ParaGard,* plus

(2) Heavy menses, dysmenorrhea, anemia, dysfunctional uterine bleeding

(3) Menopausal women using estrogen replacement therapy with intact uterus, unable to tolerate oral progestins (protects against endometrial cancer)

(4) WHO approves use with previous ectopic pregnancy; package insert advises against

(5) Allergy to copper; Wilson's disease and desires IUD

(6) Severe anemia (Levonorgestrel IUD would be a good choice)

d) **Contraindications and precautions**

(1) Same as ParaGard except **may use with menorrhagia, anemia, copper allergy, Wilson's disease**

e) **Insertion timing**

(1) Within 7 days of menses onset; if no pregnancy, other times in cycle acceptable

(2) Insertion tube is wider diameter than ParaGard; may need cervical dilation and more likely to need paracervical block, especially nullipara

(3) Counsel to expect menstrual changes

(4) NSAIDs for post insertion

IUD Myths

Do not be confused about IUDs and ectopics. Past use of an IUD does not increase a woman's risk of having an ectopic pregnancy. And current use of an IUD reduces a woman's risk of an ectopic---but only because it reduces the risk of all pregnancies. **If she does become pregnant with an IUD, she is at higher risk of ectopic pregnancy since the IUD is better at preventing an in utero pregnancy than a tubal one.**

f) Notes: same as for *ParaGard*

g) Complications: similar to *ParaGard*, plus

(1) Ovarian cysts (usually resolve spontaneously)

(2) Allergy to levonorgestrel

5) Removal of IUD

a) Generally easily performed

b) May be performed at any time

c) Physician consultation if it is not easily removed

d) Assume she is immediately fertile

e) Remove if pregnant and string is visible

6) ***Follow up is to tell a woman about the signs or symptoms of PID and pregnancy and the importance of checking the IUD strings after menses each month.***

7) Her next appointment usually is in 6 weeks (after a menses, which is the most likely time for spontaneous expulsion).

8) Complications and problems with IUDs:

a) PID within 20 days of insertion (1/1000)

(1) Risk factors include bacterial vaginosis, cervicitis, and contamination during insertion. Some do wet mount and Chlamydia/GC cultures before insertion.

(2) Management:

- BV, candidiasis: manage as usual
- Trichomoniasis: treat and reevaluate appropriateness of IUD
- Cervicitis, PID: give first dose of antibiotics before removal of IUD; removal may not be necessary if improvement occurs on antibiotics; reconsider appropriateness of IUD. Consult.
- Actinomycosis (reported on Pap smear): Consult. Evaluate for upper tract infection (may be unilateral); if signs of upper tract infection, treat with penicillin for 1 month. If asymptomatic, may manage conservatively with annual Pap smears and PID warnings, treat with antibiotics and repeat Pap smear, OR, remove IUD, treat with antibiotics, repeat Pap and if cleared reinsert IUD.
- Teach PAINS

b) **Uterine perforation** (1/1000); occurs or begins at insertion

(1) Risk factors

- Immobile, markedly anteverted or retroverted uterus, breastfeeding woman, inexperienced, unskilled provider.
- Signs are pain, loss of resistance to advancement of sound or IUD, and instrument goes deeper than expected from bimanual examination.
- Perforation by the sound usually occurs in the posterior uterine wall when the uterus is anteflexed

(2) Management

- Remove the sound
- Consult MD
- If there is no bleeding, vital signs are stable, no pain and stable hematocrit for several hours, may be sent home (provide contraception)
- If pain or signs of organ damage, call for medical help immediately; laparoscopic evaluation is needed.
- If IUD perforates acutely, attempt to remove by gentle traction on strings; if not retrieved easily, refer for medical management
- If IUD perforation is confirmed by ultrasound at a later date, refer for medical management

c) **Vasovagal reaction**, fainting with insertion (rare)

(1) Risk factors

- Stenotic cervical os
- Prior vasovagal reactions

(2) Management

- Administer oxygen if needed
- If during sounding of uterus or before IUD is placed, abort the procedure
- If IUD is in situ, do not remove as manipulation may exacerbate condition
- May administer atropine 0.5-1 mg subcutaneously or intramuscularly

d) **Expulsion**

(1) Risk factors

- Insertion during menses, or immediately postpartum
- Inadequate depth of insertion
- Nulliparous
- Previous expulsion of IUD (1/3)
- Expulsion risk decreases over time

(2) Management

- If expulsion confirmed by woman or CNM, rule out pregnancy and place a new IUD
- If expulsion is suspected, get ultrasound to locate it. Probe cervical canal and remove if IUD is found there. Replace immediately if not pregnant
- If partial expulsion, remove IUD. If no pregnancy and no infection, place new IUD

e) **Pregnancy**

(1) Risk factors

- Poor placement
- Expulsion (especially silent)

(2) Management (Consult)

- Rule out ectopic pregnancy (5-8% pregnancies with Cu IUD are ectopic). If strings are not visible and IUD found in uterus by ultrasound, advise patient she is at risk for preterm birth, but not birth defects. ***Remove with abortion or at delivery***.
- If strings are visible in first trimester, ***advise removal of IUD*** to reduce risk of spontaneous abortion and preterm labor
- If patient is aborting, remove IUD. Consider antibiotics.
- Teach PAINS

9) IUD problem management

a) Spotting, frequent or heavy bleeding, hemorrhage or anemia

(1) ***Rule out pregnancy; if pregnant, rule out ectopic pregnancy***

(2) Rule out infection, especially if post coital bleeding

(3) Rule out expulsion

(4) Assess for anemia and provide iron supplementation as needed

(5) NSAIDs

(6) Replace copper IUD with LNG IUD

b) Cramping, pain

(1) Rule out pregnancy, infection, IUD expulsion

(2) NSAIDs with menses

(3) Replace copper IUD with LNG IUD or another method

c) **Missing strings: see expulsion, above**
   (1) ***Rule out pregnancy***
   (2) **Ultrasound** to determine if IUD is still in place
      (a) If in uterus, may leave in place or remove (MD)
      (b) If pregnant, see pregnancy, above

d) Infection, see above

e) Removal
   (1) Grasp strings with hemostat close to cervix and steadily retract
   (2) If IUD is embedded, try gentle rotation of strings. If IUD cannot be removed, consult.

f. **Subdermal implants *(Norplant) Not available in US at this time for insertion; Single rod implant (Implanon)* available soon**

g. **Sterilization counseling**

1) **Female sterilization (bilateral tubal ligation or occlusion)**

a) Typical user failure rate: 0.8%-3.7% depending on procedure and timing
   (i) Younger women have higher failure rates

b) Mechanism of action: interruption of patency of Fallopian tube (preventing sperm access to ovum)

c) **Female sterilization is the most common contraceptive technique, surpassing COCs**

d) Indication: Woman wants sterilization, i.e. permanent contraception

e) Contraindications
   (1) Woman is unable to give informed consent, e.g., she does not understand the true nature of the operation due to apparent immaturity, family duress, upset over recent trauma such as unexpected cesarean section or neonatal complications, current marital discord, etc.
   (2) Woman is mentally handicapped.
   (3) Medical problems make the surgery an increased risk to the woman or make other surgeries more appropriate. Some women might have a pelvic mass and be better treated with a or alternative contraceptive methods (women with severe obesity, hypertension, lung disease)
   (4) Note: The U.S. Supreme Court has ruled that a woman need not have her spouse's consent for sterilization.

f) Advantages: possible decreased risk of ovarian cancer, permanent and highly effective contraception.

g) Disadvantages: Post tubal ligation syndrome of menorrhagia and dysmenorrhea has not been substantiated; **regret, especially among young women**. Requires surgery; expensive; not easily reversible.
   (1) Factors associated with regret: age <30, low parity, change in marital status, poverty, minority status, misinformation about permanency or risks, hasty decision, loss of a child.

h) Variety of procedures
   (1) Laparotomy approaches, including abdominal hysterectomy and mini-laparotomy.
   (2) Laparoscopy: electrocautery, bands, clips, etc
   (3) Vaginal approaches: vaginal hysterectomy, colpotomy
   (4) Specific risks and failure rates vary with procedure

2) Transcervical sterilization via polyester fibers (*Essure*)
   a) Material is introduced via the cervix to the uterine portion of Fallopian tubes
   b) Tissue growth around the polyester material causes blockage of the tubes
   c) Takes 3 months for tissue to occlude the tubes
   d) Hysterosalpingogram confirms occlusion
   e) Permanent
   f) Similar complications as IUD insertion

3) Complications and problems associated with female sterilization:
   a) **Laparotomy:** bleeding, infection, damage to internal organs, anesthetic complications, death. Managed by surgeon.
   b) **Amenorrhea: Rule out pregnancy and if woman is pregnant, rule out ectopic**.

4) Male sterilization: Vasectomy
   a) Typical user failure rate: 0.15%
   b) Mechanism of action: Blockage of the vas deferens prevents sperm passage, thus causing infertility
   c) Procedure
      (1) Vas deferens located and held in place through the scrotal sac
      (2) Through an incision the vas is identified and occluded by tying and cutting, cautery and or mechanical means
      (3) Then repeated on other side

d) Complications are rare
   (1) Bleeding, hematoma, infection
   (2) Granuloma is leakage of sperm from the occluded end and causes temporary inflammatory nodule that resolves spontaneously
   (3) Sperm antibodies developed by ½ to 2/3 of all men after vasectomy and of no pathological significance
   (4) No evidence of atherosclerosis in humans (has been found in other primates)
   (5) No evidence that prostate cancer is linked, some conflicting studies but biologically implausible

e) Advantages
   (1) Permanent
   (2) Relatively safe and easy
   (3) 20% the cost of female sterilization and far easier
   (4) No change in volume or velocity of ejaculate

f) Disadvantages
   (1) Indirect method of contraception for woman (only if one partner)
   (2) Regret 5-10%
   (3) No protection from STDs
   (4) **Not effective until sperm in vas deferens ejaculated (usually 20 ejaculations or 12 weeks)**

h. Emergency contraception

1) Indications for a woman to consider emergency contraception (EC)
   a) Unanticipated intercourse
   b) Rape
   c) Condom issue: break, slip or come off
   d) Failure to take several birth control pills
   e) Found out after sex her diaphragm had slipped, etc
2) Two oral methods—either progesterone alone or estrogen and progesterone taken within 72 hours after unprotected sexual intercourse; Copper IUD within 5-8 days of intercourse.
3) In most states, emergency contraception is not available without prescription.
4) Once implantation has occurred, EC has no effect on the pregnancy.
5) EC is not abortifacient and pregnancies carried to term have not shown adverse effects.

6) Oral methods

a) Mechanism of action: prevents pregnancy before ovulation by disrupting follicular development, blocking the LH surge, and inhibiting ovulation. Oral EC also thickens cervical mucus. If taken after ovulation, they do not affect ovarian function or endometrial maturation. They may affect tubal transport of sperm or ova.

b) Estrogen/progesterone method (slightly less effective than POPs). *(Preven®)*

(1) GI side effects: may give antiemetic prior to treatment (e.g., *Dramamine®*)

(2) Side effects: nausea, vomiting, headache, moodiness, breast tenderness, change in next menses

(3) Do not use if already pregnant or severe migraine; POPs are better for women with of history deep vein thrombosis.

(4) Yuzpe method involves taking various dosages of COCs (see box above for specific regimens); advantage is that the woman can use pills from a pack

c) Progestin only (*Plan B*)

(1) Start within 72 hours of unprotected intercourse, but it can be given up to 5 days post coital. Earlier is better.

(2) Side effects: same as COCs, but less frequent and less severe.

(3) Not teratogenic, but should not be used if woman is already pregnant because it will not be effective.

> **Quick Summary of Emergency Contraception**
>
> **PLAN B: Take 1 pill as soon as possible within 72 hours of unprotected intercourse and 1 pill 12 hours later. (progestin only)**
>
> **Preven:** Take 2 pills as soon as possible within 72 hours of unprotected intercourse, and 2 more pills 12 hours later.
>
> **Ovrette:** Take 20 pills as soon as possible within 72 hours of unprotected intercourse and then 20 pills 12 hours later per dose.
>
> **Ovral:** Take 2 pills as soon as possible within 72 hours of unprotected intercourse and then 2 more pills 12 hours later.
>
> **Levlen, Lo-Ovral, Nordette, or Tri Phasil:** Take 4 pills as soon as possible within 72 hours of unprotected intercourse and 4 more pills 12 hours later.
>
> **Alesse:** Take 5 pills as soon as possible within 72 hours of unprotected intercourse, and 5 more pills 12 hours later.

d) If the woman vomits within 1 hour of taking tablet, repeat

e) Lactating woman may use emergency contraception

f) Not to be used routinely for contraception, but multiple uses are not harmful; not as effective as other contraception

7) Emergency contraception with copper IUD (*ParaGard®*)

a) Insert within 5 days of unprotected intercourse; may insert within 8 days if ovulation date is known to have been at least 3 days after intercourse. Use standard method of insertion described earlier in chapter, and same contraindications and precautions.

b) Failure rate <1%; most effective method of post coital contraception.

c) Expensive if woman does not desire to continue use of IUD.

d) Ideal for woman who desires to continue to use the method.

e) Levonorgestrel IUS (Mirena) is NOT indicated for emergency contraception.

8) **Complications and problems associated with emergency contraception:**

a) **Emergency contraceptive pills** (IUD emergency contraception same as IUD)

(1) **Deep vein thrombosis** using combined estrogen-progestin formulas

(2) Teach ACHES

(3) Use progestin only EC pills if history venous thrombosis

b) **Pregnancy**

(1) Counsel regarding options: terminate, continue with pregnancy and adopt out

(2) Reassure that there is evidence that EC pills do not increase the risk of fetal anomalies or spontaneous abortion

9) Problem management

a) **Nausea/vomiting**

(1) POPs cause less vomiting (and they are more effective)

(2) Antiemetic before taking EC pills

(3) Repeat dose if vomiting occurred within 30 minutes to 1 hour (recommendations vary) of taking EC pills

(4) Consider IUD

b) **Amenorrhea**

(1) If no menses in 21 days (or period more than 7 days late) ***rule out pregnancy***

3. **Fertility promotion**

a. **Preconceptional counseling** (according to NIH-Content of Prenatal Care)

400 Micrograms of folic acid for all women of reproductive age as 50% of pregnancies are UNPLANNED.

1) Preconceptional health promotion offers the opportunity to provide

a) Counseling about safer sex, pregnancy planning, spacing, and contraception

b) Counseling about the availability of social programs

c) Advice regarding prescription and over-the-counter medications and herbal remedies used by the woman

d) Information on environmental hazards

2) **Interventions to reduce medical and psychosocial risk**
   a) Opportunity to intervene in medical or psychosocial risk identified by risk assessment.
   b) Treatment of disease identified, including infections
   c) Modification of chronic disease medication and regimens to decrease teratogenic risk
   d) Vaccination/Immunization
   e) Counseling regarding behaviors, including those related to HIV and other infections
   f) Nutrition counseling, supplementation, or referral (e.g. Folic Acid 400 mcg/day)
   g) Substance abuse counseling or referral for treatment programs
   h) Home visiting to treat psychosocial risks
   i) Provision of social services and financial assistance
   j) Referral to other health care providers
   k) Provision of contraception or referral for family planning
3) Risk assessment activities include
   a) History taking
   b) Physical examination
   c) Laboratory tests

> **Bottom Line**
> **Preconception counseling should be done with ALL women of reproductive age.**
> Preconception counseling allows a woman to treat herself as already pregnant—e.g. eat well, avoid illicit drugs, alcohol and tobacco.

b. **Initial assessment and diagnostic procedures/referral for infertility**
1) Infertility incidence
   a) Increased internationally
   b) Traditionally said to be approximately 5% of American couples (approx. 1 million US couples)
   c) Can debate statistics, but trend is increasing
      (1) Raised awareness of infertility among individuals
      (2) Increase in services
      (3) Delayed childbearing
      (4) 51% of primary infertility resolves spontaneously
      (5) 22% of secondary infertility resolves spontaneously
      (6) US government is interested in studying aspects of infertility

> **Note**
> Anovulation is not the most common reason for infertility, but has the highest success rate using available treatment modalities

2) Etiologies
   a) Frequently unknown
   b) Medical conditions such as endometriosis

Etiology	Incidence	Successful Treatment
Sperm Defects	32%	0-27%
Unexplained	28%	7-27%
Anovulation	21%	78-96%
Tubal Damage	14%	19%

   c) Drugs that may decrease fertility, e.g., nicotine
   d) Unknown clinical significance of potential effects of herbal remedies studied

3) Initial female workup
   a) Education about timing for pregnancy. Many people think that day 14 is the ideal day for ovulation based on books and charts. Yet few women always have 28 day cycles
   b) Education about lifestyle—e.g. influence of drugs, alcohol and even tight shorts or certain activities (e.g., competitive bicycling) for the male
   c) Thorough medical, surgical and gynecological history; careful menstrual and contraceptive history
   d) Complete physical examination (weight, blood pressure, thyroid, skin, hair for example)
   e) Pelvic examination
   f) Ovulation may be supported by history
      (1) Basal body temperature charts may assist the couple in planning sexual intercourse, and may be needed eventually if referral is needed.
      (2) See section on natural family planning for discussion of how symptothermal methods may be used for determining ovulation and enhancing the probability of conception
   g) A post-coital test (PCT) is sometimes performed to see if the man's sperm are penetrating the cervical mucus. The value of this test in the infertility work-up is controversial and it is not routinely performed. The couple is advised to have intercourse at the expected time of ovulation and the cervical mucus is examined for the presence of motile sperm 8-12 hours later.

4) Male work up
   a) In a physical examination, often the first component is simply a semen analysis.

b) Many factors can interfere with optimal sperm quality in men, including:

(1) Varicocele

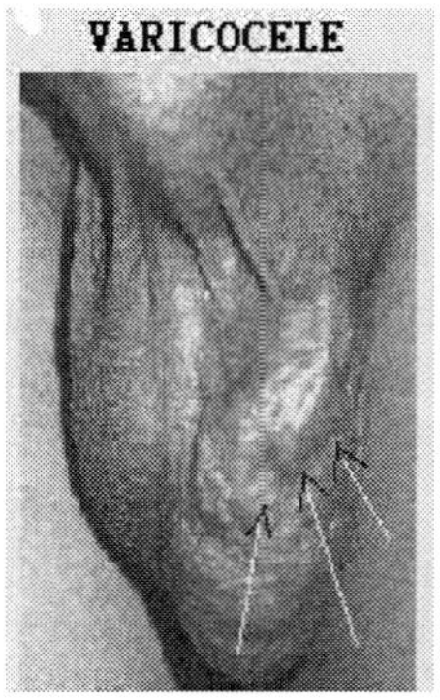

(2) Hypogonadism - a condition that results in markedly decreased levels of testosterone.

> Normal semen analysis
>
> **Total Volume**
> - **2 – 5 milliliters** is normal
> - A very low volume indicates that the seminal vesicles may not be making enough fluid or that these ducts may be blocked. It may also indicate a problem with the prostate gland.
>
> **Sperm Count**
> - **40 million to 300 million per milliliter** is normal
> - Below 10 million is poor; 20 million or more may be fine if motility and morphology are normal.
>
> **Motility and Velocity**
> - **At least 50%** sperm should be active
> - Quality of the movement **at least 2 on scale of 0-4**
>
> **Morphology**
> - **>30% normal** shape

(3) Anti-sperm antibodies

(4) Lifestyle factors (alcohol, nutrition, smoking, drugs, tight underwear, bicycling, etc)

(5) Infection

(6) Medications

(7) Retrograde ejaculation - sperm are forced into the bladder instead of through the urethra.

(8) Cancer

(9) Genetic disorders - undescended testes or congenital malformations

5) Treatments

a) Difficult when etiology is unclear

b) Some surgery has been suggested

c) Historically intertwined diagnosis and surgery (e.g. hysterosalpingogram, laparoscopy)

d) Pelvic surgical techniques not well established for efficacy

6) Pharmacological treatments (for women): use depends on suspected cause of infertility; in consultation with MD

a) Ovulatory stimulants

(1) Clomiphene citrate (*Clomid® Serophene®*)

(2) Classic drug of choice for ovulation stimulation

b) hMG (Human Menopausal Gonadotropin) (*Pergonal®)*

(1) Commercial preparation of LH and FSH

c) Follitropin beta (*Follistim®)*

(1) Used to help women/couples in assisted reproductive technology (ART) programs and induction of ovulation not due to primary ovarian failure

d) Gonadotropin Releasing Hormone (GnRH) alone or preceded by hMG or Clomiphene citrate

e) **Bromocriptine (*Parlodel®*):** Approved for use of infertility or amenorrhea associated with hyperprolactinemia in the absence of a pituitary tumor

f) **SERMs (Selective Estrogen Receptor Modulators)**

(1) Tamoxifen (*Nolvadex®)* Raloxifene (*Evista®)*

(2) Nonsteroidal antiestrogen, although has some estrogenic properties

(3) Primarily marketed for treatment of breast cancer and osteoporosis

(4) Can be used for stimulation of ovulation and correction of luteal phase defects

g) Other drugs used for induction of ovulation

(1) Thyroid stimulating hormone may be used to correct thyroid dysfunction, otherwise not useful

(2) Glucocorticoids (Prednisone, Dexamethasone) used for women with hyperandrogenic anovulation; decreases adrenal function, thus reduces androgens

(3) Estrogens to induce LH surge; not a reliable method

7) Pharmaceutical treatment of other conditions associated with infertility

a) Endometriosis

(1) Danocrine (*Danazol®):* Synthetic Steroid, derivative of testosterone with antigonadotropin properties, androgenic side effects

(2) GnRH analogues, Buserelin, Nafarelin (*Synarel®):* First nonsteroidal drugs that can reversibly suppress ovarian estrogen production

b) Luteal phase/placental defects

(1) Progesterone is not approved as "fertility" treatment

(2) However, widely used if inadequate luteal phase suspected (Crinone 8% progesterone gel is one such example from Wyeth Ayerst)

(3) Begin treatment after ovulation (by BBT or other) and continue for 8-10 weeks after that time placenta should be functional

(4) hCG has been advocated for recurrent early abortion with (insufficient evidence)

C. Well-woman/perimenopausal care

1. Laboratory tests and procedures (order/obtain/interpret)

See chapter I Primary Care for discussion of other screening tests and specific recommendations for women of different ages.

a. Screening (e.g. Pap smear)

1) Cervical epithelium

a) Stratified squamous cells on ectocervix

b) Transition into columnar epithelium in endocervix

c) Interface is squamocolumnar junction (SCJ)

d) ***Endocervical columnar epithelium should undergo metaplastic transformation to squamous epithelium*** (i.e. ***squamous metaplasia***)

(1) Squamous metaplasia is more active during adolescence and pregnancy

(2) The ***transformation zone is*** the area of metaplastic change where the tissue is ***most susceptible to oncogenic factors, principally human papillomavirus (HPV).***

(3) The ***transformation zone must be sampled*** when obtaining Pap smear.

2) HPV

a) ***HPV infection is the primary cause of precancerous cervical lesions and invasive squamous cell cervical carcinoma***.

b) More than 100 genotypes of HPV; >30 associated with anogenital lesions

(1) ***Types 6 and 11 are at low risk for cancer***, causing lesions that are condylomatous (warty), have minimal or no dysplasia (low grade intraepithelial lesions), and often regress spontaneously.

(2) ***Types 16, 18, 31, 33, and 35 are moderate or high risk for cancer***, causing lesions that are associated with higher grades of dysplasia (high grade intraepithelial lesions) and invasive carcinoma.

(3) ***High risk HPV lesions do not <u>inevitably</u> progress to invasive cancer.***

c) Diagnosis of condylomata acuminata (warts) is clinical and may be confirmed by biopsy, which is indicated if

(1) Diagnosis is uncertain

(2) Lesions do not respond to standard therapy or worsen during therapy

(3) Woman is immunocompromised

(4) Warts are pigmented, indurated, fixed, and ulcerated.

(5) No data support the use of type-specific HPV nucleic acid tests in the routine diagnosis or management of ***visible genital warts*** (CDC 2005).

3) About the **Papanicolaou (Pap) smear**

a) Cellular abnormalities can be detected and characterized based on

(1) morphologic alterations of cells created by pathologic entities,

(2) presence of inflammatory cells and/or

(3) presence of microorganisms.

b) The cervical/vaginal Pap smear is a sample of exfoliated or mechanically dislodged cells of the vagina, cervix, and in some cases, endometrium which have been smeared on a glass slide, preserved and stained, and evaluated using cytology techniques.

c) Characteristics of an adequate specimen are

- Adequate numbers of squamous epithelial cells
- Cells from the transformation zone (i.e., endocervical cells)
- Spread in a relatively even monolayer
- Epithelial cells not obscured by blood, inflammatory cells, or foreign material such as lubricant or talc
- Appropriately preserved

http://www-medlib.med.utah.edu/WebPath/TUTORIAL/CYTOPATH/CYTOPATH.html

d) Pap smear sampling

(1) Avoid contraceptive gels or creams, vaginal medications, tampons, heavy menses, sexual intercourse 24-48 hrs prior to exam. A recent study concluded that a small amount of water-soluble gel on the speculum will not interfere with Pap results. STD testing (cultures etc) was NOT researched.

(a) NB: most textbooks include the recommendation to use NO lubricants on the speculum except water, even current texts.

(b) ACOG supports collecting Pap specimen before cultures to enhance the probability of sampling abnormal cells

(c) If a wet prep is to be done during the same examination, take that sample from the posterior fornix or the lateral sidewall prior to sampling for the Pap to avoid contamination with blood

(d) ***If using spatula and brush, sample ectocervix first with spatula*** to avoid heavy contamination with blood that can occur with endocervical brush

(2) Appropriate sampling devices depend on methods used (Thin prep versus glass slide)

(3) Proper choice of speculum size to achieve good visualization

(4) Sampling devices vary according to technique used

(5) Preparing the slide depends on method used

(a) Liquid based preparation in laboratory (Thin prep) is collected with a cervical broom and swished in methanol based liquid; whole container is sent to laboratory where glass slide is prepared

Advantage: more and better preserved cervical epithelial cells

Disadvantages: Possible loss of endocervical cells and cost

(b) Clinician-prepared monolayer glass slide is conventional method

(6) Automated Pap evaluation systems select 10% of smears that are most likely to have abnormalities and need re-evaluation to increase reliability

e) Interpreting Pap smears: **Bethesda system, 2001**

(1) Includes aspects of specimen adequacy and general categorization separately

Cervical Cytology Results

- Satisfactory for evaluation
- Unsatisfactory for evaluation (no more "limited by lack of endocervical cells)
- Negative for intraepithelial lesions or malignancy (organisms consistent with infections may be mentioned)
- No endocervical cells
- Atypical squamous cells (**ASC**)
  - Atypical squamous cells of undetermined significance (**ASC-US**)
  - Atypical squamous cells: cannot exclude high grade squamous intraepithelial lesion (**ASC-H**)
- Atypical glandular cells (**AGC**)
  - AGC, favor neoplasia
  - ACG, not otherwise specified (**ACG NOS**)
- Endocervical adenocarcinoma in situ (**AIS**)
- Low grade squamous intraepithelial lesion (**LSIL**)
- High grade squamous intraepithelial lesion (**HSIL**)

Follow-Up for Abnormal pap: Bethesda Guidelines

Atypical squamous cell of undetermined significance (ASC-US)	1. Re-Pap 2 times in a period of 8 - 12 months a. Two negatives, return to annual pap b. ASC-US or greater, refer for colposcopy 2. Colposcopy as follow-up choice AND for high-risk HPV DNA a. Negative colposcopy, HPV DNA test 6 and 12 months or Pap in 6 and 12 months. b. If any of these are positive, do another colposcopy. c. Treat any CIN 3. DNA testing for high-risk HPV types. If not high-risk type, may do annual pap.
Abnormal Glandular Cell (AGC)	1. Colposcope all AGC

(2) Triage of Pap abnormalities

(a) ***Refer for colposcopy*** if any of the following are present, even during pregnancy

- **ASC-H**
- **LSIL, HSIL**
- **Squamous cell carcinoma**
- **Atypical glandular/endocervical cells whether or not neoplasia is favored**
- **Adenocarcinoma**

(3) ***CIN system (cervical intraepithelial neoplasia)***

- CIN I: mild dysplasia
- CIN II: moderate dysplasia
- CIN III: severe dysplasia, carcinoma in situ

(4) ***2001 Consensus Guidelines include HPV testing alone or in combination with a cervical cytology test to evaluate a Pap with ASC results.***

b. Diagnostic (e.g. wet mount, colposcopy)

1) Wet mount/wet prep/wet smear

a) Saline allows identification of epithelial cells, white blood cells, red blood cells, yeast, trichomonas, lactobacilli and other bacteria, and clue cells, along with other substances (e.g., oil globules).

b) KOH dissolves everything but yeast

c) Nitrazine paper allows determination of vaginal pH for diagnosis of bacterial vaginosis (BV)

d) Wet mount/wet prep findings

(1) Normal: squamous epithelial cells; lactobacilli; white blood cells; red blood cells

(a) Epithelial cells have smooth borders, few bacteria visible in the cell, and single central nuclei

(b) Lactobacilli are rod shaped organisms; indicative of normal pH; absent or decreased in bacterial vaginosis (BV)

(c) Polymorphonuclear leukocytes in numbers approximately equal to epithelial cells, or 10 per high power field (obviously will differ depending on concentration of suspension); rare in BV, high numbers indicate infection such as trichomonas, chlamydia GC, yeast

(d) If source of red blood cells is not known, further diagnostics are needed

(2) **Abnormal: trichomonads; clue cells; yeast; white blood cells in large numbers; red blood cells source unknown; no lactobacilli**

(a) **Clue cells:** epithelial cells covered with bacteria, presenting an irregular, obscured border; stippled appearance **("salt and pepper")**

(b) **Trichomonads:** motile protozoa; oval, slightly larger than white blood cells, motile; flagellae

(c) **Yeast: spores or hyphae**; spores are clear round or ovoid; hyphae are long tubular, possibly branching structures (may look like plate of spaghetti if heavy)

e) Amine or "whiff test"

(1) A small amount of discharge mixed with KOH and sniffed immediately

(2) Characteristic fishy odor noted in BV or trichomoniasis

f) Evaluating vaginal pH

(1) Normal vaginal pH is 3.8-4.2; maintained by lactobacilli; produce lactic acid and hydrogen peroxide to suppress gram negative and gram positive anaerobes.

(2) pH >4.5 is abnormal, indicating anaerobic organisms associated with BV or trichomoniasis.

2) Colposcopic examination

a) Localizes the source and extent of atypical cells detected by Pap smear

b) The colposcope is a binocular microscope with intense light and magnification

c) Indications for colposcopic examination

(1) Abnormal cervical cytology

(2) Abnormal vaginal cytology

(3) Abnormal looking cervix with or without gross lesions

(4) Post-coital bleeding

(5) DES exposure in utero

(6) Atypical genital warts

d) Colposcopic exam

(1) Systematic inspection of entire cervix and upper vagina

(2) Acetic acid in 3% solution applied to dehydrate the cell cytoplasm and intensify nuclei

(3) Findings recorded in narrative and diagrams indicating abnormal findings and sites of biopsies

(4) Endocervical curettage (not done in pregnancy)

c. Ultrasound

1) Transvaginal ultrasound

a) Determination of uterine fibroids/uterine abnormalities

b) Measurement of endometrial thickness

(1) *Indicated for perimenopausal and postmenopausal women with abnormal vaginal bleeding*

(2) Endometrial thickness correlates with the presence or absence of pathology (however, severity of pathologic changes does not correlate with measured thickness)

(3) Endometrial thickness < 5 mm is reassuring, allowing for conservative management

(4) Endometrial thickness > 4 mm requires endometrial biopsy

(5) Timing of ultrasound for women on hormone replacement therapy with sequential regimen, schedule toward the end of progestin phase or at beginning of cycle

(6) For women with endometrial thickness and atrophic endometrium on biopsy, suspect uterine polyps

(7) Persistent bleeding with normal ultrasonography

(a) Biopsy

(b) Consider hysteroscopy

c) Locate IUD with missing string

d) Evaluate pelvic masses found on bimanual examination, e.g., adnexal mass such as ovarian cyst

e) Establish location and viability of pregnancy in first trimester; establish location of placenta in third trimester

f) Assisted reproductive technology, e.g., documentation of ovulation and retrieval of ova

2) Abdominal ultrasound is used to evaluate many organs, including gall bladder and kidneys

3) Ultrasound of other sites, including evaluation of breast mass or suspected abscess, thyroid nodules, deep vein thrombosis etc.

2. Assessment and management of specific concerns

a. Vaginitis

1) Normal vaginal secretions

a) Cyclic variations in response to estrogen and progesterone fluctuations

b) Secretions begin in cells of the cervix

c) Usually clear to cloudy, nonirritating, may turn yellow after drying

d) Epithelium of vagina is usually moist, adds to cervical secretions

e) Bartholin's glands also add to secretions

f) *Normal vaginal pH is 3.8-4.2*

g) Squamous cells of epithelium contain high content of glycogen, which is metabolized in vagina by *lactobacilli* or *Döderlein's bacilli*; by-product is lactic acid

h) Amount of secretions increases with ovulation, premenstruation, pregnancy, sexual arousal

When one STD is diagnosed or you have a high index of suspicion, investigate for more

2) Normal vaginal flora

a) *Lactobacilli acidophilus* (dominant bacteria)

b) *Staphylococcus epidermidis*

c) *Corynebacteria*

d) Small amounts of *candida species*

e) Anaerobic microorganisms (*bacteroides*, anaerobic lactobacilli)

f) *Escherichia coli* can be found in about 20% of healthy women

g) Usually approximately 5-15 different species of bacteria

3) Prevention of vaginitis

a) Provide the woman with knowledge about her body, normal healthy changes, disease conditions, preventive methods, self treatments and when to seek professional care

b) Habits to increase good general health. (Decreases susceptibility to infection in general)

(1) Avoidance of vulvar and vaginal irritants (e.g. douches)

(2) Wiping anus, perineum, and vulva from front to back to decrease vaginal colonization by *E. Coli*

(3) Avoidance of anaerobic environment (cotton clothing, loose not tight)

(4) Daily bathing/cleaning of genitalia and objects (e.g. diaphragms) in contact with genitalia

(5) Avoid sexual practices that are painful or abrasive

(6) If an infection is potentially a sexually transmitted one:

(a) All partners should be evaluated for "shared" infections or other STDs

(b) Treatments should be completed before sexual activity resumed (at least without a condom)

(c) Condoms offer some protection and can adjunct contraceptive methods and should be encouraged (if she has an STD, she is at risk for others.)

4) Physical examination

a) Abdominal palpation/CVAT to rule out gastrointestinal conditions or UTI

b) Palpation for lymphadenopathy

c) Inspection of entire vulva and vagina

d) Palpation of vulva and vagina for masses and/or tenderness

e) Speculum examination, with inspection of cervix and vaginal walls

f) Wet smear, whiff test, and vaginal pH

g) Bimanual examination

5) Most common vaginal conditions

a) Physiologic secretions

b) Chemical/allergic vaginitis

c) Bacterial vaginosis (most common vaginitis)

d) Candida (Monilia) (second most common vaginitis)

e) Trichomonas vaginalis (third most common vaginitis)

f) Atrophic vaginitis

g) Desquamation vaginitis

h) Mucopurulent cervicitis

6) See table for summary of vaginitis etiology, treatment etc.

Vaginitis	Normal	Chemical/ Allergic	Bacterial Vaginosis	Trichomonas	Candidiasis	Atrophic Vaginitis	Muco-purulent
Etiology	Hormone fluctuation Sexual stimulation	Allergen or chemical exposure	Overgrowth of anaerobic bacteria	Protozoa	*Candida* species	Low estrogen milieu	May be secondary to GC/CT
Color	Clear/ cloudy	Clear/cloudy	Gray/white	Yellow/green	White/yellow	Gray/yellow	Yellow /none
Odor	None	None	"Fishy"	Malodorous	Yeasty	None	None
Consistency	Usually thin	Usually thin	Thin, homogenous	Frothy	Thick plaques	Watery, sticky	NA
Symptom	Variable amt	Burning Tenderness Dyspareunia	Malodorous discharge Pruritus None	Pruritus Burning Dyspareunia None	None Pruritus Burning Dyspareunia	Dyspareunia Burning	Asymptomatic or variable amt of discharge
Physical	None	Erythema, edema	Pooling of discharge at introitus	Erythema, edema, strawberry cervix	Erythema, vaginal plaques, excoriation	Pale, pink vagina, little rugation	Yellow exudate on endocervical swab
Ph	3.8 – 4.2	<4.5	> 4.5	5.2-7.0	<4.5	5.5-7.0	< 4.5
Micro	No pathology	No pathological organism	"Clue cells"	Trichomonad	Pseudohyphae No or few lactobacilli	Epithelial cells round	No clear pathogen
Whiff	Negative	Negative	Positive	Positive	Negative	Negative	Negative
Rx	None indicated	None usually needed	Metronidazole (CDC)	Metronidazole (CDC)	Antifungal (CDC)	Lubricant; estrogen	Depends on etiology (CDC)
Comment	Educate Reassure	Treat palliatively Remove allergen		Remember to treat partner	Ameliorate predisposing conditions	Strategies to increase endogenous lubrication	Need alternative labs (cultures etc.) to screen appropriately

Classic Descriptors For Differential Diagnosis/Treatment Of Vaginal Discharge/Vaginitis
Used with permission M. Brucker, 2003 (adapted for 2005 edition)

a) **Bacterial vaginosis (BV)**

(1) Caused by replacement of normal hydrogen-peroxide producing *Lactobacillus* sp. in the vagina with high concentrations of anaerobic bacteria, e.g., *Prevotella* and *Mobiluncus*, *G. vaginalis*, and *Mycoplasma hominis*.

(2) ACOG recommends diagnosis by presence of **3 of the following four** findings

- **pH >4.5**
- **Clue cells**
- **Positive KOH amine test**
- **Homogenous discharge**.

(3) All women who have **symptomatic disease require treatment** for symptomatic relief and to reduce the risk for infectious complications after abortion, hysterectomy, or birth. Other potential benefits include the reduction of other STDs (e.g., HIV). ***Treatment in pregnancy for asymptomatic women with a history of preterm birth may be beneficial*** (CDC 2002).

(a) ***Usual treatment is Metronidazole 500 mg PO, bid for 7 days or*** Metronidazole gel for 5 days, or
Clindamycin cream for 7 days.

(b) **Alternative treatments are not as effective** Metronidazole orally in a single dose or Clindamycin orally for 7 days or Clindamycin ovules for 3 days. Metronidazole 750 mg (*Flagyl ER)* is FDA approved but not in CDC guidelines

A large multicenter study conducted by NIH failed to find any statistically significant correlation between high or low risk women with asymptomatic BV and poor perinatal outcomes. See Carey, J. et al (2000). Metronidazole to prevent preterm delivery in pregnant women with asymptomatic bacterial vaginosis. The New England Journal of Medicine, 342(8), 534-540

Small studies have found better outcomes if women with asymptomatic BV are treated around the time of conception (as in infertility) -- and high risk women in early 2nd trimester.

Symptomatic women should be treated.

(c) **Note: creams are oil based and should not be used with condoms**

(d) **Treatment of BV in pregnancy is with oral preparations, NOT vaginal. CDC recommendation for pregnancy is**

- **Metronidazole** 250 mg orally three times a day for 7 days or
- **Clindamycin** 300 mg orally twice a day for 7 days.

(e) Metronidazole: Most common side effects are GI, including metallic taste and an ***Antabuse effect***. **Caution to avoid alcohol during treatment and up to 24 hours of completion of therapy.** It is FDA Class B drug for pregnancy and may be prescribed for the breastfeeding woman if needed. Don't use douches with metronidazole, because it works best in anaerobic conditions. Some give metronidazole intravaginally to avoid GI symptoms. Up to 10% of women report a candida infection after treatment with Metronidazole.

(4) **Treatment not recommended for asymptomatic women**

(5) Treatment not recommended for sexual partner

(6) *Advise women to return for follow-up in 1-2 weeks if no relief* after treatment: most common reason for lack of relief is another condition previously obscured by BV. Also, consider alcohol dependence screen for woman with repeated treatment failure – she may not be able to adhere to metronidazole regimen.

b) Trichomoniasis

(1) ***Recurrent infection***: establish a positive diagnosis (i.e., repeat examination and wet smear). Obtain treatment history of her and her partner(s).

- If *trichomonas vaginalis* is still present and partner(s) did not complete treatment; both (all) partners may be retreated.
- Persistent *trichomonas vaginalis* is possible but rare; resistant strains are evolving, however. Consultation with an expert for persistent treatment failures. (Repeated treatments with metronidazole should not be undertaken without consultation since leukopenia may result.)
- **Women on phenobarbital and phenytoin may detoxify metronidazole so rapidly that they need higher doses for cures, and they may be among the treatment failures.**
- Also, consider alcohol dependence as a factor in failure to adhere to treatment in woman or partner(s).

(2) Trichomoniasis and pregnancy: treatment of asymptomatic trichomoniasis in pregnancy does not prevent preterm delivery and routine screening and treatment is not recommended (Klebanoff, M. et al., (2001).

- Failure of metronidazole to prevent preterm delivery among pregnant women with asymptomatic *Trichomonas vaginalis* infection. New England Journal of Medicine, 345(7), 487-93.) ***Symptomatic pregnant women should be treated.***

(3) Treatment (CDC 2002)

- ***Recommended:*** **Metronidazole** orally in a single dose.
- ***Alternative:*** **Metronidazole orally** for 7 days

c) **Vulvovaginal Candidiasis** (Candida, Monilia, Yeast, VVC)

(1) Usually caused by *C. albicans* but may be caused by other *Candida*., e.g., *C. tropicalis* and *C. glabrata*.

(2) CDC, 2002 classifications of VVC

http://www.cdc.gov/std/treatment/5-2002TG.htm#VulvovaginalCandidiasis

Uncomplicated VVC	Complicated VVC
• Sporadic or infrequent vulvovaginal candidiasis **OR** • Mild-to-moderate vulvovaginal candidiasis **OR** • Likely to be *C. albicans* **OR** • Non-immunocompromised women	• Recurrent vulvovaginal candidiasis **OR** • Severe vulvovaginal candidiasis **OR** • Non-albicans candidiasis **OR** • Women with uncontrolled diabetes, debilitation, or immunosuppression ***or those who are pregnant***

(3) Treatment of Candidiasis:

- Treatment of asymptomatic candidiasis is not necessary; in a minority of asymptomatic *Candida* colonization, antibiotic use precipitates VVC.
- Short-course topical formulations (i.e., single dose and regimens of 1--3 days, topical or oral) for uncomplicated VVC.
- Note that pregnancy qualifies as complicated VVC.
- Examples of acceptable treatments for uncomplicated VVC (not exhaustive for regimens):
  - **Butoconazole** intravaginally for 3 days
  - **Clotrimazole** intravaginally for 7--14 days
  - **Nystatin** vaginal tablets for 14 days
  - **Tioconazole** ointment intravaginally in a single application
  - **Terconazole** cream intravaginally for 7 days

Oral Agent:

- **Fluconazole** oral tablet, one in single dose.

(4) Complicated VVC

(a) **Recurrent VVC***:* four or more symptomatic episodes per year. Most women have no apparent predisposing or underlying conditions. Vaginal cultures should be obtained to confirm the clinical diagnosis and identify non-albicans species, particularly *Candida glabrata* (***C. glabrata does not form pseudohyphae or hyphae and is not easily recognized on microscopy***). Conventional therapies are not as effective against these species.

(b) **Treatment: longer duration of initial therapy (e.g., 7--14 days of topical therapy or a 150-mg, oral dose of fluconazole repeated 3 days later).**

(c) Maintenance antifungals are given for 6 months. Patients receiving long-term ketoconazole should be monitored for toxicity.

(d) **Severe VVC:** extensive vulvar erythema, edema, excoriation, and fissure formation. Give either 7--14 days of topical azole or fluconazole in two sequential doses (second dose 72 hours after initial dose).

(e) **Non-albicans VVC: O**ptimal treatment is unknown. Longer duration of therapy (7--14 days) with a non-fluconazole azole drug is recommended as first-line therapy. For recurrence, give boric acid in a gelatin capsule vaginally for 2 weeks. Referral may be indicated if not effective. If non-*albicans* VVC continues to recur, a maintenance regimen of intravaginal nystatin has been successful.

(f) **Compromised host:** debilitating medical conditions (e.g., uncontrolled diabetes, receiving corticosteroid treatment), immunosuppressed women do not respond as well to short-term therapies. Correct modifiable conditions; more prolonged (i.e., 7--14 days) conventional antimycotic treatment is necessary.

(g) **Pregnancy:** ***Only topical azole therapies, applied for 7 days, are recommended for use among pregnant women.***

d) Desquamation vaginitis; Desquamative inflammatory vaginitis: Diagnosis of exclusion.

- May be a bacterial superinfection or a bacterial vaginitis (as opposed to vaginosis, which is not inflammatory).
- Recurrent vaginitis among predominantly perimenopausal women. Occasional vaginal or cervical spotted rash, vaginal cell exfoliation; pH is elevated.
- No pathogens can be identified.
- Pap may report increased parabasal cells; Gram stain may have increased gram positive cocci and decreased gram positive bacilli.
- Treatment is empiric with Clindamycin cream.

b. Signs/symptoms of menopause (climacteric)

1) Women in the US now live one-third of their lives after menopause

a) In 2000, it is estimated that 31.2 million women will be over age 55 and entering, or have entered menopause; increase of 85% over the last 20 years

2) Onset*: Average age of Menopause is 51:* smoking ↓ mean age of menopause

3) Definition: **loss of ovarian activity**
   a) Retrospective diagnosis--12 months usually after last menses
   b) Permanent cessation of menstruation resulting from loss of ovarian activity according to WHO.
   c) In USA, usually about the age of 49-52
   d) **Perimenopause**: loosely defined; usually associated with symptomatic events (e.g. vasomotor instability)
      (1) Some sources may suggest it is more than a decade, if one considers various physiologic changes that may be asymptomatic
      (2) Others say 4-5 years before menopause
      (3) According to WHO ends 12 months after the menopause
      (4) Massachusetts Women's Health Study found median age of inception of perimenopause (most commonly irregular menses) at 47.5 years
   e) **Postmenopause**
      (1) Period beginning 12 months after menopause
      (2) Approximately 1/3 of a woman's life

Common Perimenopausal Symptoms

- Irregular Bleeding
- Vaginal Dryness
- Heavy Bleeding
- Hot Flashes/Flushes
- Night Sweats

4) **Types of menopause**
   a) Atresia (normal biology)
   b) Surgical removal through bilateral oophorectomy (also ovariectomy), usually at time of hysterectomy and salpingectomy (debate--some surgeons will question why risk ovarian cancer by leaving ovaries behind.)
   c) Premature ovarian failure (before age 40) unknown etiology but may be autoimmune disorder
   d) Trauma (e.g. loss of blood to ovarian circulation)
5) **Factors influencing age at menopause**
   a) Smoking (inverse relationship between amount and age at menopause)
   b) Other factors less clear (including familial pattern, age at menarche, race, use of oral contraceptives, nutrition, parity)
   c) Earlier menopause for nulliparas; women exposed to toxic chemicals; and those treated medically for depression
6) **Menopausal changes/symptoms**
   a) For many women changes in menstrual cycles may be first sign of hormonal fluctuations (oligomenorrhea, dysfunctional uterine bleeding, amenorrhea)

b) Other later menstrual events
   (1) Follicles develop more rapidly in response to increased FSH
   (2) Dizygotic twinning peaks at age 37
   (3) From ages 38-42 ovulation becomes less common

c) Symptoms/signs: remember that you can find ***clinical changes anywhere estrogen receptors (alpha and beta) exist***
   (1) Reproductive system changes:
      (a) Decrease in size of uterus
      (b) Atrophy of endometrium
      (c) Vaginal epithelium becomes thinner (maturation index changes); no superficial cells, more intermediate and parabasal cells
      (d) Walls of vagina become thinner, smoother, drier and less elastic
      (e) Less rugae and paler
      (f) Dyspareunia, bleeding, irritation, dryness
      (g) Alterations in menstruation
         - Changes in cycle
         - Dysfunctional uterine bleeding
         - Sometimes first sign of perimenopause
      (h) Cervix becomes contiguous with vaginal walls and smaller in size
         - Os often stenotic
         - Transitional zone recedes
         - Mucus decreases
   (2) Vulvar changes during menopause
         - Less skin elasticity
         - Less subcutaneous fat
         - Pubic hair thins and often grays
   (3) Urinary system alterations during menopause
      (a) Atrophic distal urethritis/other bladder changes since bladder has transitional epithelial sensitive to estrogen
      (b) Cystitis symptoms
      (c) *Urge and stress incontinence*
         Urge--detrusor muscle change; more clearly linked to menopause and relationship to estrogen
         Stress--usually weakness of muscles secondary to obesity, multiparity; some link with estrogen

(4) **Bone changes** during menopause
  (a) Osteoporosis/osteopenia
  (b) Alveolar (oral) bone loss

(5) **Skin changes** during menopause
  (a) Thinning of epidermis and increase in wrinkles
  (b) 30% of skin collagen lost within first 5 years
  (c) Hyperpigmentation (senile lentigo)
  (d) Decrease in activity of sebaceous and sweat glands
  (e) Thinning of hair on head, pubis and axilla
  (f) With increased adrenocortical activity, hair follicles (e.g., on face), once stimulated will continue

(6) **Vasomotor instability: hot flash or flush, palpitations**
  (a) Hypothalamic neurons--produce GnRH and the anterior hypothalamic nuclei regulate body temperature (close proximity)
  (b) Neurotransmitter signals with GnRH release may trigger hypothalamic nuclei
  (c) Brain has estrogen receptors associated with cerebral blood flow, glucose administration and cognition
  (d) Incidence 50-85%
  (e) May be initiated by LH surge (or LH surge may be consequence of hot flush)
  (f) ***Triggered by a variety of stimuli; alcohol, spicy foods, hot weather, emotional distress or even a warm room***
  (g) Fairly common as "night sweats"

(7) **Sleep alterations** during menopause
  (a) Increased time to onset of sleep
  (b) Decreased REM sleep

(8) **Sexuality changes** during menopause
  (a) Slower and less vaginal lubrication
  (b) Decreased vaginal elasticity
  (c) Major changes occur with male sexual response, which may, in turn, affect women.
  (d) No data on aging lesbians

(9) **Migraines tend to be exacerbated** since estrogen and progesterone affect central serotoninergic and opioid neurons

(10) **Vision changes** during menopause

(a) Eye is rich with alpha estrogen receptors premenopause

(b) Not found in such abundance post menopause

(11) **Weight/metabolic changes** during menopause

(a) ***More likely to develop central obesity*** (apple versus pear shape)

(b) Less lean body mass

(c) Insulin resistance

(12) Others

(a) Some other symptoms are less clear if related to menopause or to other issues like empty nest and midlife crisis

(b) Depression: ***menopause not associated with major psychological illness***, including depression, but is associated with mood swings

(13) Breast changes--may be aging as opposed to menopause

(a) Reduced fat and lobular size

(b) More flattened appearance

d) Health risks in aging women

- **Number 1 cause of death in woman in the United States is *heart disease***
- **Cancer deaths**

Type of Cancer	**Estimated for 2003 by American Cancer Society**	
	Estimated New Cases	**Estimated Deaths**
Breast	211,300	39,800
Lung	**80,100**	**68,800**
Colon/rectal	74,700	28,850
Uterine	40,100	6,800
Ovarian	25,400	14,300
Pancreas	15,800	15,300
Bladder	15,200	3,900
Cervix	12,200	4,100

- **Diabetes Mellitus**
  - Seems to increase risk of coronary artery disease to a higher extent in women
  - Presence of diabetes is the single most powerful predictor of coronary artery disease in women
  - As women age, we become more insulin resistant (80-90% noninsulin dependent)
  - Diabetes is increasing, especially as population is aging and become more overweight

e) Some general comments for care providers for perimenopausal/menopausal women

(1) Be holistic

(2) Beware of ageism

(3) Teach health promotion

f) General health screening (see Chapter I Primary Care)

(1) Presbyopia

(2) Hearing

(3) Mammograms

(4) Dental assessments

g) Health promotion for perimenopausal/menopausal women

(1) Calcium intake 1000 mg/day between 31 and 50 years of age
1200 mg/day after age 50

(2) Add resistance training and weight bearing exercises

(3) Women at high risk for cardiovascular events (e.g. by lipid profile)

(4) Moderate alcohol consumption

(5) Remember dental health

(6) Practice Kegel exercises

(7) Vitamin D, especially if age >70 and in northern climate if diet inadequate
For all women 80 or older (800 units daily)

(8) Be aware of drug to drug interactions, including OTC

(9) Be careful—safety and injury prevention is important

(10)Sexuality is an important component of mental and physical health (70% of women aged 45 to 54 are sexually active)

(11)Avoid sun (squamous cell epithelioma is most common among older adults)

(12)Have advance directives and living wills

(13)Stop smoking!

Approximate Ages	35-45 Years	46-50 Years	51-55 Years	56-65 Years	66-75 Years
	Initial Changes	*Fluctuating Hormones*	*Short Term Effect of Estrogen Decrease*	*Long Term Effects of Estrogen Decrease*	*Longer Term Effects of Estrogen Decrease*
Physiology	Fluctuating estrogens ↑FSH Rapid follicular development	↓ Estradiol ↑ FSH Less LH surge Irregular ovulation	↑ FSH and LH No LH surge Anovulation	Anovulation	Anovulation
Menstrual Changes	Shortened cycle	Irregular cycle	Cessation	----	----
Emotional Changes	Mood Swings Irritability Anxiety	Mood swings Irritability Tension Anxiety	Mood swings Irritability Tension Anxiety	Mood depression (Somewhat controversial)	----
Sleep Disturbances	Fatigue	Fatigue Early waking	Fatigue Early waking Insomnia	Fatigue	---
Vasomotor Changes	Generalized sweating	Hot flashes/ flushes Night Sweats Palpitations	Hot flashes/ flushes Night Sweats Palpitations	---	---
Urogenital	---	Vaginal Dryness Dyspareunia	Vaginal Dryness Dyspareunia Cystitis/ Urethritis Stress incontinence Urge incontinence Vaginitis	Vaginal Dryness Dyspareunia Cystitis/ Urethritis Stress incontinence Urge incontinence Vaginitis	Vaginal dryness Dyspareunia Cystitis/ Urethritis Stress incontinence Urge incontinence Vaginitis
Other Alterations	---	---	Muscle/joint pain Paresthesias	Muscle/joint pain Paresthesias Heart Disease Osteoporosis	Muscle/joint pain Paresthesias Heart Disease Osteoporosis

Adapted from Moore, A & Noonan, M. (1996). A Nurse's guide to hormone replacement therapy. JOGNN, 25(1), 24-31

c. **Hormone replacement therapy (HRT), includes alternative therapies**

1) **Hormone replacement therapy** (HRT) = replacement of estrogen and progesterone

   Estrogen replacement therapy (ERT) = replacement of estrogen only.

   - Not appropriate for women who still have their uterus, as unopposed estrogen causes endometrial hyperplasia which may progress to endometrial cancer (whether exogenous as in ERT or endogenous as in anovulation).

2) **Potential increased health risks in women on HRT based on the Women's Health Initiative (WHI) study and others were**

   - Coronary heart disease
   - Breast cancer
   - Pulmonary emboli
   - Stroke

3) Benefits of HRT were:

- Decreased risk of colorectal cancer
- Decreased risk of endometrial cancer
- Decreased risk of hip fractures.
- Combined HRT seemed to increase the risk of ovarian cancer for the first 2 years and then ultimately decreased the risk below that for women who did not use HRT.

4) Contraindications for HRT include:

- Thromboembolic disorders
- Breast cancer
- Estrogen dependent cancer
- Liver disease
- Pregnancy

5) The upshot of the HRT studies is that long term ***combined HRT must be prescribed for individual women based on their history, needs, and risks; it should be used only for relief of vasomotor symptoms and only for the shortest time possible.*** Older women and those with heart disease, increased breast cancer risk or other chronic medical conditions might benefit from lower doses of HRT, natural hormones, or alternative therapeutic regimens for specific indications.

6) Recommendations:

- ❖ HRT is not indicated to treat/prevent coronary heart disease
- ❖ ***HRT may be indicated for certain women with vasomotor symptoms, and should be used no longer than 5 years.***
- ❖ The progestins/progesterone norethindrone acetate, norgestimate, or prometrium should be used instead of MPA.
- ❖ The lowest effective doses of hormones should be used.
- ❖ Nonhormonal therapies such as bisphosphonates and SERMS should be used for osteoporosis prevention/treatment
- ❖ Other traditional measures for osteoporosis prevention should be advised, e.g., aerobic and weight bearing exercise, calcium, vitamin D, no smoking, moderate or no alcohol
- ❖ Annual clinician breast exams and mammography are essential; women should perform BSE
- ❖ ***Local therapy for vaginal atrophy and dyspareunia***, including estrogen creams, should be used, but not systemic hormone therapy

Pharmacologic alternatives to HRT for treatment of vasomotor instability in menopause

Drug	Brand Name	Route	Side Effects	Comments
Clonidine.	*Catapres®*	Oral Patch	Nausea, vomiting, dry mouth, constipation, nervousness, agitation, hypotension, dizziness, drowsiness, fatigue, sedation, weakness, decreased libido	Antihypertensive. May be enhanced by low dose DHEA supplements. Limited evidence; side effects may outweigh benefits.
Gabapentin	*Neurontin®*	Oral	Nausea, tremor, drowsiness, blurred vision, lack of muscular coordination	Antiseizure drug. FDA approved for treatment of hot flashes; 50-70% reduction in hot flashes.
SSRIs: Venlafaxine Fluoxetine	 *Effexor®* *Prozac®*	Oral	Nausea, dry mouth, drowsiness, dizziness for venlafaxine; Nausea, decreased libido, dry mouth, weight gain, headaches for fluoxetine	50-80% reduction in hot flashes
Bellergal, danazol, tranquilizers, sedatives		Oral		

7) Therapy for vaginal dryness and urinary symptoms

- Phytoestrogens
- Kegel exercises
- Water soluble lubricants
- Calendula officinalis (English Marigold) as lubricant
- Vegetable oils

8) For lethargy, mood changes

> Warn women not to use topical estrogen as lubricant during intercourse as it can be absorbed by partner.

- Phytoestrogens
- Moderate exercise
- Stress reduction
- Anxiety has been suggested to be treated with physical exercise and evening primrose capsules
- Vitamin B (especially For irritability, mild depression)
- Chamomile tea or valerian tea for insomnia

9) For dry skin

- Moisturizing creams and oils
- Phytoestrogens
- Avoidance of direct sun (except for short periods for Vitamin D)
- Humidified air

10) For prevention or treatment of osteoporosis

- Phytoestrogens
- Calcium (questionable without estrogen)
- Exercise
- Other pharmaceuticals such as bisphosphonates and SERMs

11) For reduction of coronary heart disease
    - Phytoestrogens
    - Healthy diet, no smoking, exercise
    - Low dose aspirin
    - Vitamin E
    - Beta carotene
12) Herbs to avoid: belladonna, blue cohosh, borage, chaparral, comfrey, ephedra
13) **Some other thoughts on perimenopausal symptoms**
    a) Consider use of low dose oral contraceptives, 20-30 mcg estrogen if not smoking
    b) If so, when to move to HRT (assuming it is desired or needed)
        (1) Commonly done at age 55 since majority of women are menopausal by then.
        (2) Some providers use any of the following parameters (but none are required and or necessary)
        (3) Measure FSH annually beginning at age 50
        (4) Measure on day 6 or 7 of inert pills--or day before new cycle starts
        (5) FSH>30 mIU/mL on day 6 or 7, assume menopause
        (6) FSH/LH ratio >1:3
14) Contraceptive issues for the perimenopausal woman
    a) 21% of women in the US between the ages of 40 and 44 use no method of contraception (higher than any other age group, including adolescents)
    b) Abortion ratio (no. of abortions per 1000 live births) is second only to adolescents under the age of 15
    c) 75 % of women over age 40 who get pregnant do so unintentionally
    d) Pregnancy related mortality is directly related to age, with a jump at age 30-34 (note that birth rates among US women aged 35 to 44 years of age have doubled over the last two decades)
    e) HRT does not provide contraceptive protection
    f) A woman on a progestin only contraceptive has a pregnancy rate of 2% during the ages of 35-39; but 0.3% for 40 and over

d. Sexuality

1) Barriers to sexual health assessment
    a) Not seeing the woman's sexual history as relevant: In reality, without detailed sexual histories, conditions may go untreated or treatment options might be overlooked.
    b) Inadequate training
    c) Embarrassment
    d) Fear of offending

2) Prevalence of sexual dysfunction

a) In a survey of 1749 women and 1410 men aged 18-59, 10-52% of men and 25-63% of women reported sexual dysfunction

b) In men 40-70, 34% have moderate to complete erectile dysfunction

c) Female dysfunction is more prevalent than male

d) Sexual problems in women decrease with age

e) Increased age of men positively associated with problems

f) Non-married women 1.5 times more likely to have sexual anxiety and trouble achieving orgasm than married women

g) Men and women who are more educated have less sexual dysfunction

h) Black women tend to have higher rates of lower sexual desire

i) White women reported more sexual pain

j) Hispanic women reported lower rates of sexual problems

3) Female anatomy and physiology

a) The vagina

(1) Mucosa, muscle and fibrous layers and lined with squamous epithelium

(2) Mucosa holds blood vessels and muscular layer holds nerves

(3) Fibrous tissue contain collagen and elastin which allow for expansion of vault

(4) Uterine, pudendal and clitoral arteries provide blood supply

(5) Numerous nerves innervate-play major role in sexual function

(6) Vestibular bulbs of erectile tissue surround vaginal and introital area

b) The clitoris is composed of three parts: glans, body, and crura

(1) Composed of two corpora cavernosa surrounded by a fibrous sheath and smooth muscle

(2) Common clitoral and perineal arteries supply

(3) Pelvic nerve stimulation causes vaginal and clitoral smooth muscle relaxation which results in increased blood flow, increased cavernosal artery inflow, increased clitoral intra-cavernous pressure, tumescence and erection of the clitoris

(4) Spinal nerve innervation at L5-S1, S2-4, T12-L4

(5) Sensory pathways for clitoral stimulation from pudendal nerve

c) Stages of female sexual response (as described by Masters and Johnson; there are other models)

(1) Excitement

(2) Plateau

(3) Orgasm

(4) Resolution

d) Summary of the female sexual response cycle

According to Masters and Johnson (1966) there are three patterns of female sexual response: the single orgasm response, the multiple orgasm, and resolution without orgasm. The Kaplan Model (1979) describes the sexual response cycle in three phases: desire (mind), excitement and orgasm (genitals).

e) Sexual life cycle changes

(1) Adolescence

(a) Sexuality becomes differentiated (directed toward male or female)

(b) Masturbation becomes important expression of sexuality to boys and many girls

(c) May experience a sexual relationship with another person

(d) Statistics/trends (Youngkin & Davis, 2004)

- 8 in 10 girls are sexually inexperienced at age 15
- 40% 15-19 year olds have had sexual intercourse
- 25-42% teenage women report unwanted sexual experiences
- The younger women are at first coitus, the more likely it was to be unwanted or involuntary
- Women who begin sexual activity at an early age have more lifetime partners
- **Teens have higher rates of the most common STDs than older women**
- ***Teen pregnancy rates are declining, but 78% of teen pregnancies are unplanned***

(e) Topics to be addressed with teens

- STDs
- Contraception
- Sexual intercourse and its place in the teen's life
- Other types of sexual expression
- Satisfaction with one's sexuality
- Choosing a partner (Hatcher 2004)

(f) **Counseling considerations with adolescents (Hatcher 2004)**

- Age 12-14: very concrete, egocentric and concerned with physical appearance and acceptance. Short attention span.
- Age 14-15: Peer oriented; resist authority; limited image of future.
- Age 16-17: developing logical thought processes, goals for future.

(2) The childbearing woman: Pregnancy

(a) 1st trimester: nulliparous women reported decreased libido and decreased sexual response; parous women noted no change

- ➢ Breast tenderness, nausea, fatigue disturb contribute to decreased libido.
- ➢ Fear by both partners of harming mother or fetus

(b) 2nd trimester: arousal, sexual activity and response increased in nulliparas and multiparas

- ➢ Change in positions may be needed

(c) Frequency of coitus decreases as pregnancy approaches full term

(d) M&J reported some women orgasmic for the first time in pregnancy, probably because of increased pelvic congestion. Some orgasmic women became multiorgasmic in pregnancy.

(e) Increased vaginal discharge in pregnancy

(f) Postpartum: Initial decrease in interest due to fatigue, pain, weakness. A fear of physical harm from return to intercourse too soon was expressed. Arousal and activity increased especially among breast feeding mothers.

(g) Most women resume intercourse in 3-4 weeks after delivery

(h) Decreased steroids postpartum can decrease vaginal lubrication, so advise:

- ➢ Use of lubricants
- ➢ Kegel exercises
- ➢ Contraception

(i) Lactation may induce erotic feelings; breast stimulation and orgasm may cause let-down to occur.

(3) Early adulthood (20-45)

(a) Woman achieves maturity in sexual role and relationship tasks started in adolescence (intimacy, long term relationship)

(b) Choose sexual lifestyle, often experiment before settling down

(c) Decisions about childbearing

(d) Frequency of intercourse declines as she ages

(4) Midlife woman (45-65)

(a) Sexuality is varied; some report sex is best ever while others report sex is not as exciting or gratifying

(b) Physiologic changes of menopause may affect desire, expression and functioning; sex drive may decrease; decreased vaginal lubrication, vaginal dryness, dyspareunia, vaginal muscle spasms, diminished genital sensations and orgasms possible

(c) Other women report the opposite – increased clitoral sensitivity, increased responsiveness and more intense orgasms

(d) When fear of accidental pregnancy is gone, may be less inhibited; also having no child care and privacy in the home may enhance expression

(5) Older adulthood (after age 65)

(a) Sexual frequency may decline, though many continue to be sexual and enjoy sexual activity

(b) Availability of a partner is an important factor that limits many older women's sexual function

(c) Stressors that may decrease libido include role changes

(d) Societal expectations may negatively affect sexual expression

(e) Irritation or discomfort with penetration may reduce desire (vaginal dryness, genital atrophy, loss of fat pad on mons and labia); orgasm may be painful

(f) More time available for sexual expression with reduced family and career responsibilities

(g) Drugs for chronic conditions may alter sexual response

(6) Masters and Johnson

(a) Women can remain sexually active entire life and have no decline in orgasmic potential

(b) *The best insurance for sexual activity in later years is frequent sexual activity between 20-40*

(c) Sexual activity mitigates many involutional changes caused by decreased sex steroids

(d) Changes in sexual response with aging do not mean decreased functioning

(e) Longer foreplay is required in aging women for clitoral response.

(7) Lesbian women

(a) 2% to 12% of women are lesbian

(b) Many are bisexual and approximately 80% have had heterosexual experience

(c) Compared to general female population, lesbians have a decreased risk for HIV, CIN, and STDs like chlamydia, gonorrhea and syphilis. Should still check for STDs.

(d) Same risk for BV, monilia and herpes

(e) 5 to 7 times increased risk for alcohol abuse

(f) Many have history of sexual abuse

(g) Management

- Create a supportive environment
- Use gender-free language
- Do not forget to screen for current domestic or partner abuse
- Discuss safer sex techniques as well as sex toy maintenance and sanitation.

f) Cultural factors

(1) Be aware that there are differences among cultures regarding sexual practices, expectations, and comfort in discussing sexuality

(2) Examples – earlier marriage and childbearing, arranged marriages, prohibitions regarding contraception, coitus during menses and postpartum, female circumcision/genital mutilation, role expectations for men and women, religious proscriptions, etc.

g) **Sexual problems and concerns**

(1)***Desire phase***

(a) Differences in sexual interest levels of partners

(b) Psychiatric disorders such as depression

(c) Deviance from the norm-aversion or addiction

(d) Physical or emotional stress

(e) Medications

(f) Poor nutrition

(g) Alcohol and substance abuse

(h) Illness

(i) Body image

(j) Social conditioning

(k) Fatigue

(l) Hostility

(m) Monotony or boredom

(2) ***Arousal phase:*** Inability to achieve physiologic arousal

(a) Anxiety and depression are major contributors

(b) Longer foreplay is required in aging women

(3) Organsmic phase: Inability to experience orgasm

(a) ***Primary anorgasmia-*** an individual who has never experienced orgasm under any circumstances, despite normal sexual arousal. Could be physical; i.e. a condition of the pubococcygeus muscle or hormonal.

(b) ***Secondary anorgasmia-*** absence of orgasm that occurs after a history of orgasmic response. May be situational (orgasm occurs during masturbation, but not with partner; or random-not having orgasm with enough regularity to satisfy their own sense of what is desirable). According to Morokoff, the various physiological and psychological factors that affect a woman's ability to achieve orgasm cannot be separated from the cultural expectations of the ways in which orgasm will occur, if it is expected to occur at all.

(c) ***Determinants of female orgasm include***

a. Educational and social level

b. Religious background

c. Childhood experiences

d. Sexual techniques

e. Illness, depression

f. Medication, alcohol

g. Hormonal changes

(4) Sexually associated pain

(a) Vaginismus: painful involuntary spasm of pubococcygeal muscles upon attempted vaginal penetration

(b) Dyspareunia-painful intercourse considered to physiological in nature until proven otherwise

(c) Pain causes loss of vaginal lubrication which causes further pain

(d) Physical causes include scarring, imperforate hymen, genital infection, endometriosis, pelvic masses, PID, ectopic pregnancy, episiotomy pain and hormonal insufficiency

h) Sexual health assessment

(1) Past problems with sex, risk of acquiring the HIV, present sexual satisfaction, and questions. (Hatcher states that if you have time for only one question the **most important question to ask every woman is "What do you do to protect yourself from AIDS?")**

(2) Setting and confidentiality-utmost importance

(3) Attitude of midwife

(a) **Legitimization**-the midwife establishes her right to ask questions of a sexual nature

(b) **Acceptance-**Do not make judgments about what people do or do not do.

(c) Maintain eye contact with client

(d) Maintain facial expressions of approval

(e) Maintain an even tone of voice

(f) Maintain a posture showing interest (lean toward woman not away from her)

(g) Use open-ended questions that begin with what, how, when and who.

(h) **Universalization-**demonstrating in your questions that there is a wide range of sexual expression

(i) Language-Do not use gender specific language

(j) Avoid slang and medical jargon-use simple words and phrases that would not be misunderstood

(k) Use language that matches the level of woman

(l) Inform woman in advance that she will be asked questions about sexuality and sexual expression and that she may "pass" on anything she chooses not to answer.

4) **Responding to an identified sexual problem**

a) Obtain a thorough health and sexual history

b) Perform physical and pelvic exam to rule out infection, abnormal anatomy, etc.

5) **The PLISSIT Counseling Model** was developed for health care workers who are not trained counselors or sex therapists.

P **Permission** Giving: Allows the woman to discuss her concerns in a nonjudgmental atmosphere.

LI **Limited information**: The health care provider provides basic information addressing the woman's concerns, such as anatomy and dispelling sexual myths

SS **Specific suggestions**: Providing specific suggestions, such as use of vaginal lubrication or position changes.

IT **Intensive therapy**: Refer unless qualified to address problems identified; intensive therapy is indicated when severe emotional or psychological issues underlie a sexual concern or dysfunction.

e. **Sexual abuse/sexual assault**

1) **Sexual harassment:** unwelcome sexual advances, requests for sexual favors, and other oral or physical conduct or written communications of an intimidating, hostile, or offensive nature or action taken in retaliation for reporting such behavior regardless of where such conduct may occur (US Equal Opportunities Commission, 2002 in Youngkin and Davis)

a) Many women do not report because they would rather stop the behavior than punish the perpetrator.

b) Woman may have inability to concentrate, reduced confidence, decreased job motivation, stress, anger, fear, helplessness

c) Physical complaints: nausea, anorexia, headaches, chest pain, chronic fatigue, alcohol abuse or abuse of prescription or non prescription drugs to relieve stress.

d) Do complete history and physical

e) Differentials: depression, chronic fatigue syndrome, gastroenteritis, dyspepsia, ulcers, migraine or cluster headaches, panic or anxiety attacks, stress

f) Plan: give information about effects of harassment, including impact on marital and family life. Validate and support self esteem. Discuss options. Encourage assertiveness training. Refer for psychotherapy or legal assistance if needed.

2) **Sexual abuse; sexual assault; rape**

a) **Rape: forced sexual intercourse perpetrated against the will of a person. Force may be physical violence, coercion, or threat of harm.**

(1) **Acquaintance rape** usually occurs in a dating context and is perpetrated by someone the victim knows and trusts.

(2) **Sexual assault involves actions other than rape,** e.g., sodomy (forced anal intercourse), oral copulation (forced copulation of the victim's mouth with the sexual organ or anus), rape with an object (forced penetration of vagina or anus with a foreign object), and sexual battery (unwanted touching of an intimate body area for sexual arousal).

b) **Midwife may be required by law to report rape/sexual assault**

c) **Incidence**: one of most frequently committed and underreported violent crimes in the US
    (1) More likely to report the rape if assailant is a stranger
    (2) Occurs at all ages, but very young, adolescents, very old and mentally handicapped are the most vulnerable
    (3) **600,000 Sexual Assaults per year in the US** (FBI statistics 2005)
    (4) 5-10% result in pregnancy

d) **Rape-trauma syndrome**: Response of women to assault
    (1) Similar to post-traumatic stress disorder (PTSD); 2 or 3 phases depending on author
    (2) **Acute Phase:** Immediately after assault or disclosure of assault. Lasts hours to 3-6 months; lifestyle is disrupted; anxiety, fears, phobias, suspiciousness, depression, feelings of inferiority, cognitive dysfunction; guilt, shame, embarrassment, self blame are common. Disturbances of eating, sleeping, GI function, sexual intimacy. Physical trauma in 67%, so woman may need medical care. Needs safety and to regain control over life.
    (3) **Readjustment phase:** period of transmission; woman rationalizes that she might have been able to prevent the assault and makes unrealistic plans to prevent another.
    (4) **Reorganization Phase:** may last 2 years or more; flashbacks and nightmares; survivor deals with the reality of her experience and may make lifestyle changes, including relationships and work.

e) Acute stress disorder is similar to PTSD but is confined to a time period of at least 2 days and not longer than four weeks following the traumatic event.

3) Components of care

a) **Explore history of sexual abuse any time woman presents with multiple physical complaints**

b) **If assault occurred within 72 hours, *refer to designated sexual assault center with trained sexual assault examiners for assessment***

c) **Symptoms of sexual assault may be:** headaches, sleep disturbance, weight gain or loss, eating disorder, GI symptoms, sexual dysfunction, menstrual irregularities, vaginitis, urinary symptoms. Relationship, work, school problems.

d) Record details of assault
    (1) Use anatomical drawings
    (2) Document penetration, digital manipulation, use of foreign objects
    (3) Document use of foam or condoms

(4) Ejaculation; also document any victim activities that may have altered the findings (e.g. douching, bathing, wiping, dental hygiene)

e) Past medical history with immunizations and HIV status, alcohol or drug dependence

f) Ob and gyn history with sexual activity. The forensic exam should be done with someone who has specialized training.

g) Social history with living situation, support system, need for legal, social, psychiatric assistance etc

h) Thorough physical exam and STD testing (obtain consent prior to the exam).

(1) Disrobe standing on a sheet to collect evidence

(2) Put clothes in a labeled paper bag

i) Inspect entire body; use Wood's Lamp to examine for body fluids; photograph trauma

j) Treat injuries

k) Diagnose and treat STDs, including vaginitis

l) Vaginal smear for sperm

m) Collect Fingernail scrapings, hair samples, blood or fluid on the body

n) **Emergency contraception as appropriate** (i.e., within time frame, no contraindications and pregnancy does not already exist)

o) Offer antibiotic prophylaxis for chlamydia, gonorrhea, syphilis, trichomonads; if refused, be sure to do follow up cultures

p) Follow up in 24-48 hours with phone call, in a week to evaluate psychological status, and at 4-6 weeks for repeat testing for STDs and pregnancy. Refer as needed for community services and mental health care.

D. Assessment and management of deviations from normal; indications for consultation, co-management or referral

1. Amenorrhea: absence of menses

a. Definitions

1) Primary amenorrhea:

a) No menses by age 14 in the absence of growth or development of secondary sexual characteristics

b) No menses by age 16 regardless of the presence of normal growth and development with the appearance of secondary sexual characteristics

2) Secondary amenorrhea: In a woman who has been menstruating, the absence of a period for 3 cycle intervals or 6 months duration.

b. Causes of amenorrhea:

1) Physiologic: pregnancy, lactation, menopause
2) Anatomic defects (patency and continuity of outflow tract; development of endometrium lining)
3) Genetic disorders

➢ **Turner's syndrome**

- Absence of one X chromosome
- 45 XO
- Congenital ovarian failure ("streak ovaries")
- Short stature, broad chest, webbed neck
- Infertile; secondary sex characteristics do not develop

➢ **Testicular feminization (androgen insensitivity syndrome)**

- Results from absence of androgen receptors
- 46XY
- Absence of uterus and blind pouch in vagina
- Gonads are testes
- Normal breast development
- Scant pubic and axillary hair
- Male testosterone levels

4) Endocrine disorders
5) Defective enzyme systems
6) Autoimmune diseases
7) Tumors
8) Eating disorders
9) Excessive exercise
10) Medications
11) Past surgery

➢ **Asherman's syndrome**

Etiology

- Destruction of the endometrium
- Vigorous curettage
- Abortion complicated by infection
- Tuberculosis endometritis
- Uterine surgery

Clinical consequences

- Amenorrhea
- Spontaneous abortion
- Infertility
- If not amenorrheic, still may have hypomenorrhea and dysmenorrhea

ASHERMAN SYNDROME

Acquired **A**nomaly
Secondary to **S**urgery
Hysterosalpingogram confirms diagnosis
Endometrial damage/ **E**ugonadotropic
Repeated uterine trauma
Missed **M**enses
Adhesions
Normal estrogen and progesterone

12) Ovarian disorders

13) CNS disorders

c. History and physical

1) Psychological/stress
2) Family history of anatomic/genetic
3) Signs of physical problems (e.g. malnutrition; galactorrhea, decreased peripheral acuity)
4) Abnormal growth and development
5) Normal reproductive tract, evidence of estrogen (e.g. Rugated vagina, cervical mucus ferning)
6) Evidence of CNS disease
7) Lower genital tract: labial agglutination; imperforate hymen, transverse vaginal septa
8) ***Cervical stenosis post-surgery, electrocautery or cryosurgery***

d. Management for amenorrhea: *#1 Rule out pregnancy*

1) Measure TSH and assesses thyroid
2) Prolactin <100 ng/mL usually rules out pituitary tumor
3) Implement a progesterone challenge
   a) Parenteral progesterone in oil (200mg)
   b) Oral micronized progesterone (300mg)
   c) Medroxyprogesterone acetate (10mg for 5 days)
   d) If bleeding (any amount beyond a few spots) results within 2-7 days:
      - Anovulation is diagnosed
      - Outflow tract patency and reactive endometrium prepared by estrogen is confirmed
      - If TSH and prolactin are normal further systemic evaluation is unnecessary

> **Note:** progesterone challenge may trigger ovulation in a previously anovulatory female and this will present as bleeding that occurs 14 days after the progestational challenge (Speroff, p. 427).

4) **Possible diagnoses are**
   - Polycystic ovarian syndrome
   - Hormone producing ovarian tumor
   - There is risk of unopposed estrogen leading to hyperplasia & then carcinoma
5) **Therapy for amenorrhea:**
   - Monthly administration of medroxyprogesterone acetate, 10 mg, daily for the first 10 days of the month
   - COCs when contraception desired

6) ***A positive withdrawal bleed in response to progesterone, in the absence of galactorrhea, and a normal prolactin level together rules out the presence of pituitary tumor***
7) **If no bleeding from progesterone challenge**
    a) Out flow tract problem
    b) Inadequate estrogen proliferation of the endometrium
    c) Refer for MD management

2. **Dysmenorrhea: painful menses, usually described as cramps in the lower abdomen, back and thighs.**
    a. **Primary:** painful menstruation without demonstrable pathology.
        1) More common in younger women; typical onset is several months after menarche, when regular ovulation begins, and abates in severity in the 20s.
        2) Associated symptoms with abdominal cramps may be backache, headache, fatigue, nausea, vomiting, diarrhea, and syncope.
        3) May begin a day or 2 prior to menses and usually lasts for the first 2-4 days of the period.
        4) Management
            a) Lifestyle changes such as exercise, orgasm by sexual intercourse or masturbation to relieve pelvic congestion; local heat.
            b) Pharmacologic management: nonsteroidal anti-inflammatory drugs, e.g., ibuprofen; oral contraceptives suppress ovulation and prevent endometrial growth.
            c) Other methods include transcutaneous electrical nerve stimulation and even surgical interruption of nerves. Complementary measures include homeopathy, acupuncture, black cohosh, blue cohosh, chamomile, cramp bark, ginger pasque flower, and wild yam (Sinclair, p. 451-452).
    b. **Secondary**: painful menstruation in the presence of a pelvic disease.
        1) More common in women older than 20 years.
        2) May be associated with adenomyosis, uterine fibroids, endometrial polyps, cervical stenosis, congenital malformations, endometriosis, chronic PID, pelvic congestion syndrome, ovarian cysts or tumors, Asherman's syndrome, uterine prolapse, IUD.
        3) Management
            a) Rule out infection with cultures, rule out fibroid tumors with ultrasound.
            b) Refer for definitive diagnosis of endometriosis, adenomyosis, Asherman's syndrome etc.
            c) Remove copper IUD (consider replacing with progestin IUD).

d) Comfort measures as for primary dysmenorrhea. See specific deviations for further discussion (e.g., pelvic mass, infection, IUD complications, endometriosis etc).

3. **Dysfunctional uterine bleeding (DUB)**

a. A variety of bleeding patterns representing anovulatory cycles when **pathology and systemic causes have been ruled out**.

1) ***Oligomenorrhea***: menses occurs at intervals >35 days.

2) ***Polymenorrhea:*** menses at intervals of <21-24 days

3) ***Hypermenorrhea/menorrhagia***: regular bleeding excessive in duration and flow (>80 mL per cycle or longer than 7 days)

4) ***Metrorrhagia***: irregular bleeding

e) ***Menometrorrhagia***: excessive, prolonged bleeding at frequent and irregular intervals

6) ***Hypomenorrhea:*** regular bleeding with less than normal amount

7) ***Intermenstrual bleeding***: bleeding at any time between otherwise normal menses

8) Types of dysfunctional uterine bleeding

a) Estrogen withdrawal (after oophorectomy, radiation or midcycle when estrogen dips prior to ovulation)

b) Estrogen breakthrough (with low dose COCs, generally spotting)

c) Progestin breakthrough (when high ratio of progesterone to estrogen; e.g. Depo-Provera)

b. **Normal menses**

- Cycles from 24 to 35 days
- Length 2-7 days
- Amount: <80mL

c. **Menorrhagia**

1) Incidence is approximately 9-14% of women

2) Symptoms

a) ***Heavy bleeding at regular intervals suggests ovulation***

b) Heavy bleeding at irregular intervals suggests anovulation

c) Pattern and character of bleeding and associated activities should be recorded

3) Diagnosis

a) Woman's self reports: wide range; both over and under estimations

b) Counting the number of days: **More than 7 days usually classified as menorrhagia**. However only 45% of women with menses of 7 days duration have blood loss in excess of 80 mL

c) Counting the number of sanitary products: Not accurate; women vary widely in their use and frequency of use.

4) Pathophysiology of DUB

a) **Pregnancy!**

b) **Common:** anovulation, endometrial hyperplasia, uterine leiomyomas, endometrial polyps and adenomyosis

c) Others: Carcinoma; Infections (PID), Endometritis

d) Systemic: Thyroid and liver disorders, coagulopathies, Cushing's Disease, Adrenal hyperplasia

e) **Medications:** corticosteroids, psychotropic medications

f) **Anovulatory cycles:** perimenarchal; perimenopausal; polycystic ovary syndrome (PCOS): result in high sustained levels of estrogen; endometrium overgrowth (e.g. PCOS). At the maximum point of overgrowth the endometrium begins to slough but is disorganized because of the lack of progesterone.

5) Diagnosis of DUB: *Rule Out Pregnancy!*

a) Systems review

b) Complete history, physical, pelvic and laboratory assessments

c) History: menstrual; thyroid; bleeding/bruising; sexual abuse

d) Physical exam: thyroid, skin changes, pelvic exam (trauma, infection, lesions, foreign bodies), bimanual exam (refer if uterus larger than 10 weeks or presence of mass or tenderness)

e) Labs: Pregnancy test; Pap smear (only 50% will be positive with endometrial cancer); GC and chlamydia cultures; coagulation studies with bleeding times; CBC with platelets in adolescents

f) Diagnostic tests (e.g. sonography, endometrial biopsy); D & C only when endometrial biopsy can not be done or tolerated.

g) Women with diabetes mellitus, obesity or hypertension are at increased risk of endometrial carcinoma; with a threshold value of 5mm for endometrial thickness, transvaginal ultrasonography had a positive predictive value of 9 percent for detecting any abnormality, with 90 percent sensitivity, 48 percent specificity, and a negative predictive value of 98 percent.

6) Treatment of DUB

a) First make a diagnosis because treatment is focused on the cause

b) Outpatient treatment if hemodynamically stable

c) For menorrhagia due to DUB, pharmaceutical and surgical options are tried respectively

d) With pharmaceutical options, instruct woman to keep record of bleeding for 3 months, then return for follow-up

e) Pharmacological treatments for DUB

(1) ***Intense estrogen and progesterone*** therapy for 7 days.

- Example COCs (35mcg) up to four times daily for 5 days
- Or three times a day for 5 days, or three times a day for 7 days

(2) ***If bleeding stops***, she stops the COCs and will bleed 2-4 days

(3) If she needs contraception, begin COCs again; if not give MPA, 10 mg for 12 days each month.

- Alternative: Conjugated estrogen 10mg/day (2.5mg four times daily); after bleeding stops, add MPA, 10mg, for 12 days each month

(4) Other agents

- NSAIDs: 12-50% effective by influencing prostaglandins, platelet aggregation; administer during first three days of menses; reduces bleeding 40-50%.
- Antifibrinolytic drugs: Tranexamic acid (do not give to women with a history of thromboembolism); side effects include nausea and headaches

f) Surgical options

(1) D&C: not very effective but can be used to treat acute episodes that do not respond to combined estrogen and progesterone therapy

(2) Endometrial ablation: Use with thermal balloon most effective 90% improvement; 40-50% become amenorrheic; 22% require subsequent hysterectomy. Estimated 9% hysterectomy rate after endometrial ablation and a five-year follow-up period. Two to six percent post-operative complications rate. ***Women still need contraception but IUD's are contraindicated.***

(3) **Hysterectomy: Only definitive treatment** for DUB

Disadvantages:

- 35% reported fatigue 3 months post-op; 25-50% morbidity rate including infection, hemorrhage; transfusion reactions, atelectasis, myocardial infarction, cardiopulmonary arrest, DIC, anaphylactic reactions.
- Negative responses include fatigue, weight change, nervousness, insomnia, difficulty concentrating or remembering, periods of crying, loss of appetite, constipation or diarrhea, sadness, and changes in sexual behavior.

When faced with a hysterectomy, women want….

- To know physical effects after hysterectomy
- To know body parts involved
- To discuss sexuality and femininity issues
- Information about HRT and participation in the decision
- More support from groups/hot lines

❖ Physical, mental, and sexual improvement reported.

4. **Uterine fibroids (myomas/leiomyomatas)**
   a. Affects approximately 30% of reproductive aged women; higher in African American women.
   b. Composition
      1) ***Benign tumors*** made up of smooth muscle and an extracellular matrix of proteins collagen and elastin
      2) **Intramural** are within the uterine wall
      3) **Serosal** extend externally or internally into the endometrial cavity (i.e. submucus)
   c. **Signs and symptoms**
      1) **Menorrhagia: most common sign**
      2) Non-cyclic pelvic pain presenting as dyspareunia or dysmenorrhea
      3) Urinary frequency and urgency
      4) Incontinence
      5) Rectal pressure
      6) Constipation
      7) Menorrhagia that is progressive
   d. **Physical findings:**
      1) Enlarged, firm, nontender, irregularly shaped uterus-12 week sized uterus possible
      2) Increased abdominal girth
   e. **Management (consult if symptomatic or uterus >12 week size)**
      1) Check Hematocrit or Hemoglobin, pap and endometrial biopsy if menses irregular
      2) Ultrasound only helpful if the bimanual is difficult (e.g. when the woman is obese)
      3) Non-surgical: Fibroid embolization.
      4) Hysterectomy not indicated if the uterine size is 12 weeks or less
      5) NSAIDs initially on a scheduled basis
      6) Iron for anemia
      7) COC's or Depo Provera aid in decreasing size of fibroid
      8) ***GnRH agonists to shrink the fibroid, efficacy 50%***

9) Surgical management: Hysteroscopic resection with or without endometrial ablation; laparoscopy. Hysterectomy or myomectomy when medical management fails; anemia unresponsive to medical therapy; chronic pain and dysmenorrhea, dyspareunia; urinary symptoms; rapid enlargement and inability to exclude a uterine sarcoma.

f. Agency for Healthcare Research and Quality (AHRQ) Evidence-Based Report (2001)

1) Quality in studies lacking
2) Effect of myomectomy on long-term symptomatic relief unknown
3) Favorable outcomes associated with hysterectomy for up to 2 years
4) No support for prophylactic hysterectomy with asymptomatic fibroids
5) ***GnRH agonist therapy is the only pharmaceutical intervention with evidence related to efficacy***
6) Use of GnRH agonist prior to surgery decreases blood loss.
7) Uterus conserving treatments may be better in perimenopausal women than in premenopausal women.
8) Fibroids are associated with increased risks for preterm labor, abruption, C/S and breech presentation
9) Hysterectomy does not seem to adversely affect sexual functioning

5. Polycystic ovarian syndrome (PCOS)

a. Although ***not always present***, PCOS traditionally is characterized by

1) Obesity
2) Android obesity: Central body fat
3) Amenorrhea
4) Hirsutism
5) Acanthosis nigricans: a gray-brown velvety discoloration of the skin, usually on the neck, groin, axillae or under the breasts. Marker for insulin resistance.

b. Pathophysiology: includes persistent anovulation which results in a non fluctuating hormone pattern

- The LH level is higher in these women which stimulates the follicle without releasing an egg.
- Cysts are formed in the ovaries because an egg cannot be released which then leads to theca cell hyperplasia.
- Many small cysts on the ovaries can be seen on an ultrasound. Looks like a string of pearls.
- Increase in stromal tissue.
- This active stromal tissue contributes to increased secretion of androstenedione and testosterone, the usual products of theca cells which leads to the anovulation, hirsutism etc.

- Sex hormone binding globulin (SHBG) is reduced due to increased testosterone and hyperinsulinemia. This decrease in SHBG also increases the level of circulating testosterone.

c. Differential diagnosis

1) Cushing's syndrome

2) Adrenal hyperplasia

3) Hyperprolactinemia

4) Androgen-producing tumors

d. Diagnosis of PCOS

1) 25% ovulatory women have "cystic ovaries, so U/S is not an effective tool for diagnosis."

2) For women with hyperandrogenism

a) Fasting glucose/insulin ratio less than 4.5 is consistent with insulin resistance

b) 2-hour glucose test with75g glucose load; normal is <140 mg/dL

c) If free testosterone level in non-hirsute women is elevated proceed to glucose testing

d) Always R/O pregnancy with a sensitive pregnancy test

e) Check thyroid function

f) LH should be elevated with PCOS- 3:1 LH:FSH

e. Treatment (in consultation or by referral MD)

1) Increase FSH to androgen ratio with clomiphene citrate (*Clomid*)

2) Wedge resection to remove testosterone producing stromal tissue.

3) Treatment with flutamide, an antiandrogen

4) Oral diabetic drugs e.g. metformin (*Glucophage)*, 500 mg three times daily

5) Weight loss may be the underlying effect responsible for success with metformin

6) For women not seeking pregnancy, MPA (*Provera)* 5-10mg daily for the first 10 days every month; or COCs which also improve the lipid profile

f. Sequelae of PCOS

1) Infertility

2) Dysfunctional uterine bleeding

3) Endometrial hyperplasia leading to endometrial cancer

4) Cosmetic concerns: hirsutism, alopecia, acne

5) Increased risk for cardiovascular disease

6) Diabetes Mellitus

6. Breast problems; breast cancer

If you palpate a breast mass, CONSULT

a. Breast problems

Breast variations and deviations

Breast Condition	**Comments/Definition**
Amastia	Lack of Breast Development
Macromastia	Extreme Enlargement
Micromastia	Development only to prepubertal state
Polymastia	More than two breasts
Supernumerary nipple (Polythelia)	Extra nipple along the mammary line Incidence approximately 1%
Asymmetry	Normal finding during adolescence Over time, breasts become similarly sized

1) Nipple discharge

a) Description

(1) Milky, multicolored, sticky, purulent, watery, serous, serosanguinous, bloody

(2) Presenting symptom in 3.4% of malignant disease

b) Serous, serosanguinous, sanguinous & clear watery more likely associated with malignancy; biopsy should be scheduled

c) 75% caused by intraductal papillomas

d) 4% unilateral bloody discharge is linked to cancer

2) Fibrocystic changes

a) Physiologic nodularity, exaggeration of normal tissue response of the breast; results from fluctuation of ovarian hormones

b) Histologic findings

(1) Cysts lined with columnar epithelium

(2) Microcysts: ≤1mm

(3) Macrocysts ≥2-3mm (more common in women 45 yrs or older)

(4) Duct ectasia: dilation of duct system close to areola; more common peri and post menopausal

(5) Hyperplastic epithelial changes

(a) Increase in acini (adenosis); Increase in the cells lining the ducts and acini (hyperplasia); also referred to as sclerosing adenosis

(b) Changes increase in incidence approximately 10-15 years prior to menopause

(c) Hyperplasia is associated with an increase risk of cancer, especially when classified as “atypical hyperplasia.

c) By age 35-50, 90% of women have fibrocystic changes

d) Signs and symptoms

(1) Lumpiness and premenstrual pain

(2) Generalized lumpiness commonly in the upper outer quadrants

e) Risk of cancer

(1) Atypia: Increases risk of cancer approximately six-fold, especially in women 45 years and older

(2) Atypical epithelial hyperplasia

(3) Atypical lobular hyperplasia

(4) Diffuse papillomatosis with atypia

f) Treatments

(1) Non-pharmacologic

(a) Palliative

- Warm compresses
- Supportive bra

(b) Dietary (not evidence-based)

- Low salt diet
- Methylxanthine restriction (60% reduction)
- Caffeine restriction

(c) Vitamins

- Vitamin E, 800ug/day needed
- Side effects include hypertension, thrombophlebitis, fatigue and gynecomastia.

(d) Herbal

- Evening primrose oil
- Ginseng tea

(2) Pharmacologic

(a) Danacrine (*Danazol®*) (androgenic)

- Side effects include bone loss
- Redevelop symptoms in 12 months (60% improve with 800mg/day)

(b) Diuretics

- Small doses
- Usually spironolactone

(c) Estrogen antagonists

- ***Tamoxifen (70% report pain relief)***

(d) Ergot

- Bromocryptine *(Parlodel®)*
- Antiprolactin action
- Nausea and vomiting are side-effects

3) Benign neoplasms

- 1 in 12 breast lumps are malignant in premenopausal women; 50% are malignant in post-menopausal women.

a) Cysts

(1) Fluid filled sacs of variable size with or without pain

(2) Mobile, soft, round

(3) Aspiration usually reveals clear or dark green fluid

(4) If lump persists, biopsy is indicated.

b) Fibroadenoma

(1) Third most common lesion of the breast

(2) Common during ages 20-40

(3) Painless with no cyclic changes

(4) Circumscribed, mobile, round dumb-bell shape usually 2-2.5 cm

(5) Caused by proliferation of fibrous and glandular tissue

(6) 10-20% reoccurrence rate

(7) Diagnosis by tissue biopsy and examination

(8) Treatment surgical

c) Cystosarcoma phyllodes

(1) Type of fibroadenoma

(2) Grows rapidly and causes skin changes

(3) Treatment is surgical excision

d) Intraductal papilloma

(1) *Over age 40*

(2) Wart-like growth in mammary duct usually near the nipple

(3) Causes ***bloody discharge*** from specific duct via round clock evaluation

(4) Diagnosed by mammogram, sonogram, needle aspiration

(5) Treatment is surgical excision

e) Multiple papilloma

(1) Associated with an increased risk of cancer

(2) Women over 40 are higher risk

(3) Diagnosis by biopsy

(4) Treatment by excision

f) Galactocele

(1) Obstruction of breast duct usually beneath areola

(2) Common after recent lactation

(3) Treatment is to excise and drain

4) **Breast inflammation**

a) **Mondor's disease**

(1) Breast thrombophlebitis requiring no treatment

(2) NSAIDs may be helpful

(3) Usually resolves in 2-3 weeks.

b) **Mammary duct ectasia**

(1) Dilation of sub-areolar ducts that causes breasts to become red and hard and have palpable lumpiness below the areola

(2) Perimenopausal age-related

(3) Bloody, sticky green nipple discharge may be present

(4) Diagnosis by biopsy

c) **Paget's disease**

(1) 0.7% incidence

(2) Peak occurrence in women 60 & older

(3) Eczema like velvety patch.

d) **Lactational mastitis (see Chapter IV Postpartum Care)**

b. **Breast cancer**

1) **1 in 8 lifetime risk.** This represents the cumulative lifetime risk for a newborn who lives to be 90 years of age. The odds change as a woman ages. At age 50, 1 out of 50 women (2%) get breast cancer. By age 80, 5 out of 50 women (10%) get breast cancer. **Eighty percent of all breast cancer occurs in women over 50 years of age.** Early detection has increased the risk statistics but breast cancer is on the rise due to unexplained causes; diet and environmental pollutants may play a role.

2) **Mortality**: Less than 5% of US women die from breast cancer. Fifty percent die from cardiovascular disease (e.g. heart attacks and stroke). Among cancers, breast cancer is the second leading cause of death (lung cancer is first).

3) **Prevention**

a) Self Breast Examinations (SBE): not really prevention, but may assist in early detection

b) Mammography: early detection rather than prevention

c) Lifestyle factors

(1) Dietary fiber: Studies consistently associate high fiber diets with decreased breast cancer risk.

(2) ***Obesity has consistently been associated with breast cancer***; dietary fat has been studied; results conflict about its association with breast cancer.

(3) Phytoestrogens in soy and green tea and antioxidant vitamins are inconclusive.

(4) Exercise: 4 hours or more a week during the reproductive years reduces risk. Exercise lengthens menstrual cycles (decreases overall exposure to hormones)

(5) Breastfeeding: Reduction in premenopausal women who have breastfed.

- Breastfeeding before the age of 20 decreases the risk of breast cancer by 50%
- 25% reduction if one breast feeds between 20-24
- No reduction for breastfeeding after age 30

4) Risk factors

a) Female gender, though males may also develop breast cancer.

b) Only about 25% of the women who have risk factors develop breast cancer.

c) **Factors to consider in a work-up of a breast mass**:

- ➢ Age
- ➢ History of breast cancer
- ➢ History of proliferative changes
- ➢ Family history of breast cancer.

d) Family history

- ➢ Family history is the greatest of the known risk factors
- ➢ 5 - 20% of all breast cancer cases are associated with a family history. When a first degree relative has a history of breast cancer, the RR is increased two-three fold.

e) Genetic

5-10% incidence in women with breast cancer

❖ BRCA1 and BRCA2

- ➢ One faulty gene predisposes the women to an increased risk of both breast and ovarian cancer.
- ➢ Both men and women carry the gene and have a 50:50 chance of passing on a faulty gene.
- ➢ On average, one defective gene gives a woman an 85% chance of developing breast cancer in her lifetime.
- ➢ With BRCA1 mutation, the risk for ovarian carcinoma is 40-65%
- ➢ With BRCA2 mutations, the risk is 10-20%.

- **The average age of diagnosis is 45 years.**
  - Men with BRCA1 or BRCA2 mutations face an increased risk of prostate cancer. Men with BRCA2 mutations, however, face an increased risk of breast cancer (6% incidence).
  - Begin mammograms 5-10 years before the onset of cancer in a family member or at age 25 (various recommendations)
  - Prognosis much poorer with BRCA mutations and breast cancer regardless of lymph-node status. This is in direct contrast to BRCA negative cases.
- **HER-2 is a normal gene over-expressed in cases of breast cancer**

f) **Age:** breast cancer is a disease of aging

g) Personal history of benign breast disease

h) High socioeconomic status

i) History of ovarian or endometrial cancer

j) **Early age of menarche (<12) and late menopause (>55)**

k) Term child birth before age 19 reduces risk by 50%.

l) **Race**
  - Black women have an overall decreased risk (10% less likely to get breast cancer) compared to white women, but ***black women are more likely to die from the disease than white women***.
  - Reasons for this include: later diagnosis, more aggressive tumors, and lower tumor responsiveness to treatment.
  - Latina women have lower rates but the reason is not known.

m) **Hormone replacement therapy**
  - Associated with an increase in breast cancer over time
  - Relative Risk (RR) of 1.35 for women who used HRT for 5 or more years. However, breast cancer mortality is decreased in HRT users.

n) **Oral contraceptives** are associated with increased ***diagnosis*** of breast cancer incurrent OCP users, but not with women ten years after OCP use. (Hatcher 2004)

o) **Alcohol consumption:** Two drinks daily or more increase the risk of breast cancer by 2.5 times as compared to nondrinkers. Less than 1 1/2 drink a day was not associated with an increased risk.

p) **Breast implants**: no documented increased risk

q) **Environmental**: contradictory, especially regarding polychlorinated biphenyls (PCBs). National information can be obtained at 800 422 6237

5) **Diagnostic tests for breast mass (by MD); the midwife should probably consult regarding any breast mass.**
   a) The great majority of breast masses are benign; some reports say 95%
   b) Ultrasound distinguishes the difference between a cystic and a solid mass
   c) PET (Positron emission tomography) identifies the higher metabolism of malignant tumors; investigated as a noninvasive test to eliminate falsely positive mammograms.
   d) Aspiration: If fluid is not aspirated, send for ultrasound. Fluid aspirated tends to be yellow to dark gray-green.
   e) Fine needle biopsy: 18% false positive; 35% false negative
   f) Core biopsy: Outpatient procedure: 96% accurate; like ear piercing
   g) Excisional biopsy removes the entire lump
   h) Sentinel Node Mapping Biopsy/Resection: Radioactive substance or a blue dye is injected into the area around the tumor; later the ipsilateral axilla is explored through a small incision and the node that has taken up the dye is excised. If histologically negative, 95% predictive value, if positive, 100% predictive value.
   i) Histology is definitive diagnosis.
6) Reasons for delay in diagnosis (number of claimants)
   - Poor exam by physician/health care provider (50)
   - Inadequate examination (51)
   - ***Failure to order mammogram*** (54)
   - Repeat exam did not arouse suspicion (55)
   - Distracted by other health problems (55)
   - Failure to react to mammogram (60)
   - ***Delay in or failure to consult*** (75)
   - Failure to do proper biopsy (110)
   - Mammogram misread (110)
   - Negative mammogram report (125)
   - ***Failure to follow-up with woman*** (150)
   - Physical findings failed to impress (169)

from Medscape Women's Health: online, 9/21/98

7) **Types of breast cancer**

a) **Carcinoma in situ of the breast** is an accumulation of cells that look cancerous but do not have the capacity to move beyond the borders of the breast tissue where they originated. Can be ductal (DCIS) or lobular (LCIS)

b) **Invasive or infiltrating:** cancer cells beyond the walls of the ductal or lobular tissue. Usually associated with a mass; can spread to the lymph nodes.

c) **Staging**

Tumor, Nodes, Metastases (TNM) Breast Cancer Classification System: Columbia Clinical Classification System	
Stage 0	DCIS or LCIS
Stage I	Tumor <2cm, with no node involvement
Stage II	Tumor >2cm up to $\leq$5cm with or without nodal involvement
Stage III	Advanced
IIIA	>5cm and/or spread to nodes
IIIB	Any size and spread to skin, or chest wall
Stage IV	Metastasis

8) **Treatments for breast cancer**

a) Modified radical mastectomy (MRM) versus Breast Conserving Treatment (BCT)

b) Suggest to woman to obtain second or third opinion; take 2-4 weeks to do research.

c) Tumor size a major determinant of prognosis.

d) Tumors less than 1 centimeter with unaffected lymph nodes have a 90% cure rate without any systemic therapy.

e) Tumors larger than 2 centimeter warrant systemic therapy

f) Mastectomy versus Lumpectomy: Lumpectomy (BCT) requires radiation with Stage 1 or Stage II.

g) Without radiation the reoccurrence rate is 30-45% higher. Same reoccurrence rate as mastectomy; Mastectomy for lesions $\geq$4 centimeters

h) Chemotherapy

7. Adnexal masses

a. Benign

1) Functional cyst (follicular and corpus luteum, theca cysts)

2) ***Follicular cysts are the most frequently encountered type of ovarian cyst.*** They form in the first half of the menstrual cycle if the dominant follicle fails to ovulate and continues to grow, or if other follicles fail to undergo atresia. Corpus luteum cysts are small, less than 3 centimeters.

> If you palpate an adnexal mass, CONSULT.

3) **Theca cysts are usually associated with pregnancy and often bilateral.**

4) Other functional cysts usually unilateral

5) Often large but less than 10 centimeters

6) No ascites

7) Any cyst >4cm should be ruled out for neoplasm

8) ***Cysts are more likely to be cancerous as the size of the cyst and the age of the woman increases.***

b. Malignant

1) Often bilateral

2) Often associated with ascites

c. Diagnosis (in consultation with MD)

1) Ultrasound best for diagnosis

2) Complex cysts that are large and painful, or if US reports multiloculations, septa, papillae and increased blood supply, the suspicion for cancer is heightened and exploratory laparotomy is indicated.

d. CA 125

1) A cell surface antigen.

2) Naturally elevated in pre-menopausal women during menses, with fibroids and with a history of PID.

3) Use with postmenopausal women with adnexal masses -- not premenopausal women.

8. Vulvar variations

a. White lesions

1) Lichen sclerosus

a) Most common of all white lesions

b) May occur at any age

c) May resolve at puberty or during pregnancy

d) Possible precursor to malignant transformation (0-9%)

e) Signs and Symptoms of lichen sclerosus

(1) Adhesions between minora and clitoral structures

(2) Itching

(3) Epithelial thinning; "cigarette paper" appearance

(4) Progressive destruction of vulvar architecture

f) Etiology

(1) Autoimmune

(2) Metabolic

(3) Infectious

g) Differential diagnoses

(1) Vitiligo

(2) Leukoderma

(3) Cancer

h) Management

(1) Biopsy

(2) Estrogen cream for labial agglutination

(3) Betamethasone valerate (Valisone) 0.1% twice a day for 2-3 weeks

(4) Taper to Clobetasol .05% twice a day

(5) Testosterone proprionate 2% in petroleum

(6) Follow-up visits every 6 months

(7) Lifetime maintenance

2) Vitiligo

a) Etiology unknown

b) Lack of skin pigmentation

c) Autosomal dominant disorder

d) Associated with thyroid dysfunction, pernicious anemia, and diabetes mellitus

e) Depigmented areas may be seen as lesions

f) Lesions have well defined edge

g)May see dark hairs from a depigmented area

3) Leukoderma

a) Temporary or permanent loss of cutaneous pigment due to physical trauma

b) Differential includes Vitiligo and Lichen Sclerosis

c) Look for cause of trauma

d) No treatment is indicated

b. Ulcerations

1) Behcet's Syndrome

a) Rare inflammatory disorder of unknown etiology

b) Characterized by recurrent oral and genital ulcerations

c) Monoarticular arthritis and CNS manifestations can occur when severe

d) Lesions are multiple and painful

e) Treatment

(1) No specific treatment. Only palliative.

(2) Burrow's solution three times daily for 15-20 minutes

(3) Topical and systemic corticosteroids provide most dependable reprieve.

(4) Colchicine

2) Syphilis: Chancre

3) Herpes Simplex: Herpetic vesicles progressing to ulceration

c. Papular and nodular lesions

1) Endometrioma

a) Implanted in a tear or episiotomy site

b) Varies in size from a few millimeters to a few centimeters

c) Sensitive, mobile lesions

d) May enlarge during luteal phase

e) Treatment: Excision is both diagnostic and curative

2) Cysts

a) Epidermal cysts

(1) Multiple

(2) Most common cystic tumor of the vulva

(3) Composed of cellular debris

(4) Solid and firm to palpation

(5) Yellow in color

(6) May stay the same size or slowly enlarge

(7) Asymptomatic

(8) If diagnosis is obvious, no treatment is necessary

b) Bartholin's cysts

(1) Obstruction of Bartholin's gland

(2) Cause of obstruction is obscure

(3) Usually occurs between the ages 23-50

(4) May remain dormant or become acutely infected

(5) Prompt treatment required if infected (often incision, drainage and even marsupialization)

c) Hidradenoma

(1) Incidence highest in sexually mature

(2) Caucasian women

(3) Majority are single lesions

(4) Secondary infection may occur

(5) Originate from apocrine sweat glands

(6) Excision is diagnostic and curative

d) Hidradenitis suppurativa

(1) Genetic predisposition

(2) Blockage and infection of apocrine sweat glands

(3) Usually over lower abdomen, mons, labia, inner thighs and axilla

(4) Hot, red, painful nodule that swells and forms abscess; leaving scars

(5) Often recurrent

(6) May become chronic

(7) Treat with broad spectrum antibiotics

e) Fox-Fordyce

(1) Characterized by chronic pruritus and eruption of small papules/cysts

(2) Occurs in postpubertal and premenopausal women

(3) Apocrine sweat gland disorder

(4) Glands become plugged with keratin

(5) Leads to formation of retention vesicles

(6) Multiple flesh-colored lesions

(7) Responds to hormones

(8) Treat with anti-acne medication

d. Pigmented lesions

1) 10% of vulvar lesions

a) Biopsy needed for definitive diagnosis

b) Melanomas account for less than 2% of all vulvar lesions

c) 8-10% of melanomas occur on vulva

2) Lentigo

a) Most common vulvar dark lesion

b) Asymptomatic, light brown in color, resemble freckles

c) Appears early to mid life

d) Flat circumscribed macules from 1-10mm

e) Appears on skin and mucous membranes

(f) Excision is diagnostic and curative

3) Nevi

a) Not common on vulvar skin

b) Color ranges from tan to dark brown

c) Biopsy needed to confirm diagnosis

d) Should not be treated by destructive techniques

e. Inflammation symptoms

1) Vulvodynia (pain of the vulva)

a) Chronic vulvar discomfort with burning, stinging, irritation, and rawness.

b) Includes

- **Vulvar vestibulitis**
- **Vulvar dermatoses** (lichen planus and lichen sclerosus,),
- **Cyclic vulvovaginitis**
- **Dysesthetic ("essential") vulvodynia.**
- Multiple conditions may coexist

2) Vulvar vestibulitis syndrome

a) Usually premenopausal, age 20-30

b) Almost exclusively Caucasian women

c) Acute onset

d) Three criteria for vulvar vestibulitis

(1) Entry dyspareunia

(2) Erythema or inflammation of the vestibule, frequently involving the posterior fourchette

(3) Pain reproduced by pressure with a cotton tipped applicator on the vestibule

(4) May have history of some type of vulvar therapeutic procedure

(5) Becomes a chronic problem

e) Etiology of vulvar vestibulitis unknown

(1) May be provoked by yeast infection

(2) Use of chemical irritants

(3) History of therapeutic procedures

(4) May present as vaginal burning or discharge.

National Vulvodynia Association

f) Treatments for vulvar inflammation

- Refer to a support group/ biofeedback
- Sitz baths, topical lidocaine gel
- Vulvar hygiene, avoid allergens
- Treat underlying pathology (HPV, candida etc)
- Topical estradiol cream for atrophy
- Tricyclic antidepressant
- Psychological and behavioral pain management; biofeedback
- Interferon for HPV
- Low oxalate diet with calcium citrate
- Surgery

LOW – OXALATE DIET

Low-oxalate foods have less than 2 mg of oxalate per serving.
Moderate-oxalate foods have 2 to 6 mg of oxalate per serving. Patients should eat no more than three of these foods per day.
• **High-oxalate foods** have more than 7 mg of oxalate per serving. Avoid these foods.

3) Cyclic vulvovaginitis

a) Pain is worse just before or during menses

b) Pain is exacerbated by intercourse

c) Some relatively symptom-free days

d) History of frequent use of antibiotics for other conditions

e) Physical findings

(1) Variable erythema and edema

(2) Minimal vaginal discharge

f) Treatment

(1) Refer to support group

(2) Fluconazole 150 mg weekly for 2 months, then bi weekly for 2 to 4 months

(3) Biofeedback

(4) Low-oxalate diet

(5) Oral calcium citrate

4) Dysesthetic vulvodynia

a) Typically occurs in women who are peri-or post menopausal

b) Pudendal neuralgia

(1) Diffuse, unremitting, burning pain that is not cyclic

(2) Less point tenderness

(3) Urethral or rectal discomfort

c) Physical findings: Usually no erythematous cutaneous changes

d) Treatment

(1) Refer to support group

(2) Tricyclic antidepressants in gradually increasing amounts (6 or more months of therapy)

(3) Biofeedback

4) Evaluation of vulvodynia (vulvar pain)

a) History

b) Pelvic exam

c) Fungal and bacterial culture

d) Wet prep

e) Biopsy any suspicious lesions

5) Vulvar intraepithelial neoplasia (VIN): Usually pigmented or discolored lesions

a) *Associated with HPV and/or extramammary Paget's disease*

b) *VIN containing Paget's cells*

c) Oozing ulcerations or eczema-like patches with crusting or scaling

d) Biopsy

6) Vulvar biopsies

a) Under sterile conditions

b) Topical antiseptic solution

c) Local infiltration (Lidocaine 1%)

d) Punch biopsy from the deepest part of lesion or the darkest area in a flat lesion

e) Monsel's solution for hemostasis

Differential Diagnosis by Signs and Symptoms

Itching	*White*	*Ulcer*	*Pigmented*	*Papules/Cysts*
Lichen sclerosus Fox-Fordyce Pediculosis pubis Scabies	Lichen sclerosus Vitiligo Leukoderma	Herpes Behcet's disease Lichen planus Syphilis	VIN Nevi Lentigo	Epidermal cysts Bartholin's cyst Folliculitis Hidradenitis suppurativa Inclusion cysts Skene's duct cyst

f. Ectoparasitic infections

1) Pediculosis Pubis (Lice)

a) Signs and Symptoms: Pruritus; nits on pubic hair

b) **Treatment of pubic lice**

- Permethrin 1% crème rinse applied to affected areas and washed off after 10 minutes (Pregnancy Class B)
- Lindane 1% shampoo applied for 4 minutes then washed off.
- Lindane not recommended use in pregnancy, lactating women or children less than 2 years of age

c) Cautions

- Do not apply treatment to eyes.
- Use an occlusive ophthalmic ointment to eye lashes

d) Follow-up

Re-evaluate woman in 1 week if symptoms persist

2) Scabies

a) Signs and Symptoms: Pruritus, burrow tracts

b) Treatment

- Lindane 1%, 1 ounce of lotion or 30g of cream applied thinly to all infected areas from neck down. Wash off after 8 hours.
- Sulfur (6%) precipitated in ointment applied thinly to all areas nightly times three. Wash off previous applications before re-applying.

c) **For both pediculosis pubis and scabies**:

- Bedding and clothing should be decontaminated by machine washing in hot cycle or dry cleaned or all removed from body contact for at least 72 hours.

9. Pelvic relaxation

a. Etiologic factors

1) Congenital

2) Chronic Stress

3) Childbirth

4) Physical injury

5) Aging (loss of estrogen leads to atrophy and loss of collagen and elastic tissue)

6) Aerobic exercise

b. Structures

1) Pelvic diaphragm: coccygeus and levator ani support urethra, anus and abdominal contents

2) Urogenital diaphragm: bulbocavernosus, ischiocavernosus

c. Types of pelvic prolapse

1) Urethrocele: weakening of pubocervical fascia and herniation of urethra into vagina

2) Cystocele: same as urethrocele except the bladder herniates into the vagina; stress incontinence; complaints of urgency, incomplete emptying, pelvic fullness.

3) Rectocele: protrusion of the rectum into the posterior vaginal lumen; constipation, rectal fullness, incomplete emptying

4) Enterocele: herniation of the small bowel into the vaginal lumen

d. Examination

1) For cystocele and urethrocele: Visualize with posterior blade of the speculum depressed onto posterior vaginal wall. Palpate for bladder neck when cystocele present. Have woman cough.

2) For rectocele: speculum anterior, ask woman to bear down

3) For enterocele: have woman stand and do a rectovaginal exam by palpating the small bowel between the thumb and index finger.

e. Cystocele

1) Differentials

a) Inflamed Skene's gland

b) Urethral diverticulum

c) UTI

d) Tumor

e) Anterior enterocele

2) Classifications of cystocele

a) ***First degree:*** anterior vaginal wall from urethral meatus to the anterior fornix descends halfway to the hymen.

b) ***Second degree:*** Anterior vaginal wall and bladder extend to hymen.

c) ***Third degree:*** Anterior vaginal wall and underlying structures are outside the hymen.

3) Nonoperative therapy for cystocele

a) Hormone/estrogen therapy

b) Kegel exercises

c) Pessaries (the largest size, comfortable and retained with valsalva). The vagina needs to be well estrogenized; the woman should be given specific education and instruction and re-evaluation should occur (e.g. every 3-4 months)

f. Uterine (descensus) and vaginal vault prolapse

1) ***First degree:*** prolapse into upper barrel of vagina

2) ***Second degree:*** prolapse to the introitus

3) ***Third degree (total):*** prolapse through the introitus (i.e. procidentia)

g. Rectocle

1) ***First degree:*** Protrusion half way to the hymen

2) ***Second degree:*** Protrusion descends to the hymen

3) ***Third degree:*** Protrusion beyond the hymen.

10. Urinary incontinence

a. Incidence

1) 8-10% in women 15-64 years

2) 12-15% in women 65 years and older

3) 50% of all urinary incontinence occurs in women 65 years and older

4) Fewer than 50% of woman seek advice

b. **Physiology of urinary incontinence**

1) To fill the bladder, intravesical pressure must stay low and urethral pressure high (i.e. contracted) for continence.

2) The pubourethral muscles and ligaments, the anterior vaginal wall and the endopelvic fascia support the urethra and aid in continence.

3) Bladder and urethra are smooth muscle. Innervation is derived from fibers originating at T10-L2.

- Sympathetic stimulation relaxes the bladder and contracts the urethra, resulting in continence.
- Parasympathetic stimulation contracts the bladder but has no effect on the urethra or bladder neck. The smooth muscles of the urethra are under alpha-sympathetic control. Intraurethral pressure is supplied by muscle and vascular supply.

c. Risk factors for urinary incontinence:

1) Ingestion of certain foods: caffeine, acidic fluids, alcohol, artificial sweeteners
2) Voiding habits
3) Low estrogen milieu
4) Neurological
5) Medications (antihypertensive agents)
6) Smoking
7) Diabetes Mellitus

d. Screening

1) All women should be screened
2) Ask several different questions because often not admitted to on first inquiry
   a) Do you ever leak urine/water when you don't want to?
   b) Do you ever leak urine when you cough, laugh or exercise?
   c) Do you ever leak urine on the way to the bathroom?
   d) Do you ever use pads, tissue, cloth in your underwear to catch urine?

e. Important points for a medical history

- Respiratory — COPD/Bronchitis
- CV — Hypertension, Heart Failure
- GI — Constipation, Rectal Soiling
- CNS — Multiple Sclerosis, Spinal trauma, CVA/neoplasms, Disc lesions
- Endocrine — Diabetes Mellitus
- Psychiatric — Mental state, dementia

f. Differential diagnosis

1) Genuine stress incontinence (GSI)
2) Urge incontinence (detrusor instability) versus cystitis
3) Mixed
4) Fistulas and neurogenic bladders
5) Overflow

g. Diagnostic procedures for urinary incontinence:

1) History and physical exam
2) Urinalysis and culture
3) Test for residual urine (less than 50 mL is normal)
4) Test for bladder capacity and first urge (400-500 mL and 150-200 mL respectively)

5) **Stress test**

A bladder volume of 300ml is achieved and then the woman is asked to cough, first in lithotomy and then upright.

- ***Urine leakage with cough suggests stress incontinence.***
- ***Delayed leakage or persistent leakage suggests detrusor instability.***

6) The pad test determines presence of urinary incontinence but not cause

h. Genuine stress incontinence (GSI)

1) Involuntary loss of urine in the absence of detrusor contraction when the intravesical pressure exceeds the maximum urethral pressure. Women with GSI usually have low urethral closure pressure.
2) Etiology: Bladder neck and proximal urethra are not adequately supported due to scarring following pelvic surgery or bladder suspension operations or denervation due to injuries (e.g. vaginal delivery)
3) Predisposing factors
   a) Childbirth (one vaginal delivery yields a 2.5 greater risk than nulliparity)
   b) Aging
   c) Loss of estrogenic milieu
   d) High impact physical exercise
   e) Diuretics
   f) Morbid obesity

> Behavioral methods including Kegel exercises and biofeedback should be utilized before drugs and surgery for urinary incontinence.
>
> Information about Kegel can be found at http://www.incontinet.com.

4) **Symptoms of GSI:** leaking of urine when coughing, sneezing, running or jumping
5) **Treatment of GSI:**
   a) Life-style modification
   b) Reduce caffeine intake; weight loss; smoking cessation; prevention of constipation; use of tampons for exercise-induced incontinence
   c) Kegel exercises
      (1) A 67% improvement has been reported
      (2) Better outcome when Kegel's started before incontinence.
      (3) Teaching Kegel's needs to be frequent with several opportunities to reinforce.
      (4) **Women should be instructed to perform 10-20 a day, each for 10 seconds.**
      (5) Thirty a day is the goal.
      (6) Six weeks is needed to achieve beneficial effects.

d) **Pelvic floor muscle training (PFMT)**

(1) More specific than Kegel's.

(2) Daily minimum of 30-45 PFMT contractions for 10 seconds each.

(3) Relax 10 seconds between.

(4) Sets can be divided into 2 to 3 times or done all at once.

(5) Correct technique demonstrated by descent of the clitoris and an upward, inward contraction of the anus.

e) **Bladder training includes education, scheduled voiding, and systematic delay of voiding and positive reinforcement.**

f) **Estrogen .625mg/ day improves intrinsic vascular and muscular tone of bladder neck**. Estrogen may also stimulate alpha-adrenergic receptors which lead to urethral contraction (e.g. increase bladder outlet resistance).

(1) Surgery to elevate the bladder neck, retropubic and needle bladder neck suspension recommended over anterior vaginal repair.

(2) Alpha adrenergic agents, e.g., pseudoephedrine 15-30mg po, three times daily; not to be use in individuals with hypertension. Increases tone of the urethral smooth musculature. Side effects problematic

(3) Pelvic floor electrical stimulation; biofeedback. Effective for both stress and urge. Uses electronic instruments to relay information to women about bladder activity (e.g. stimulus/response). Biofeedback can also help women determine if they are doing PFMT correctly. The latter has been shown to be more effective with urge incontinence than oxybutynin

i. **Urge incontinence**

1) ***Painless loss of urine with a strong desire to void often due to detrusor instability***. Frequency and nocturia are common. The norm for voiding in women is 5-7 times a day.

2) Etiology: low estrogen milieu, demyelinating disease, stroke, diabetes mellitus, thyroid disease

3) **Symptoms of urge incontinence:**

- Can not stop urine flow
- Trouble holding urine until they can get to the bathroom
- Urinary frequency greater than 7 times during the day and twice at night
- Spontaneous loss of urine/control including enuresis (loose urine while sleeping)

4) **Treatments for urge incontinence:**

a) **Bladder training** teaches the individual how to resist voiding, voiding on a time schedule, and how to postpone voiding.

b) **Anticholinergic agents** (oxybutynin, dicyclomine hydrochloride and propantheline) block contraction of the normal bladder and probably the unstable bladder as well. ***Contraindicated in individuals with glaucoma.***

(1) Oxybutynin (1st choice): Use 2.5-5.5mg three or four times daily Anticholinergic and direct smooth muscle relaxant properties. Side effects include dry skin, blurred vision, and change in mental status, nausea, constipation and dry mouth.

(2) Tricyclic antidepressants (imipramine, doxepin, desipramine and nortiptyline). Limited application. Used for nocturnal enuresis.

(3) Estrogen assists with detrusor control by stimulating alpha adrenergic receptors.

11. Endometriosis

a. Presence outside of the endometrial cavity of endometrium, which responds to cyclic hormone influences by swelling and producing local inflammation.

b. Reported sites of endometriosis

1) Classically, endometriosis was reported in the deep pelvis

2) Ovarian cysts ("chocolate cysts") are endometriomas

3) Endometrial tissue has most commonly been found in: ovary, cul de sac, uterine ligaments, peritoneum, rectovaginal septum, cervix. Lesions may occur anywhere in the body.

4) "Powder burns" identified upon laparoscopy or laparotomy are usually implants of endometriosis (although the disease may have a range of visual manifestations.

c. Etiology of endometriosis is unknown, but there are several theories

1) Retrograde menstruation (no longer leading theory as most menstruating women have some reflux of menstrual fluid)

2) Genetic influences; perhaps polygenic or multifactorial

3) Hematogenous or lymphatic spread of endometrial tissue.

4) Metaplasia of peritoneal tissue induced by hormones or menstrual fluid combined with abnormal immune response

d. Incidence

1) 3-10% reproductive age women; 25-35% infertile women.

2) Most common single gynecologic diagnosis causing hospitalization of women aged 15-44 (DeCherney 2003).

e. Diagnosis

1) Differential diagnosis includes inflammation (PID, salpingitis), ectopic pregnancy, ovarian cysts, pelvic adhesions, ovarian cancer, or other GI/GU pathology

2) Diagnosis is difficult. Symptoms could be related to another condition or several other conditions occurring simultaneously.

a) Physical exam is usually nonspecific; a tender nodule at the uterosacral ligament has been considered pathognomonic.

b) Definitive diagnosis is only by surgery with subsequent histology confirmation of the endometrial tissue

c) No single lab test

(1) Assays of endometrial antibodies being studied, CA 125 has been suggested but high rate is not definitive

(2) Sonograms and MRI of some help, but not definitive

f. Risk factors that have been identified for endometriosis:

- Early menarche
- Short menstrual cycles
- Long duration of menstrual flow
- Asian race
- First degree relative with endometriosis (x7 risk)
- Uterine abnormalities that obstruct flow
- IUD use
- Sexual intercourse during menses

g. Signs/symptoms of endometriosis:

- ***Dysmenorrhea and Dyspareunia*** are the most common presenting complaints.
- ***Chronic pelvic pain***
- GI or GU symptoms; constipation caused by avoidance of defecation due to associated pain (dyschezia)
- Abnormal vaginal bleeding
- ***Infertility***.
- Rectal bleeding,
- Hematuria
- Post coital bleeding
- Cyclic sciatica
- Spontaneous abortion
- Pain may be non existent, mild, or incapacitating.

h. American Society for Reproductive Medicine in 1996 classified pelvic endometriosis as minimal, mild, moderate, and severe based on size, location of endometriomas, depth, extent of adhesions, and ovarian/tubal enclosure or obliteration.

i. Goals of treatment of endometriosis:

1) Arrest disease progression
2) Alleviate pain or other symptoms
3) Restore fertility if desired
4) Maintain psychological wellbeing of woman/couple

j. Treatment (in consultation with MD)

1) Medical interventions
    a) **Oral contraceptives**
    b) **Nonsteroidal antiprostaglandins** for dysmenorrhea is palliative
    c) **Danocrine (*Danazol*)** is a synthetic steroid. Majority of women experience amenorrhea after 6-8 weeks of use. Anabolic and androgenic side effects (weight gain, acne, oily skin); often reserved for women with severe disease. Does not seem to be superior to surgery for treatment of infertility.
    d) **GnRH analogues:** buserelin and nafarelin (*Synarel*). Nonsteroidal drugs that reversibly suppress ovarian estrogen production by down regulation of gonadotropins. Suppression of FSH and LH results in a fall in estrogen levels, and pseudomenopause results. Avoids androgenic side effects and serum lipid alterations observed with danocrine. May have "flare effect" shortly after beginning course of treatment-- a temporary worsening of condition and usually lasts about two weeks. Side effects include hot flashes, vaginal dryness, osteoporosis (usually after six months of therapy and can be reversible after therapy discontinued), amenorrhea and other symptoms of a hypoestrogenism.

RLQ pain: AEIOU

Appendicitis/ **A**bscess
Ectopic pregnancy/ **E**ndometriosis
Inflammatory disease (pelvic)/ **I**rritable bowel
Ovarian cyst (rupture, torsion)
Uterine colic/ **U**rinary stones

***What is down regulation*?**

- Normally, the hypothalamus secretes one pulse of GnRH every 60-90 minutes into the pituitary portal circulation.
- Each pulse causes the pituitary to release a pulse of LH and FSH into the peripheral circulation, stimulating follicle development and eventually ovulation.
- After ovulation the corpus luteum secretes estradiol and progesterone. The pulses of GnRH are essential to this process.
- Administration of a GnRH analogue means the pituitary is exposed to a chronic continuous infusion, probably culminating in desensitization of the pituitary receptors and down regulation.

2) **Surgical interventions**

   a) In a randomized study of chronic pain, long term outcomes of women treated medically (not surgically) were better. Extensive endometriosis probably culminates in hysterectomies, although pain may continue. Hysterectomy with ovariectomy is <u>almost</u> 100% curative.

   b) Treatment for mild or moderate endometriosis is laparoscopy with laser treatment of lesions or adhesions (at the risk of causing more adhesions)

   c) Effectiveness of surgical interventions not well established.

k. **Psychological interventions for chronic disease**

   1) Referral to gynecologist (often specialist in infertility)
   2) May have feelings of inadequacy/anger at body/powerlessness
   3) All the associated issues of infertility
   4) Need psychological support
   5) Anticipatory guidance about procedures/treatments

12. **Sexually transmitted diseases/infections (STD)**

   a. STDs are among the most common infectious diseases in the US today. More than 20 STDs have now been identified, and they affect more than 13 million men and women each year. The annual comprehensive cost of STDs is estimated to be well in excess of $10 billion. STDs affect men and women of all backgrounds and economic levels. Complications tend to be more severe and more frequent for women than for men because of the increased frequency of asymptomatic infections. Having STDs other than AIDS increases one's risk for becoming infected with HIV.

   b. Factors that influence STDs

      1) Earlier reproductive maturity and increased longevity - longer sexual life span
      2) Greater sexual freedom
      3) Changing roles of women
      4) Increasing use of drugs - correlation between drug use and STDs
      5) Increased travel etc
      6) Antibiotic resistance
      7) Treatment delay
      8) Contraception

         a) ***Condoms are the only contraceptives that offer protection against STDs***
         b) Oral contraceptives are linked to increase in chlamydia (but not PID)
         c) IUDs, injectables, implants and patches offer no protection
         d) Spermicides may actually increase risk of STDs because of irritation

Bacterial vs. Viral STDs

Bacterial	Viral
Often symptomatic	Asymptomatic
Early presentation	Delayed presentation
Rapid diagnosis	Diagnostic tests may be unreliable
Effective treatment available	Symptomatic treatment
Curative	Usually non-curative
Reservoirs can be controlled	Life-long

c. Syphilis

1) Causative organism is *Treponema pallidum*
   a) Extremely fragile and destroyed by drying, heating and washing.
   b) Organism enters the body through small breaks in the skin or mucous membranes that occur during sexual intercourse
   c) Approximately 1/3 of those exposed acquire the disease
   d) Also spread through contact with infected lesions and sharing of needles
   e) The incubation period ranges from 10 - 90 days
   f) Enhances risk of HIV transmission

2) Clinical manifestation - stages of syphilis
   a) **Primary syphilis:** ***chancre***--*painless indurated lesion* found on the penis, vulva, vagina, rectum, mouth and lips (anywhere the organism enters the skin); discharge from chancres highly infectious; duration 3-8 weeks. The primary chancre is not often observed in women, as it is likely to be on the cervix.

   - ***Darkfield microscopic exam reveals Treponema spirochete. Early testing may be false negative. Darkfield testing is more reliable in males with primary syphilis.***

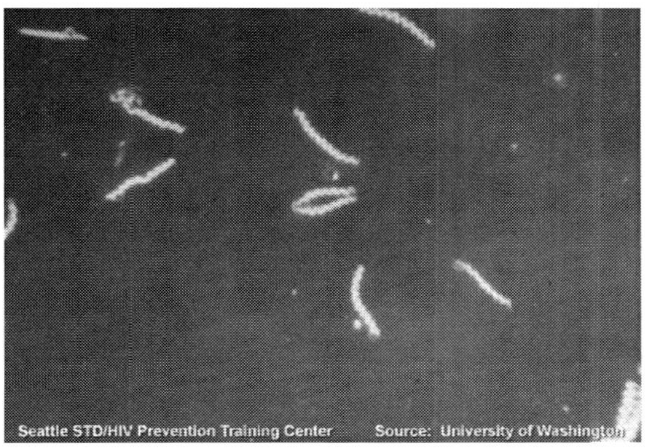

b) **Secondary syphilis – systemic**: Blood borne bacteria spread to all major organs.

- Hair loss and adenopathy
- ***Skin rash may involve the palms and soles.***
- Patches in mouth, anogenital area.
- Malaise, arthralgia, headache, occasionally liver and kidney dysfunction.
- ***Condylomata Lata are flat warty lesions that are highly contagious***
- Stage lasts 1-2 years. Testing should be accurate.

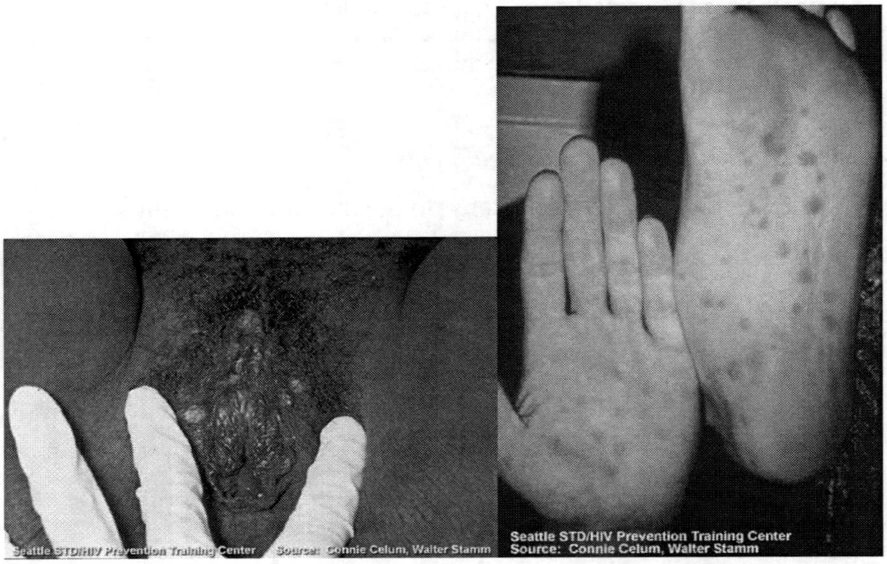

Condylomata lata (L) and rash (R) of secondary syphilis

c) **Latent syphilis follows the secondary stage** – the immune system suppresses the disease.

- Probably non infectious after 4 years but still placental transmission is still possible.
- Asymptomatic.
- Diagnosis is by blood test.
- A person may be in this stage her entire life

d) **Tertiary syphilis -- most severe stage and least common today.**

- Destructive skin, bone and tissue lesions develop.
- Cardiovascular damage - aneurysms, heart valve damage and heart failure.
- Personality changes minor to psychotic; tremors, mental deterioration; ataxia, paresthesia, damaged joints
- Irreparable damage to bone, liver, skin.
- Neurosyphilis causes loss of vision and dementia.

3) **Diagnosis of syphilis**
   a) Detailed history
   b) Physical examination
   c) Spirochetes on micro from tissue scrapings of chancre (more likely to be positive in men than in women)
   d) ***Screening is done with nontreponemal test.***
      - VDRL (Venereal disease research laboratory test)
      - RPR (Rapid plasma reagin titer)
      - Many factors, including undiagnosed lupus, may cause false positive
   e) ***Diagnosis is with treponema specific test***
      - TPHA (Treponema pallidum hemagglutination)
      - MHATP (microhemagglutination treponema pallidum)
      - FTA ABS (fluorescent treponemal antibody screen)
4) **Treatment regimen depends on stage of syphilis:**
   a) Benzathine penicillin (*Bicillin®*)
   b) Doxycycline 100 mg twice daily for 14 days
   c) Erythromycin 500 mg every 6 hours for 14 days
   d) All sexual contacts within the last three months are screened and treated even if their RPR is negative
   e) ***If pregnant and penicillin allergic—desensitize***

Jarisch-Herxheimer Reaction

- ❖ Reaction caused by dying spirochetes releasing toxins.
- ❖ Incidence varies depending on stage (Primary Syphilis: 50%, Secondary Syphilis: 90%, Latent Syphilis: 25%).
- ❖ It should not be confused with an allergic reaction, especially since fever is one of the major signs.
- ❖ Other signs and symptoms include adenopathy, rash and arthralgia.
- ❖ It usually occurs 2-6 hours after treatment is started; symptoms may last for 24 hours.

d. **Gonorrhea**
   1) Causative organism is ***Neisseria gonorrhoeae***, which infects columnar epithelium.
   2) This tissue is found in the urethra in men, the cervix in women, the rectum and oropharynx.
   3) The disease is spread through direct physical contact usually during sexual activity or to the newborn during birth

4) The incubation period is 3 to 4 days
5) The disease offers no immunity to subsequent reinfection
6) Gonococcal infections - inflammatory response - if untreated - fibrous tissue and adhesions
7) **Clinical manifestation in women**
   a) Most women are asymptomatic or have minor symptoms
   b) A few women may complain of vaginal discharge, dysuria or urinary frequency
   c) After the incubation period redness and swelling occurs at the site of contact (usually the cervix or urethra; may be the oropharynx)
   d) A purulent exudate often develops
   e) ***The disease may remain local or can spread to the uterus, fallopian tubes and ovaries, causing pelvic inflammatory disease (PID).***
   f) The vulva and vagina are usually involved only when little estrogen is present e.g. post menopausal women.
8) **Clinical manifestation in men**
   a) Heterosexual infection is usually via the urethra
   b) Men generally seek medical attention quickly because symptoms are uncomfortable; complications are less likely. Complications are prostatitis, urethral strictures, and sterility from orchitis and epididymitis.
   c) Symptoms are dysuria, profuse purulent urethritis 2-5 days after infection
9) **General considerations regarding gonorrhea:**
   a) Anorectal gonorrhea occurs from anal intercourse or contamination from infected vaginal secretions
   b) Gonococcal pharyngitis is the result of oral/genital contact
   c) Sequelae may be **ectopic pregnancy, infertility**, disseminated gonococcal infection with fever, skin lesions, arthralgia, and arthritis.
   d) Infected neonates develop **ophthalmia neonatorum**, which may cause blindness; prevention is timely administration of prophylactic topical antibiotic, e.g., erythromycin ointment, at birth
10) **Diagnosis of gonorrhea:**
    a) The immediate identification of gonococcal infection is usually made with a gram stain of the discharge
    b) ***Confirmation is by isolation of Neisseria gonorrhoeae in culture.***
    c) Cultures can be interpreted within 24-48 hours
    d) In men presumptive diagnosis is made if there is a history of sexual contact with an infected person followed within a few days by purulent discharge.

e) **In women, the only definitive diagnosis is by culture** as they are usually asymptomatic. Swabs need to be taken from the cervix, urethra, and anus

f) GenProbe: 2 results from 1 sample. Increases lab efficiency with single tube testing.

g) Gonorrhea and chlamydia screening may be done in conjunction with ThinPrep Pap smear.

11) **Treatment**

a) Treat sexual contacts before culture results even if asymptomatic

b) Treat sexual contacts simultaneously to prevent reinfection.

c) The individuals must abstain from sexual intercourse

d) If chlamydial infection is not ruled out, treat for chlamydia also.

e) Follow up re-culture may be done 4-7 days after treatment (not required by CDC for uncomplicated GC).

f) Traditional treatment is with penicillin; many strains are penicillin resistant

- **Drugs of choice** for uncomplicated cases of cervicitis, pharyngitis, urethritis, and proctitis are parenteral **ceftriaxone**, ciprofloxacin, cefixime, or ofloxacin *plus* oral doxycycline or azithromycin for presumed chlamydia coinfection.
- Disseminated infections (bacteremia, meningitis, endocarditis, septic arthritis) are treated with ceftriaxone, cefotaxime or ceftizoxime.

12) Prevention is better education, proper reporting, follow-up of women and their contacts, use of condoms, and chemoprophylaxis to prevent neonatal gonococcal conjunctivitis.

e. **Chlamydia**

1) Extremely common - some suggest the **most prevalent STD worldwide**

2) Causative organism is *Chlamydia trachomatis*, which causes urogenital infections in men and women, ocular trachoma, and lymphogranuloma venereum. In newborns it may cause ophthalmia neonatorum and pneumonia.

3) Incubation period is 1-3 weeks

4) **Risk factors**

a) ***Age less than 25***

b) Multiple sex partners

c) Sex partners with multiple partners

d) History of STD

e) Use of non barrier contraception

f) Gonorrhea infection

5) **Clinical manifestations**
   a) Men
      (1) Urethritis: dysuria, urethral discharge
      (2) Epididymitis: scrotal pain, swelling, tenderness, fever
      (3) Proctitis: rectal discharge, painful defecation
   b) Women
      (1) ***Cervicitis***: mucopurulent discharge, cervical edema
      (2) ***Urethritis***: dysuria, frequency
      (3) ***PID:*** abdominal pain, nausea, vomiting, fever, abnormal vaginal bleeding
      (4) ***Perihepatitis***: fever, nausea, vomiting, right upper quadrant pain
6) **Complications**
   a) ***Infertility***
   b) Reiter's syndrome (urethritis, conjunctivitis, arthritis)
   c) Cervical erosion
   d) Salpingitis
   e) Transmitted to newborns - conjunctivitis and pneumonia
7) Diagnosis is by culture or DNA probe
8) Treatment
   a) Doxycycline 100 mg po twice a day for 7 days
   b) Tetracycline 500 mg po four times daily for 7 days
   c) ***Erythromycin or*** azithromycin ***in pregnancy***

f. Human Immunodeficiency Virus (HIV)/Acquired immune deficiency syndrome (AIDS)

1) Incidence
   a) Estimated one million Americans are infected with HIV
   b) 16,000 new cases <u>daily</u> in the world
   c) ***One in 100 sexually active adult is infected; only 1 in 10 of them knows***
2) Causative agent is a retrovirus (see pathophysiology section in Chapter I)
3) Screening
   a) Need consent, and in some states the consent must be written
   b) Need program in place for counseling about results
   c) Screening for HIV antibodies is with a sensitive screening test (e.g., the enzyme immunoassay [EIA])
4) Diagnosis
   a) Reactive screening tests must be confirmed by Western blot or an immunofluorescence assay (IFA).

b) If confirmed, a positive antibody test indicates that a person is infected with HIV and can transmit the virus to others.

c) HIV antibody may be detected by 25 days, and is detectable in at least 95% of patients within 3 months after infection.

d) While a negative antibody test result usually indicates that a person is not infected, ***antibody tests cannot exclude recent infection.***

5) **Acute retroviral syndrome:** fever, malaise, lymphadenopathy, skin rash occurs in the first few weeks after HIV infection, ***before antibody test results become positive.*** If suspected, a test for viral load should be done in addition to the confirmatory HIV tests.

6) **Treatments – refer unless working under protocol**

a) Pharmaceutical treatments

(1) No single approach to antiviral therapy for the HIV infected individual has ever been agreed upon, even when AZT was the only drug available. As more drugs are introduced, even more numerous strategies

(2) *Major drug classifications used for HIV infections include*

- Antivirals
- Reverse Transcriptase Inhibitors
- Nucleoside Analogues
- Non-nucleoside Reverse Transcriptase Inhibitors
- Protease Inhibitors
- Antimicrobials
- Alpha Interferon
- hCG
- Interleukin-2
- Some drugs used for opportunistic infections common with HIV are designed specifically for HIV positive women--e.g. CMV and cidofovir

7) HIV and pregnancy

a) Pregnancy itself does not appear to influence the rate of progression of HIV disease; however, it clearly impacts treatments

b) Protocol 076 outlines current guidelines for HIV positive woman in pregnancy.

c) Circumcision and breastfeeding are both discouraged in developed countries

d) ZDV administered during 2nd and 3rd trimester, during labor and for 6 weeks to the newborn has shown a decrease in vertical transmission from 25-30% to 5-8%.

8) HIV and the newborn: In perinatally infected babies, HIV-1 RNA levels are high and slowly decline during the first two years of life

9) One of the future approaches to HIV is prevention of STDs in general, as STDs increase an individual's risk of contracting HIV if exposed.

10) Factors that affect susceptibility to HIV by the exposed person
    a) Lack of condom use
    b) High risk partner
    c) Genital ulcers
    d) Other sexually transmitted diseases
    e) Multiple sexual partners
    f) Traumatic sexual practices (e.g., anal sex)
    g) Cervical ectopy (adolescence, pregnancy, OCPs)
    h) Presence of foreskin (based on African studies)
    i) Sex during menstruation
    j) Use of nonoxynol 9 as contraceptive or lubricant

11) Factors that increase the potential for transmitting HIV from infected person
    a) Acute primary infection (just seroconverting)
    b) Advanced clinical disease (e.g. CD_4 below 200 per cubic mm)
    c) Elevated plasma viral levels
    d) Genital ulcers
    e) Other STDs
    f) Cervical ectopy

If a laboring woman is HIV positive

Recommendations used to call for Cesarean Section delivery of HIV positive women. Recent data suggests that the risk of vertical transmission is directly proportionate to the viral load. Definitely schedule a c-section with Viral Load >1,000 copies per mL.

Contraceptive Method and HIV

METHOD	EFFECT ON HIV	RATIONALE	COMMENTS
Combined oral contraceptives	May increase risk	Perhaps due to cervical ectropion as entry point; Estrogen and progesterone may modify cell mediated immune system, making individual more susceptible	Less blood loss to avoid anemia and exposure to others Interactions with other drugs
Norplant and Depo Provera	Do not decrease the risk of HIV, may increase shedding of virus from cervix	May be related to abnormal bleeding--especially with women who use tampons during the light bleeding (more like to microabrasions) More female to male HIV transmission if intercourse during menses Low estrogen may result in more vaginal fragility which might increase male to female transmission	Good low maintenance method for contraceptive effectiveness
Intrauterine Devices	May have increased risk of HIV during first three weeks after insertion; Questionable degree of increase thereafter	May be associated with irritation of uterine lining Increased bleeding or spotting may increase female to male transmission	Increased days of bleeding, and anemia
Condoms	Reduce risk of GC by 50%; most researchers extrapolate those results to HIV but no good study exists	When used for pregnancy protection if it fails, only a problem at certain cycle times; when used for STD protection, failure is always a problem Failures seem to be associated with dryness of vagina	Requires partner cooperation and correct technique
Spermicides (N-9)	Some data suggests N-9 may increase transmission. No published studies comparing different spermicides	Can increase risk if woman has allergic irritation or if they are not allowed to dissolve (gritty and more likely to cause microabrasions)	
Contraceptive Sponge (N-9)		Probably more harmful than other methods because of high level of spermicide (increasing irritation) and length of time it remained in vagina	
Diaphragm and Cap with (N-9)		Should be advised to remove device as soon as possible to reduce risk of irritation	
Sterilization	No effect No STD protection or HIV protection	Note: These women seek preventive care less often	Good efficacy for contraception
Hysterectomy	Women > 45 have higher rate than younger women of male to female transmission of HIV	Discussion of lubrication, possible estrogen replacement	

g. Herpes simplex virus (HSV); genital herpes

1) Strains
   a) **Type 1** – associated with infection of gums, dermis, CNS
   b) **Type 2** – associated with infection of anogenital area
   c) Either strain can cause disease on mouth and genitals

2) **Primary infection**
   a) Herpes simplex virus is established in the sensory nerve ganglion.
   b) The virus remains dormant
   c) Upon activation the virus moves down the nerve to the skin or to the mucous membrane
   d) Once infected the virus usually persists for decades, if not for life

3) **Clinical manifestation**
   a) Incubation period 1-45 days
   b) Burning or tingling
   c) Vesicles on penis, scrotum, vulva, perineum, perianal, vagina, cervix
   d) Vesicles rupture and form ulcerations
   e) Primary infections - local inflammation and pain, fever, headache, malaise, myalgia, dysuria; purulent discharge with cervical lesions.
   f) ***Many (if not most) HSV infections are asymptomatic***
   g) Primary lesions are usually present for 17-20 days
   h) After the first infection, the virus remains latent in the sacral ganglia

4) **Diagnosis**
   a) Clinical diagnosis of HSV is insensitive because many do not have the typical lesions.
      - Confirmed by culture and type-specific serologic tests since the prognosis for infection with HSV-1 differs from the prognosis of HSV-2 with respect to recurrence.
   b) In the presence of ulcers, HSV culture is indicated; sensitivity declines as lesions heal, within a few days of onset.
   c) Cytologic detection of cellular changes of herpes virus infection is insensitive and nonspecific, both in genital lesions (Tzanck preparation) and cervical Pap smears. Should not be relied on for diagnosis of HSV infection.
   d) Type-specific and nonspecific antibodies to HSV develop during the first several weeks following infection and persist indefinitely.
   e) Rapid-result blood tests have been developed; false negatives occur with early infection and false positives occur. Results need to be confirmed.
   f) Type specific serum tests are useful to diagnose women with unrecognized infection and to manage sex partners of people with HSV. For example, a woman with no history of herpes whose husband has a positive history may benefit from being tested preconceptionally or during pregnancy. Chances are that she too is HSV positive and does not have to fear a primary outbreak during pregnancy.

5) **Management**
   a) Pain management
   b) Keep lesions clean and dry
   c) Discuss the role of stress, tiredness, poor nutrition
   d) Safer sex practices, including counseling re risks of oral sex and transmission
   e) Counsel regarding transmission risks, therapy, and implications for pregnancy
   f) Psychological response may be a grief reaction, with resolution and acceptance of HSV as a chronic condition over time. Counseling may be indicated

6) **Treatment**

   Antiviral drugs do not cure HSV; they decrease the length of symptomatic infection and viral shedding.

   a) Oral acyclovir, valacyclovir, and famciclovir are used with various regimens.
      - Valacyclovir and famciclovir are better absorbed than acyclovir.
      - ***Topical antiviral drugs are not recommended.***
   b) Treatment should begin as soon as possible in the primary episode and with prodromal symptoms for recurrences.
   c) **Offer suppression therapy if ≥6 recurrences per year.** Frequency of outbreaks diminishes over time, so suppressive therapy should be discontinued every year to determine the need. Safety of suppressive (daily) antiviral therapy for several years has been established. Suppressive antiviral therapy reduces ***but does not eliminate*** subclinical viral shedding.
   d) For severe or systemic infections, acyclovir is given intravenously

7) **Complications**
   a) Immunosuppressed women (e.g. HIV infected)
   b) Pregnancy
      (1) Neonates: serious systemic disease that can be fatal
      (2) ***Cesarean section if lesion or prodrome present***
      (3) More likely to be problematic if primary outbreak during the pregnancy; recurrent disease has less viral load
      (4) ***Most authors recommend suppression therapy with acyclovir after 36 weeks.***

8) Recurrence

a) Recurrence occurs in about 80% of cases

b) Stress

c) Sexual activity

d) Sunburn

e) Fever

f) HSV can be transmitted at any time - condoms should be used at all times

g) When lesions are present the woman should avoid sexual activity

h. Human papilloma virus (HPV) -- genital warts

1) Clinical manifestation of infection with human papillomavirus (HPV). Warts are benign hyperplastic growths of squamous epithelium of the skin or mucous membranes. Genital warts differ in that they are primarily transmitted sexually. Infection with HPV is thought to occur following minor trauma to the epithelium. The incubation period is about 3 months. Some studies have suggested a greater incubation period (years)

2) Clinical characteristics

a) On moist surfaces warts appear as **cauliflower-like lesion.**

b) On dry surfaces keratotic and smooth warts are seen.

c) *If untreated most lesions resolve spontaneously.*

d) Latent or subclinical infection persists indefinitely

e) Most cases of genital warts are asymptomatic but occasionally they are pruritic

f) Presence can cause psychological distress and in some cases loss of sexual function.

> **Remember**
> Condylomata Acuminata is a common perineal manifestation of HPV (cauliflower growth)
>
> Condylomata Lata is an uncommon perineal manifestation of secondary syphilis (so-called flat warts)

3) Complications

a) Rapid growth during pregnancy - an infected mother may transmit the virus to her newborn during birth

b) Although visible warts are usually caused by HPV types 6 and 11, with a low potential for invasive cancer, other strains can coinfect visible lesions

4) Diagnosis

a) Clinical appearance of lesions on the external genitalia, perianal skin, cervix, vagina, urethra, anus, and mouth. Intra-anal warts are seen predominantly in people who have had receptive anal intercourse; perianal warts can occur in without anal sex. HPV types 6 and 11 may occur in the conjunctiva, nasal, oral and laryngeal mucus membranes.

b) ***Confirmed by biopsy if the diagnosis is uncertain e.g.,*** lesions do not respond to standard therapy; disease worsens during therapy; patient is immunocompromised; or warts are pigmented, indurated, fixed, and ulcerated.

c) Type-specific HPV nucleic acid tests in the routine diagnosis or management of visible genital warts is **not recommended.**

5) **Treatment of genital warts:**

a) Cryosurgery with liquid nitrogen, electrocautery

b) Topical treatments

(1) TCA or BCA (trichloroacetic/bichloroacetic acid)

(2) Podophyllin (not in pregnancy)

(3) Patient applied topical treatment, e.g., imiquimod (not in pregnancy)

c) Surgical excision

d) Condylomata recognized early in pregnancy should be treated early enough to allow healing prior to delivery. If treatment not successful, contemplate c-section if lesions are large enough to interfere with vaginal delivery.

2002 CDC STD Treatment Guidelines:

STD	Infecting Organism	Treatment
Genital Herpes	Virus: HSV-1 or HSV-2	Acyclovir 400 mg TID 7-10 days (initial attack) or 200 mg, 5 X day for 7-10 days Famciclovir 250 mg tid X 71-10 days Valacyclovir 1 gram bid X 7-10 days Recurrent: Acyclovir 400 mg TID for 5 days or Famciclovir 500 mg bid X 5-10 days or Valacyclovir 1 gram bid X 5-10 days or Acyclovir 200 mg 5 times a day
Granuloma Inguinale Endemic in tropics Painless ulcer, red, bleed easily	Gram negative Calymmatobacterium granulomatis	Trimethoprim-sulfamethoxazole: one DS tab BID for 3 weeks Or Doxycycline 100mg BID for 3 weeks Pregnancy: Erythromycin with Gentamycin
Lymphogranuloma Venereum	*Chlamydia trachomatis*	Doxycycline 100mg BID for 21 days Or Erythromycin base, 500mg QID for 21 days
Syphilis	*Treponema pallidum*	Primary, Secondary and Early Latent: Benzathine PCN G 2.4 mill. U. IM X 1 Late Latent or unknown: Benzathine PCN G, 7.2 mill U total, adm. as 2.4 mill/U IM each at one week intervals Primary or Early Latent, PCN allergy (non pregnant): Doxycycline 100 mg BID for 4 weeks or Tetracycline 500 mg qid X 4 weeks If Pregnant and PCN allergic: desensitize Administer above for 4 weeks for Late Latent
Non-gonococcal Urethritis (NGU)	Possible Chlamydia or Gonorrhea	Azithromycin 1g po, X 1 Doxycycline 100mg BID for 7 days Erythromycin ethylsuccinate 800 mg QID for 7 days
Chlamydia: often asymptomatic	C. trachomatis	Azithromycin 1G X1 Or Doxycycline 100mg BID for 7 days (equally efficacious) Erythromycin base (less efficacious) 500mg/QID for 7 days or Erythroethylsuccinate (requires test of cure) or Ofloxacin or Levofloxacin Pregnancy: E-base, amoxicillin, or azithromycin
Gonococcal Infection ***Note***	N. gonorrhoeae	Cefixime 400 mg po, X 1 Ceftriaxone 125 mg, IM, X 1 (most effective) Ciprofloxacin 500 mg, po, X 1 Ofloxacin 400 mg po X 1 Levofloxacin 250 mg po X 1 For patients who cannot tolerate cephalosporins or quinolones: Spectinomycin, 2G IM, X 1 (but not in pregnancy) *: Always treat for Chlamydia when you treat for gonorrhea unless ruled out by highly sensitive CT test*
Chancroid: co-factor of HIV;	H. ducreyi	Azithromycin 1g X 1 Erythromycin 500 mg TID X 7 days Ceftriaxone 250 mg, IM X1

i. Pelvic inflammatory disease (PID)

1) Pelvic inflammatory disease is the **clinical syndrome resulting from the ascending spread** of microorganisms from the vagina and endocervix to the endometrium, the fallopian tubes and/or to contiguous structures. Caused by multiple organisms. May include endometritis, salpingitis, tubo-ovarian abscess, and pelvic peritonitis.

2) Etiology
   - **a) C. trachomatis most common**
   - b) N. gonorrhoeae
   - c) Anaerobic bacteria (e.g. bacteroides)
   - d) Facultative gram negative rods (e.g. E. coli)
   - e) Mycoplasma hominis
   - f) Actinomyces israelii (associated with prolonged IUD use).

> **PID complications**
> **I FACE PID**
>
> **I**nfertility
> **F**itz-Hugh-Curtis syndrome
> **A**bscesses
> **C**hronic pelvic pain
> **E**ctopic pregnancy
> **P**eritonitis
> **I**ntestinal obstruction
> **D**isseminated: sepsis, endocarditis, arthritis, meningitis

3) Epidemiology
   - a) In the U.S. about 850,000 women, requiring more than 212,000 hospital admissions and 115,000 surgical procedures are reported each year.
   - b) Risk factors
     - (1) Multiple sex partners
     - (2) History of previous PID
     - (3) IUD use (oral contraceptives decrease the risk)
     - (4) Marital status (single women are at higher risk)
     - (5) Asymptomatic gonococcal infection in either sexual partner.

4) Symptoms and signs
   - a) Moderate fever (generally above 99°F)
   - b) Bilateral lower abdominal pain maximal in the region of the fallopian tubes and generally lasts no longer than 14 days.
   - c) Increased vaginal discharge
   - d) Irregular bleeding
   - e) Cervical motion tenderness
   - f) Tender adnexal mass(es)
   - g) Purulent endocervical discharge
   - h) Nausea and vomiting
   - **i) NOTE:** Only about 20% of the women with PID show all these signs. They are similar to other pathologic conditions such as appendicitis, ectopic pregnancy, septic abortion, rupture of an ovarian cyst, pyelonephritis, etc.

5) **Sequelae of PID**

   a) ***The most common cause of involuntary infertility in women.***

   b) Dissemination to liver resulting in a perihepatitis.

   c) ***Fitz-Hugh-Curtis*** syndrome; "Violin Strings" form between the abdominal wall and liver capsule (may occur in both gonococcal and nongonococcal types of PID).

   d) Unilateral or bilateral ovarian ***abscesses*** .

   e) Tubal occlusion, scarring, and adhesions with chronic abdominal pain.

   f) Death due to rupture of the ovarian abscesses.

6) Diagnosis

   a) **Definitive diagnosis consists of direct visualization of inflamed fallopian tube(s) on laparoscopy, laparotomy, or biopsy evidence of salpingitis.** Only a confirmed culture of a biopsy of the fallopian tube positively identifies the etiology of salpingitis.

   b) Presumptive diagnosis can be made on clinical grounds alone.

   c) Laboratory findings useful in diagnosis of PID

      (1) Positive culture for *N. gonorrhoeae* or *C. trachomatis* (or DNA probe) from the endocervix.

      (2) Positive Gram stain for intracellular gonococci from the cul-de-sac or endocervix.

      (3) Elevated white blood cell count.

      (4) Elevated erythrocyte sedimentation rate

7) **Treatment**

   a) Consultation/referral

   b) Major decision is whether or not to hospitalize

   c) Can be treated on an outpatient basis only if temperature is <38°C, WBC <11,000/mm^3, there is minimal evidence of peritonitis, active bowel sounds, and they are able to tolerate oral nourishment and treatment.

   d) **Hospitalize the woman if:**

      - ***She is pregnant***
      - Diagnosis is uncertain
      - Surgical emergencies such as appendicitis and ectopic pregnancy must be excluded
      - A pelvic abscess is suspected
      - Severe illness precludes outpatient management
      - She is unable to follow or tolerate outpatient regimen
      - The clinical follow-up after 48-72 hours of starting antibiotics cannot be arranged

e) No single antibiotic will be active against all possible pathogens.

f) Hospitalized patients

(1) *Parenteral cefotetan or Cefoxitin AND doxycycline*

(2) *OR clindamycin and gentamicin.*

g) Ambulatory therapy

(1) *Ceftriaxone and doxycycline 14 days for both*

(2) *OR Ofloxacin and metronidazole 14 days for both*

h) **Follow-up**

- Close medical follow-up
- **Evaluation of woman 2-3 days after start of therapy for symptomatic improvement, drug reactions, and compliance--must demonstrate significant improvement--although may still have some signs/symptoms**
- Repeat exam and endocervical and rectal cultures 4-7 days after completing therapy
- Confirmation of clinical resolution by repeating exam and endocervical culture 4-6 weeks after completing therapy.
- Sex partners should be evaluated for STDs.
- Removal of IUD if in situ (this can take place during therapy). Recommendations to remove IUD differ; consult.

j. Less common sexually transmitted diseases

Hint—do not spend excessive time on these, they are important, but their incidence is quite small in the general population

Condition	Etiology	Clinical Picture	Diagnosis	Treatment	Comments
Lymphogranuloma Venereum	Chlamydia trachomatis Incubation 3 days-3 weeks	Anorectal lymphedema making bowel movements painful. Blood stained stool. Vaginal Narrowing and Dyspareunia	LGV complement fixation test for antibodies Rule out other STDs	Doxycycline 100 mg po bid for 21 days or Alt: E Base 500 mg po qid for 21 days	Treat pregnant women with erythromycin Azithromycin may prove useful but no published data
Granuloma Inguinale (Donavanosis)	Calymmato bacterium granulomatis Incubation approximately 5-12 weeks	Painless papular or ulcerative lesions on vulva, vagina, urethra and anus Inguinal adenopathy	Donavan bodies found on Giemsa stained smears	Doxycycline 100 mg) po bid for 21 days or TMP/SMZ one (800mg/160mg) po bid for 3 weeks Alt: Ciprofloxacin 750 mg po bid for 3 weeks, OR Erythromycin base 500 mg po qid for 3 weeks, OR Azithromycin 1 g po once per week for 3 weeks	Complications include genital scarring, scar carcinoma. Pregnant and lactating: erythromycin and consider adding parenteral aminoglycoside (e.g., gentamicin). Azithromycin may prove useful but published data are lacking. Doxycycline and ciprofloxacin are contraindicated in pregnant women
Molluscum Contagiosum	Unknown Incubation 14-40 days	2-5 mm fleshy growths in genital or other area. Often dimpled in center	Usually based on visual examination	No treatment if not sexually active. TCA, Podophyllin, Cryotherapy	Watch for secondary staph infection
Chancroid	H. ducreyi Incubation 3-10 days	Painful macule Kissing ulcers (autoinoculation)	Clinical exam, although can order culture with special media	Azithromycin 1 g po in single dose, OR Ceftriaxone 250 mg (IM) in single dose, OR Ciprofloxacin 500 mg po twice a day for 3 days, OR Erythromycin base 500 mg po tid for 7 days	Also may have bubo, although more commonly associated with LGV Remember Cipro contraindicated in pregnancy

13. Ovarian cancer

a. Incidence

1) **Epithelial ovarian cancer is the leading cause of death from <u>gynecologic</u> cancer in the US**
2) Approximately 30,000 annual cases, and 15,000 deaths
3) 5 percent of all cancer deaths in women in the US
4) More women die of this disease than from cervical and endometrial cancer combined, though fewer women get it.

b. Epidemiology and risk factory

> **BRCA-1** is associated with cancers of the:
> Breast
> Ovaries
> Colon

1) Age related; peaks in eighth decade
2) Uncommon before age 40
3) Higher incidence in industrialized nations
4) More common among women who have infertility, nulliparity, frequent
5) miscarriages, and who use ovulation-inducing drugs such as clomiphene (frequent ovulation).
6) **Each pregnancy reduces the ovarian cancer risk by about 10 percent**;
7) Breast feeding and tubal ligation also appear to reduce the risk.
8) ***Oral contraceptives reduce the risk*** of ovarian cancer in women with a familial history of cancer and in the general population.
9) Estrogen replacement after menopause may or may not increase the risk of ovarian cancer.
10) Familial cases account for about 5 percent of all ovarian cancer
    a) Theorize it is autosomal dominant
    b) Likely associated with BRCA-1

> **Tip**
> Suspect ovarian cancer with a palpable ovary in a postmenopausal woman
>
> Therefore, consult in this situation

c. Clinical presentation and differential diagnosis of ovarian cancer:

1) Most are first diagnosed when the disease has already spread beyond the true pelvis.
2) The occurrence of abdominal pain, bloating, and urinary symptoms usually indicates advanced disease. **Localized ovarian cancer is generally asymptomatic.**
3) The diagnosis of early disease usually occurs with palpation of an asymptomatic adnexal mass during routine pelvic examination.
4) ***Adnexal masses in premenarchal or postmenopausal women are more likely to be pathologic: consult.***

d. Screening/Diagnosis

1) **Measure serum levels of the tumor marker CA-125.** 80 – 85% of women with epithelial ovarian cancer have high levels of CA-125, ***but it does not have good sensitivity as screening test.***

2) Transvaginal sonography is also better for diagnosis than screening

Stage	Description	5 year Survival
0	--	--
1	Confined to Ovary	90
2	Confined to Pelvis	70
3	Intra-abdominal Spread	15-20
4	Spread Outside Abdomen	1-5

e. **Treatment: Surgical excision and chemotherapy**

14. Cervical cancer

a. ***Most frequently begins at the squamocolumnar junction.*** Transformation zone is term for area of squamous metaplasia, where the most rapid cellular changes occur.

b. **Dysplasia:** abnormal maturation of the cells, usually in the transformation zone area.

- ➢ Significant features for the diagnosis of intraepithelial neoplasia include immature cells, disorganized cells, nuclear abnormalities, and increased mitotic activity.
- ➢ Dysplasia may be mild, moderate or severe with carcinoma in situ as the next most ominous finding without having a diagnosis of invasive carcinoma.
- ➢ These terms, though replaced in the Bethesda system with new terminology may still appear on Pap reports.

c. **Metaplasia** is the conversion of normal tissue cells into another cell type in response to chronic stress or injury. With prolonged exposure to the stimulus, cancer may occur.

d. **Cervical intraepithelial neoplasia (CIN)** as Pap reporting terminology has also been replaced by the Bethesda system (see also section C.1.a).

- ❖ CIN may be suspected by the Pap smear cytologic results, but this diagnosis is made on the basis of histological study of the biopsy.

CIN I mitoses and immature cells in lower one-third of epithelium

CIN II involvement of the lower half of the epithelium

CIN III involvement up to the upper third of the epithelium

Changes in Terminology for Reporting Pap Results

Bethesda System	CIN Classification	Papanicolaou
ASC-US	ASC-US	Atypia
ASC-H		
AGC, AGC-NOS, AIS	AGC-US	
Low grade SIL (LSIL)	HPV change	Koilocytotic, warty condylomatous atypia
	CIN I	Mild dysplasia
High grade SIL (HSIL)	CIN II	Moderate dysplasia
	CIN III	Severe dysplasia, carcinoma in situ

CIN: Cervical intraepithelial neoplasia
ASC-US: Atypical squamous cells of undetermined origin
ASC-H: Atypical squamous cells, cannot exclude high grade lesion
ACG: Atypical glandular cells
ACG-NOS: Atypical glandular cells, not otherwise specified
AIS: Endocervical adenocarcinoma in situ
SIL: squamous intraepithelial lesion
Table was constructed using information from Hatcher 1998, Sinclair 2004, and DeCherney 2003.

e. ***Human papilloma virus (in the presence of co-factors such as smoking) plays a major role in the development of dysplasia and cervical cancer.***

1) >30 HPV types occur in the anogenital area
   - Low risk HPV types for cervical cancer: 6, 11, 42, 43, 44 (associated with condylomata and low grade lesions)
   - Moderate risk HPV types for cervical cancer: 33, 35, 51, 52 (in higher grade lesions that persist but rarely progress to cancer)High risk HPV types for cervical cancer: 16, 18, 31, 39, 45, 56, 58, 59, 68 (associated with high grade lesions and invasive cancer)
   - Most common is type 16

2) ***<1% of women with HPV actually develop cervical cancer***

3) Co-factors with HPV for cervical cancer:
   - Multiple sexual partners over a lifetime
   - High risk sexual partners (history of multiple partners, HPV infection, exposure to partner with cervical neoplasia)
   - Smoking***
   - History of condylomata acuminata
   - History of STDs
   - Early age of first intercourse (<20 years.)
   - Immunodeficiency***
   - Multiparity
   - Long term oral contraceptive pill use

f. ***Cervical cancer screening test is Pap smear; diagnosis is by biopsy, usually colposcopically directed.***

1) Begin screening three years after initiating sexual intercourse, but no later than at 21 years old. Some cell changes are transient and insignificant during these 3 years; it takes years for cervical cancer to develop. Cervical cancer is extremely rare under the age of 25.
2) After age 21, Pap test at least every three years (more often if at risk). ACOG still advocates annual Pap tests.
3) Women 65 - 70 years of age with at least three normal Pap tests and no abnormal Pap tests in the last 10 years may stop cervical cancer screening.
4) Women who have had a total hysterectomy do not need cervical cancer screening unless the surgery was done as a treatment for cervical precancer or cancer.

g. **Midwifery management of abnormal Pap smear is referral to a qualified colposcopist**. Women with biopsies positive for CIN or invasive disease are managed by a physician

15. Adenomyosis

a. ***Growth of endometrial tissue in the myometrium***

b. Average age of symptomatic women is usually 40 years or older

c. Symptoms

1) ***Menorrhagia: heavy or prolonged menstrual bleeding***
2) ***Dysmenorrhea, often beginning up to 1 wk. prior to onset of menses***

d. Signs

1) ***Diffusely enlarged uterus, usually <14 cm***
2) ***Soft, tender uterus, especially at time of menses***
3) ***Anemia possibly***

e. Management

1) Initial consultation depends on practice agreements
2) Depends on age and desire for future fertility
3) NSAIDs for dysmenorrhea
4) Iron for anemia
5) Oral contraceptives for control of bleeding
6) Menstrual suppression with progestins or continuous oral contraceptives for control of bleeding
7) Refer for possible hysterectomy if severe

NOTES

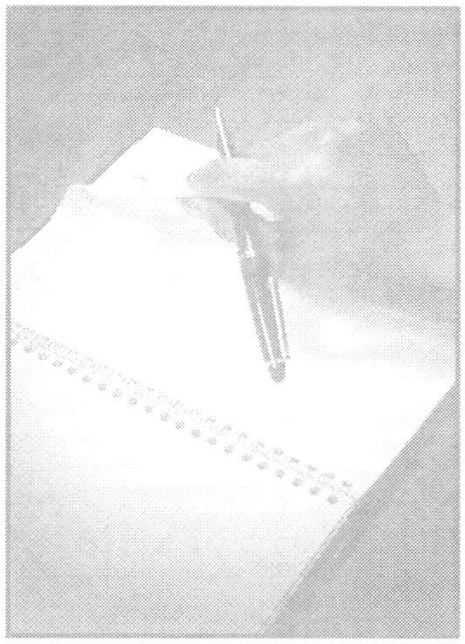

Chapter VII

Professional Issues

VII. Professional Issues (up to 5%)

A. **Midwifery practice**

1. Scope of practice
2. Development of clinical practice guidelines
3. Development of patient education materials
4. Patient records/charting
5. Interdisciplinary relationships
6. Ethics: **ACNM Code of Ethics 2004**

B. **Health care system and its relationship to midwifery practice**

1. Equal access to health care/cultural sensitivity
2. Administrative structure of agencies (hospitals, birth centers, HMOs)
3. National health care policy (e.g. WHO Baby Friendly Hospital Initiative)
4. Barriers to midwifery practice (restraint of trade, limited access, reimbursement issues)

C. **Legal issues**

1. Statutes/regulations that affect midwifery practice
2. Medical malpractice/legal liability issues
3. Birth registration

D. **Maintaining standards of care**

1. Evidence-based practice/review of practice-related literature
2. Peer review/quality improvement
3. Continued competency activities

ACNM Standards for Midwifery Practice 2003

ACNM Philosophy 2004

NOTES

A. Midwifery practice

1. Scope of practice

The American College of Nurse-Midwives (ACNM), as the professional midwifery organization, publishes documents that address the clinical boundaries of midwifery practice. The documents have evolved over the years, as has midwifery practice. All midwives who expect to be licensed and credentialed for hospital privileges and reimbursement in the United States today should be familiar with such documents as:

- Definition of Midwifery Practice (2004)
- ACNM Philosophy (2004)
- ACNM Code of Ethics (2005)
- ACNM Standards for the Practice of Midwifery (2003)
- ACNM Core Competencies for Basic Midwifery Practice (2002)

a. Definition of Certified Nurse-Midwife (CNM): An individual educated in the **two disciplines of nursing and midwifery**, who possesses evidence of **certification according to the requirements of the ACNM**.

b. Definition of Certified Midwife (CM): An individual educated in the **discipline of midwifery**, who possesses evidence of **certification according to the requirements of the ACNM**.

c. "Certification according to the requirements of the ACNM" means that the individual has successfully **passed the national certification examination** administered by the ACNM or its designee, currently the American Midwifery Certification Board (AMCB) (formerly named ACNM Certification Council, Inc [ACC]), including requirements for maintaining that certification. Prerequisites for sitting the exam include successful **completion of a program** of midwifery education **accredited by the ACNM Division of Accreditation (DOA)** and, in the case of the **CNM, current licensure as a Registered Nurse** (RN). Requirements for continuing certification are set by the organization granting the credential, i.e. ACNM or AMCB.

d. Midwifery practice (ACNM 2004) is:

1) **Independent management of women's health care** focusing particularly on common primary care issues, family planning and gynecologic needs of women, pregnancy, childbirth, the postpartum period and the care of the newborn.
2) **Within a health care system that provides for consultation, collaborative management or referral** as indicated by the health status of the client.
3) In accord with the **Standards for the Practice of Midwifery**, as defined by the American College of Nurse-Midwives.

e. Scope of practice: refers to the range of activities and their boundaries within which midwives may provide health care i.e., practice their profession.

1) Delineates what a midwife may or may not do in her particular practice, i.e., what aspects of care may be provided by the midwife independently, under which conditions she must consult, what conditions may be managed collaboratively, and under what circumstances the midwife is expected to refer the client.

2) The individual midwife's scope of practice may depend on (not an exhaustive list):

a) Experience, knowledge, skill, philosophy

b) Education, both basic and continuing

c) State and federal laws that regulate practice and health care institutions

d) National standards

e) Policies and procedures of the site or institution

f) Professional standards, e.g., ACNM

g) Scope of practice of employing or consulting physician

h) Practice guidelines developed and agreed to by the CNM/CM and employer/consultant physician (or institution).

2. Development of clinical practice guidelines

a. ACNM Standards for the Practice of Midwifery (2003) **STANDARD V: M***IDWIFERY CARE IS BASED UPON KNOWLEDGE, SKILLS, AND JUDGMENTS WHICH ARE REFLECTED IN WRITTEN PRACTICE GUIDELINES.* The midwife:

1) **Describes the parameters of service for independent and collaborative** midwifery management **and transfer** of care when needed.

2) **Establishes practice guidelines for each specialty area** which may include, but is not limited to, ***primary health care of women, care of the childbearing family, and newborn care***.

3) Includes the following information in each specialty area:

a) ***Client selection criteria***

b) ***Parameters and methods for assessing health status***

c) ***Parameters for risk assessment***

d) ***Parameters for consultation, collaboration, and referral***

e) ***Appropriate interventions including treatment, medication, and/or devices.***

4) Resources for developing clinical practice guidelines (not exhaustive)

a) Literature reviews on particular clinical issues, especially evidence-based medicine databases (e.g., Cochrane)

b) ACNM position statements

c) Clinical bulletins and committee opinions of the American College of Obstetricians and Gynecologists (ACOG), American Academy of Pediatrics (AAP), American Academy of Family Physicians (AAFP), Association of Women's Health, Obstetric, and Neonatal Nurses (AWHONN) and others

d) National guidelines published by federal organizations such as Center for Disease Control and Prevention (CDC), Agency for Healthcare Research and Quality (AHRQ)

e) Other organizations' guidelines as indicated, e.g., National Association of Childbearing Centers (NACC)

3. Development of patient education materials

a. Considerations

1) Patient population targeted (e.g., language, comprehension, education, cultural/ethnic group)

2) Purpose of the material (e.g., education, persuasion, screening)

3) Research (evidence) base (e.g., consistent with current research findings, recommendations and practice guidelines)

4) Quality of education materials (e.g., formatting, readability etc)

5) Health literacy is the capacity to obtain, interpret, and understand basic health information and services and the competence to use them effectively. (Joint Committee on National Health Education Standards, 1995)

a) Ability to understand instructions on prescription drug bottles, appointment slips, health education brochures, directions and consent forms, and the ability to negotiate complex health care systems.

b) Varies by context and setting and is not necessarily related to years of education or general reading ability.

c) Involves processing complex information and making treatment decisions.

d) Skills needed for health literacy

(1) Visual (understand graphs or other visual information)

(2) Computer, including internet

(3) Information (obtain and apply relevant information)

(4) Numerical or computational (calculate or reason numerically)

(5) Oral language skills

(6) Others (legal, negotiation, assertiveness)

4. Patient records/charting
   a. ACNM Standards for Midwifery Practice 2003, Standard VI: *MIDWIFERY CARE IS DOCUMENTED IN A FORMAT THAT IS ACCESSIBLE AND COMPLETE.* The midwife:
      1) Uses records that facilitate communication of information to clients, consultants, and institutions.
      2) Provides prompt and complete documentation of evaluation, course of management, and outcome of care.
      3) Promotes a documentation system that provides for confidentiality and transmissibility of health records.
      4) Maintains confidentiality in verbal and written communications.
   b. Charting/record keeping may also depend on national, state, and practice or institution policies
   c. Health Insurance Portability and Accountability Act of 1996 (HIPAA)
5. Interdisciplinary relationships
   a. Per the joint statement on collaborative practice relations between obstetrician-gynecologists (ob/gyns) and CNM/CMs (ACNM 2002)
      1) The quality of collaborative practices is enhanced by a working relationship characterized by mutual respect and trust as well as professional responsibility and accountability.
      2) Collaborating ob/gyns and CNM/CMs should concur on clear mechanism for consultation, collaboration and referral based on the individual needs of each patient.
      3) ACOG and ACNM affirm their commitment to promote appropriate standards for education and certification of their respective members, to support appropriate practice guidelines, and to facilitate communication and collegial relationships between obstetrician-gynecologists and certified
   b. **Definitions of collaborative management for medical, gynecological and obstetrical conditions (ACNM 1997)**
      1) **Consultation** is the process whereby a CNM or CM, who maintains primary management responsibility for the woman's care, seeks the advice or opinion of a physician or another member of the health care team.
      2) **Collaboration** is the process whereby a CNM or CM and physician jointly manage the care of a woman or newborn who has become medically, gynecologically or obstetrically complicated. The scope of collaboration may encompass the physical care of the client, including delivery, by the CNM or CM, according to a mutually agreed-upon plan of care. When the physician must assume a dominant role in the

care of the client due to increased risk status, the CNM or CM may continue to participate in physical care, counseling, guidance, teaching and support. Effective communication between the CNM or CM and physician is essential for ongoing collaborative management.

3) **Referral** is the process by which the CNM or CM directs the client to a physician or another health care professional for management of a particular problem or aspect of the woman's care. The woman may return to the midwife for continued care after resolution of the problem or she may remain in the care of the physician following referral.

6. **Ethics: ACNM Code of Ethics (2005)**

The Code of Ethics sets forth values, ethical principles, and standards to which professionals aspire and by which their actions can be judged. The purpose of this code is to identify the moral obligations of all certified nurse-midwives and certified midwives inherent in their professional roles. Specifically, midwives are obligated to support and maintain the integrity of the profession of midwifery in order to promote the health and well-being of women and newborns within their families and communities.

Midwives in all aspects of professional relationships will:

1. ***Respect basic human rights*** and the dignity of all persons.
2. ***Respect their own self worth***, dignity, and professional integrity.

Midwives in all aspects of their professional practice will:

3. Develop a ***partnership with the woman*** in which each shares relevant information that leads to ***informed decision making***, ***consent*** to an evolving plan of care, and ***acceptance of responsibility*** for the outcomes of their choices.
4. ***Act without discrimination*** based on factors such as age, gender, race, ethnicity, religion, lifestyle, sexual orientation, socioeconomic status, disability, or nature of the health problem
5. Provide an environment where ***privacy is protected*** and in which all pertinent ***information is shared*** without bias, coercion, or deception.
6. ***Maintain*** confidentiality except where disclosure is mandated by law.
7. Maintain the necessary knowledge, skills, and behaviors needed for ***competence***.
8. ***Protect women***, their families, and colleagues from harmful, unethical, or incompetent practices by taking appropriate action that may include reporting as mandated by law.

Midwives as members of a profession will:

9. Promote, advocate for, and strive to ***protect the rights, health, and well-being*** of women, families, and communities.
10. ***Promote just distribution of resources*** and equity in access to quality health services.

11. ***Promote and support the education*** of midwifery students and peers, standards of practice, research, and policies that enhance the health of women, families, and communities.

B. Health care system and its relationship to midwifery practice

1. Equal access to health care/cultural sensitivity:

a. Equal access to health care: ACNM Position Statement on Health Care For All Women And Families (2004)

1) ACNM supports a health care system that enables women and their families to receive appropriate care based on need, regardless of their ability to pay, socioeconomic status, race, ethnicity, culture, religion or sexual orientation.

2) ACNM supports legislation that maintains the balance between controlling the cost of health care and ensuring that consumers receive adequate and accessible quality health care. Consumers of health care should have access to the full spectrum of qualified health care professionals and providers, including CNMs/CMs.

3) ACNM supports legislation that ensures consumers have the following basic rights of access and choice when participating in a health plan:

a) Adequate number and variety of health care providers within reasonable distance of the consumer's home or workplace

b) Direct access to women's health care services in a variety of settings by a variety of health care providers that are accessible, community based and culturally competent.

c) Comprehensive health care benefits for all women and families.

b. Cultural sensitivity: ACNM Position Statement On Ethnic and Cultural Diversity (1999)

1) **Every individual has the right** to safe, satisfying health care with **respect for human dignity as well as ethnic and cultural variations**.

2) Midwifery care is focused on the needs of the individual and family for physical care, emotional and social support, active involvement of significant others **according to cultural values and personal preferences**.

3) **Educational preparation** of CNM/CMs includes experiences that promote cultural competency and proficiency; students should demonstrate professional standards of practice in keeping with these beliefs.

4) ACNM promotes **education for its membership** which will develop respect for ethnic and cultural variations.

5) ACNM actively seeks to recruit and retain persons from ethnic and cultural minorities into educational programs and the general membership and encourages diverse representation at all levels within the organization.

2. **Administrative structure of agencies (hospitals, birth centers, HMOs)**

   a. Resources available from ACNM:

      1) *Guidelines for Establishing a Nurse-Midwifery* provides general information on the business and administrative aspects of establishing a midwifery practice.

      2) **Nurse-Midwifery Service Directors Network (SDN) is** an organization (separate from the ACNM) of CNMs and CMs who administer midwifery practices. Provides a network for sharing ideas and concerns that are unique to the administration of midwifery practices. Open to any CNM/CM who directs a practice, regardless of the size.

      3) ***Administrative Manual for Nurse-Midwifery Services (2nd edition)*** provides information regarding administering a midwifery practice. Topics include: Models of Practice, Financial Management, Quality Management, Human Resources, and Students.

      4) The Midwifery Business Institute (MBI) or University of Michigan Service/Practice Director's Institute has been held annually for several years, frequently at the same time and place as meetings of educational and service directors. Presentations and workshops include productivity, billing, negotiating and managing managed care contracts, appealing to managed care administrators, team building, collaborative practice, strategic planning, legal pitfalls and marketing.

      5) **The ACNM Business Committee** within ACNM provides support on business issues. A curriculum for midwifery programs was initially written. Members of the section provide educational topics as well as consultation on various topics to the membership.

      6) At the regional level, the ACNM sponsored workshops on leadership during the past couple of years.

3. **National health care policy (e.g., WHO Baby Friendly Hospital Initiative)**

   a. **The Baby Friendly Hospital Initiative- USA: an international program of The World Health Organization (WHO) and The United Nations Children's Fund (UNICEF).**

      1) Ten Steps to Successful Breastfeeding; recognizes hospitals and birth centers that have taken steps to provide an optimal environment for the promotion, protection and support of breastfeeding.

2) In the US, the Baby-Friendly Hospital Initiative is implemented by the non-profit organization, Baby-Friendly USA. Interdisciplinary committees in hospitals desiring certification complete an application, which is reviewed by a committee.
3) The **Ten Steps to Successful Breastfeeding** are
   a) Have a written breastfeeding policy that is routinely communicated to all health care staff.
   b) Train all health care staff in skills necessary to implement this policy.
   c) Inform all pregnant women about the benefits and management of breastfeeding.
   d) Help mothers initiate breastfeeding within an hour of birth.
   e) Show mothers how to breastfeed and how to maintain lactation, even if they should be separated from their infants.
   f) Give newborn infants no food or drink other than breast milk unless medically indicated.
   g) Practice "rooming in" by allowing mothers and infants to remain together 24 hours a day.
   h) Encourage breastfeeding on demand.
   i) Give no artificial teats, pacifiers, dummies, or soothers to breastfeeding infants.
   j) Foster the establishment of breastfeeding support groups and refer mothers to them on discharge from the hospital or birthing center.

b. **The ACNM MCH Providers Partnership** is funded by the Maternal and Child Health Bureau of the Health Resources and Services Administration.
   1) Goals are improving the health status of, and systems of services for, pregnant women and infants and building a unified health care system responsive to current challenges through 1) a re-examination of the roles and responsibilities of public and private providers, and 2) implementation of strategies to strengthen their complementary nature.
   2) Provides communication link between maternal and child health programs, nurse midwives, and other health providers serving pregnant women. The Partnership has fostered the development of a number of activities to promote collaboration and increase dialogue between public and private providers.

c. **The Coalition for Improving Maternity Services**
   1) Coalition of individuals and national organizations with concern for the care and well-being of mothers, babies, and families.
   2) Mission is to promote a wellness model of maternity care that will improve birth outcomes and substantially reduce costs.

3) Evidence-based mother-, baby-, and family-friendly model focuses on prevention and wellness as the alternatives to high-cost screening, diagnosis, and treatment programs.

4) **Ten Steps of the Mother-Friendly Childbirth Initiative for Mother-Friendly Hospitals, Birth Centers, and Home Birth Services.** (To receive CIMS designation as "mother-friendly," a hospital, birth center, or home birth service must carry out our philosophical principles by fulfilling the Ten Steps of Mother-Friendly Care):

   a) Offers all birthing mothers:
      - Unrestricted access to the birth companions of her choice, including fathers, partners, children, family members, and friends;
      - Unrestricted access to continuous emotional and physical support from a skilled woman-for example, a doula or labor-support professional;
      - Access to professional midwifery care.

   b) Provides accurate descriptive and statistical information to the public about its practices and procedures for birth care, including measures of interventions and outcomes.

   c) Provides culturally competent care -- that is, care that is sensitive and responsive to the specific beliefs, values, and customs of the mother's ethnicity and religion.

   d) Provides the birthing woman with the freedom to walk, move about, and assume the positions of her choice during labor and birth (unless restriction is specifically required to correct a complication), and discourages the use of the lithotomy (flat on back with legs elevated) position.

   e) Has clearly defined policies and procedures for:
      - collaborating and consulting throughout the perinatal period with other maternity services, including communicating with the original caregiver when transfer from one birth site to another is necessary;
      - linking the mother and baby to appropriate community resources, including prenatal and post-discharge follow-up and breastfeeding support.

   f) Does not routinely employ practices and procedures that are unsupported by scientific evidence, including but not limited to the following:
      - Shaving
      - Enemas
      - IVs (intravenous drip)
      - Withholding nourishment
      - Early rupture of membranes
      - Electronic fetal monitoring

g) Other interventions are limited as follows:
- Has an induction rate of 10% or less;
- Has an episiotomy rate of 20% or less, with a goal of 5% or less
- Has a total cesarean rate of 10% or less in community hospitals, and 15% or less in tertiary care (high-risk) hospitals
- Has a VBAC (vaginal birth after cesarean) rate of 60% or more with a goal of 75% or more.

h) Educates staff in non-drug methods of pain relief and does not promote the use of analgesic or anesthetic drugs not specifically required to correct a complication.

i) Encourages all mothers and families, including those with sick or premature newborns or infants with congenital problems, to touch, hold, breastfeed, and care for their babies to the extent compatible with their conditions.

j) Discourages non-religious circumcision of the newborn.

k) Strives to achieve the WHO-UNICEF "Ten Steps of the Baby-Friendly Hospital Initiative" to promote successful breastfeeding (see above):

Source: The Coalition for Improving Maternity Services (CIMS).

4. **Barriers to midwifery practice (restraint of trade, limited access, reimbursement issues)**: Barriers identified by ACNM (2001) are:

a. Managed Care Consumer Protections
   1) Gag rules for licensed health professionals' patient communications
   2) Lack of direct access to women's health providers for female enrollees
   3) Lack of use of quality assurance measures with increased emphasis on maternal child health indicators.
   4) Lack of consumer choice of provider: discrimination against "classes" of providers, including consumer designation of midwives as primary care providers

b. Compensation for Services
   1) Medicare has restricted midwifery payment to 65% of the physician fee schedule. CHAMPUS and many private third-party payers have implemented the Medicare payment policies.
   2) Free standing birth center facility costs are not covered in numerous state Medicaid programs. In other federal programs (exception: CHAMPUS), there is no payment policy for reimbursement of facility costs.

c. State Laws and Regulations
   1) State laws are inconsistent with national standards of practice: some states prevent midwives from legally practicing to the full extent of their educational training and clinical preparation.

2) State laws are inconsistent with national standards; some impose physician supervision requirements and limit midwives' scope of practice, including prescriptive authority.
3) Inconsistency across states: the hodge-podge of state laws functions is a barrier to midwives' practice mobility, including telehealth practice.
4) Federal ERISA law inconsistent with state laws guaranteeing consumer access to midwives, preempting the state laws under ERISA.

d. Practice Issues
   1) Midwives are not recognized as licensed independent practitioners providing the full range of reproductive health services by selective requirements for billing through a physician.
   2) Clinical privileges for midwives: Discrimination by MCOs and hospitals; State and federal antitrust laws through the Federal Trade Commission, the Department of Justice and state Attorneys General are not consistently enforced.
   3) Transportation Act regulations require a physician to verify in person that it is safe to transport a maternity client by air.
   4) Indian Health Services regulations require direct supervision of a midwife by a physician in all cases. This regulation has prohibited the IHS from placing midwives in areas of need. Collaboration and consultation are needed rather than direct supervision.
   5) Medicare program requires that all histories and physical exams be performed by a physician. The Joint Commission on Accreditation of Healthcare Organizations (JCAHO) has adopted this as their standard for accreditation, thus causing problems for midwives seeking hospital admitting privileges.

e. Support for Midwifery
   1) Deficiency of National Health Service Corps placement sites and scholarships available for graduate midwives in full scope practice.
   2) Deficiencies in education funding: Midwifery programs also need funds for clinical training (e.g., Graduate Medical Education [GME funds are not available to midwifery programs).
   3) Lack of access to professional liability insurance: the costly insurance market limits adequate coverage for a variety of settings/practices; further, some insurance underwriters place restrictions and/or surcharges on MD policies that prohibit or discourage collaborative arrangements.

C. Legal issues

1. Statutes/regulations that affect midwifery practice: following are excepts from 2002 testimony of ACNM Executive Director Deanne Williams submitted in response to proposed regulations on midwifery licensure in the state of New Jersey, in which she described Basic Principles for Midwifery Licensure.
   a. Successful completion of a formal education program accredited by a nationally recognized agency
   b. Pass a national certification examination
   c. The scope of practice that is recognized by law or regulation should be consistent with the content of the education process and the certification examination.
   d. Laws and regulations related to health care professionals should facilitate consultation, collaboration and referral between professionals, thus assuring the client access to a provider of choice and access, in a timely manner, to care that is appropriate for her condition and personal needs.
   e. Representation on decision making body. When decisions are made regarding licensure, the number of votes offered to the profession being licensed should be equal to the number of votes assigned to any other profession represented on the decision making body.
   f. Status of graduate midwives. Graduates of accredited midwifery education programs who have qualified to take the certification examination should have a mechanism to begin their career, under supervision of a licensed midwife or physician, prior to successful completion of the certification examination.
   g. Title protection. CNMs and CMs should be able to maintain their license and credential without a requirement for clinical practice. For example, educators, administrators and policy makers should be recognized for their clinical preparation.
   h. Prescriptive authority. The practice act should create a mechanism for CNMs and CMs to prescribe medication, including Schedule 2 and above controlled substances, without a formulary.
   i. Licensing body. ACNM supports the development of boards of midwifery as the ultimate decision maker regarding the licensure and practice of midwifery.
   j. Qualified attendants in all settings. ACNM believed that women should have information about and the opportunity to choose the licensed health care professional and birth setting that best match the current health status of the mother and baby and the personal values of the mother/family. Informed decision making and safe practice begin with access to qualified health care professionals who work collaboratively within a health care system that promotes seamless access to the appropriate level of care.

2. Medical malpractice/legal liability issues
   a. **Occurrence policies** cover a midwife for claims made during and *after* the policy is in force (that is, forever), as long as the claims are due to malpractice occurring while the policy is in force.
   b. A **claims-made policy** covers a midwife only for claims and lawsuits made while the policy is in force. That is the way many insurance companies cover professionals--including the largest writer of insurance for health care practitioners.
      1) Claims-made is like renting your coverage instead of permanently buying it. If you cancel or fail to renew your policy at its annual expiration date, your coverage stops. If you are sued just a day later (even though the suit is for alleged malpractice while the policy was in force), you are not covered for that action.
      2) A **tail** is an attachment to the expired policy and extends the coverage for alleged malpractice occurring during the policy period for a length of time after the policy expiration date.
      3) When the practitioner relies on the employer's coverage and leaves the position for new employment, he/she has no control over whether the tail is purchased. For example, several years after changing jobs the CNM is served with suit and finds out his/her former employer is now deceased and the estate did not bother (nor was it obligated) to purchase a tail for the employer or any of the former employees.
      4) Some tails are longer than others. An *unlimited* tail (also called unlimited "extended reporting" or "ERP endorsement") is desirable.
   c. **The Myth of Vicarious Liability: Impact on Barriers to Nurse-Midwifery Practice (Abstract),** Jenkins SM. *Journal of Nurse-Midwifery*, volume 39, no. 2, March/April, 1994

Lack of understanding of the legal concept of vicarious liability may underlie certain barriers to nurse-midwifery practice. Malpractice insurance surcharges, denial or restrictive limitation of clinical privileges, and physician "supervision" requirements may all be premised, at least in part, upon an assumption that physicians who work with, and hospitals that grant clinical privileges to, nurse-midwives will automatically be liable for any negligent actions or omissions of CNMs. This article examines the basis for such assumptions and, based upon research into the current case law on this subject concludes that popular assumptions regarding physician/CNM or hospital/CNM vicarious liability are unfounded. According to the author's research, no reported cases exist to support that assumption. Vicarious liability arises from the relationship between two parties and is imposed solely on the basis of the relationship. An employer is almost always vicariously liable for the negligent actions or omissions of his employee. If a nurse-midwife is the bona fide employee of a hospital or physician, the latter will most likely be subject to vicarious liability. Absent of any employment relationship, however, such liability will not necessarily be imposed. Rather, the result will vary depending upon the facts of each case, and each professional's relative degree of fault would be determined upon the basis of his or her own actions. Hospital liability for nonemployee nurse-midwives who hold clinical privileges should be no different from hospital liability for physician members of its medical staff--that is, in most cases the hospital will not be vicariously liable for the negligence of its nonemployee staff, but will be directly liable for its own negligence if it failed to credential or monitor the performance of its staff members properly. A malpractice surcharge case, and the insurance principles and data that may be derived from that case, are also discussed. (article is available at www.midwife.org)

3. **Birth registration**
   a. Birth certificates yield most reliable information about the mother, the birth attendant, and the place of birth.
   b. Birth certificates contain information on many demographic, social and medical risk factors, procedures used during labor and delivery, the birth attendant, and outcomes (e.g. weight, APGAR, infant transfer)
   c. U.S. Standard Certificate of Live Birth was created in 1989
      1) Separates CNMs from other midwives
      2) Identifies homebirths and freestanding birth center births
      3) Data are compiled in each state and then aggregated by the National Center for Health Statistics (NCHS) which publishes annual reports of natality data at the national level.
      4) Mother's work sheet (race, age, etc) and facility worksheet (details of prenatal care and birth)
      5) Facility has a manual to guide completion of birth certificates
      6) Almost all births are registered electronically
   d. Advantages of data
      1) Any observed differences are real (i.e. no sampling error or need for statistical significance)
      2) Can be used to describe the entire population of women or an entire specific population (e.g. out-of-hospital birth in a certain geographic area)
      3) If data for the entire country are used, the findings are stable.
   e. Limitations of data
      1) Most states did not distinguish among midwives before 1989
      2) Some states identify births by student nurse-midwives as "other midwives"
      3) Some midwives do not sign the birth certificates for the babies they deliver.
      4) All of the above lead to underreporting of CNM attended births.
      5) Can not distinguish between births that occur at home by intention and births that occur at home by accident. This undermines attempts to use national natality data to determine the safety of home births.
      6) It takes NCHS about two years to aggregate, analyze, and report the national data.

D. Maintaining standards of care

1. Evidence-based practice/review of practice-related literature

a. Evidence-based practice

1) Evidence based practice is the conscientious, explicit, and judicious use of current best evidence in making decisions about the care of individual patients, integrating individual clinical expertise with the best available external clinical evidence from systematic research.
(Sackett DL, Rosenberg WMC, Gray JAM, Haynes RB, Richardson WS. Evidence based medicine: what it is and what it isn't. BMJ. 1996 Jan 13; 312 (7023): 71-2.)

2) Research is systematically reviewed and assigned categorized by level according to the validity of results.
The following table shows the hierarchy of studies, where Level I is deemed to be the most quality assured, robust (least biased), and thus the best evidence. Note, there are refinements of this synoptic table: see http://www.cebm.net/index.asp

Level I	Evidence obtained from a systematic review or meta-analysis of all relevant randomized controlled trials
Level II	Evidence obtained from at least one properly designed randomized controlled trial
Level III-1	Evidence obtained from well-designed pseudo-randomized controlled trials (alternate allocation or some other method)
Level III-2	Evidence obtained from comparative studies with concurrent controls and allocation not randomized (cohort studies), case control studies or interrupted time series with a control group
Level III-3	Evidence obtained from comparative studies with historical control, two or more single-arm studies or interrupted time series without a parallel control group
Level IV	Evidence obtained from case series (either post-test or pre-test and post-test), opinions of respected authorities (narrative reviews), descriptive studies, reports of expert (i.e. consensus) committees, case studies

3) Recommendations for clinical practice are graded from A to D based on this

A	consistent level 1 studies
B	consistent level 2 or 3 studies ***or*** extrapolations from level 1 studies
C	level 4 studies ***or*** extrapolations from level 2 or 3 studies
D	level 5 evidence ***or*** troublingly inconsistent or inconclusive studies of any level

"Extrapolations" are where data is used in a situation which has potentially clinically important differences than the original study situation. For more information and a detailed list of resources, go to http://www.cebm.net/index.asp

4) Several online resources maintain databases of systematic reviews of medical literature for practicing clinicians.

   a) UpToDate Clinical Reference - UpToDate® is a database of clinical topic reviews that synthesize clinical evidence and practice expertise. The authoring clinicians review the journal literature in their field and related fields to offer current practice recommendations supported by high-quality evidence.

   b) EBM Reviews - Cochrane Database of Systematic Reviews - This database comprises full-text systematic reviews of the medical literature conducted by the international Cochrane Collaboration. Cochrane groups conduct rigorous appraisal and synthesis of the literature to answer focused clinical questions of interest to both clinician and researcher.

   c) EBM Reviews - ACP Journal Club - ACP Journal Club contains enhanced abstracts of methodologically sound and clinically relevant research studies published in major clinical journals, along with commentary of the applicability of each study's results in clinical practice.

   d) EBM Reviews - Cochrane Central Register of Controlled Trials (CCTR) - The Cochrane Controlled Trials Register (CCTR), part of the EBM Reviews collection in Ovid, contains 300,000 bibliographic records for controlled clinical trials in healthcare.

   e) EBM Reviews - Database of Abstracts of Reviews of Effects - DARE is a full-text database that contains brief critical assessments of systematic reviews and meta-analyses in areas such as diagnosis, prevention, rehabilitation, screening, and treatment.

   f) Clinical Evidence - Updated monthly, Clinical Evidence provides summaries of current knowledge on medical treatment for a range of conditions, developed through literature searching and assessment of systematic reviews.

   g) InfoRetriever - InfoRetriever allows users to search multiple databases for condition overviews, practice guidelines, clinical rules, calculators, drug treatment, and other topics in evidence-based medicine.

   h) GIDEON - GIDEON is an online diagnosis and reference tool for the tropical and infectious diseases, including epidemiology, microbiology and antimicrobial chemotherapy information. Comprised of four modules, GIDEON allows users to select among different criteria such as symptoms or agents in order to find information to assist with patient diagnostic and care decisions

i) bmjupdates+, from the BMJ Publishing Group and McMaster University, provides users with access to a searchable database of best evidence from the medical literature and email alerts of selected articles from specified disciplines. After creating a free account, users can access featured articles and headlines. Email alerts can be customized to reflect individual clinical areas of interest, relevance ranking, and frequency preferences.

j) HealthGate Clinical Guidelines (formerly EBM Solutions) - HealthGate offers comprehensive evidence-based, clinical guidelines that support evidence-based clinical decision-making and patient education. These guidelines are designed to provide crystallized information in a practical, usable format for clinicians and patients.

k) Evidence-Based Medicine Journals, e.g., Evidence-based HealthCare, Evidence-based Medicine, Evidence-based Mental Health, Evidence-based Obstetrics and Gynecology

l) Additional Evidence-based Medicine Resources

(1) National Guideline Clearinghouse - The National Guideline Clearinghouse™ (NGC) is a comprehensive database of evidence-based clinical practice guidelines, providing physicians, nurses, and other health care providers with objective and detailed information.

(2) Agency for HealthCare Research & Quality - AHRQ, a department of the United States Department of Health and Human Services, is the lead agency charged with supporting research designed to improve the quality of health care, reduce its cost, and broaden access to essential services.

(3) Health Services/Technology Assessment Text- Developed by the National Library of Medicine, Health Services/Technology Assessment Text (HSTAT) is a searchable collection of large, full-text clinical practice guidelines, technology assessments, quick-reference guides for clinicians, consumer health brochures, evidence reports, and health information.

b. Review of practice-related literature

1) Databases such as PubMed, MEDLINE, CINAHL, OVID

2) Subscriptions to online news services such as Kaiser Foundation Daily Newsletter, MedScape

3) Peer reviewed journals in print and online, such as

a) *Journal of Midwifery and Women's Health* (formerly Journal of Nurse-Midwifery)

b) *Journal of Obstetric, Gynecologic and Neonatal Nursing* (JOGNN)

c) *Obstetrics and Gynecology* ("green journal")

d) *American Journal of Obstetrics and Gynecology* ("gray journal")

e) *Pediatrics*

f) *Journal of the American Public Health Association*

g) *Birth*

2. Peer review/quality improvement

a. Peer review

1) 1997 ACNM Position Statement on Quality Management: Peer review is the assessment and evaluation of midwifery practice by other midwives to measure compliance with ACNM standards. In the peer review process, a midwife's practice undergoes scrutiny for the purpose of professional self-regulation. All participants in the peer review process have the opportunity to enhance professional knowledge and skills.

2) **National Practitioner Data Bank** (NPDB)

a) The databank is an information clearinghouse to collect and release certain information related to the professional competence and conduct of physicians, dentists and, in some cases, other health care practitioners (including CNM/CMs).

b) The NPDB was created by the Health Care Quality Improvement Act of 1986 to improve the quality of health care by encouraging hospitals, state licensing boards and other health care entities, including professional societies, to identify and discipline those who engage in unprofessional behavior. It is intended to restrict the ability of incompetent physicians, dentists and other health care practitioners to move from State to State without disclosure of previous incompetence.

c) **Information reported to the NPDB:**

(1) Medical malpractice payments (**only category for which there is mandatory reporting of CNM/CMs)**

(a) The law recognizes that a malpractice claim may be settled for reasons that do not reflect negatively on professional competence.

(b) There is no intent to construe a payment in settlement of a complaint or claim as medical malpractice.

(2) Adverse licensure actions (voluntary reporting of CNM/CMs)

(3) Adverse clinical privileges actions (voluntary reporting of CNM/CMs)

(4) Adverse professional membership actions (voluntary reporting of CNM/CMs).

(a) Since the ACNM does not participate in professional review actions which affect membership, this category of reporting is not applicable for CNMs/CMs.

d) A CNM/CM can "self-query" the NPDB at any time, free of charge. If you submit a Request for Information Disclosure form you will receive either a notification that no information exists in the NPDB, or information as it was reported. One should know if she has been reported; a notification is sent to the practitioner whenever the NPDB processes a report.

e) If information is inaccurate, practitioner must contact the reporting entity to request that a Correction be filed.

f) State licensing boards, hospitals and other health care entities have access to the NPDB. Plaintiff's attorneys may query under certain circumstances. The NPDB is prohibited by law from disclosing information on a specific practitioner to a medical malpractice insurer, defense attorney or member of the general public.

b. Quality improvement:

1) Quality Management in Midwifery Care (from 1997 Position Statement)

a) Promotion and evaluation of high quality care are a priority for the midwifery profession, and ACNM strongly recommends that practicing midwives participate in all aspects of quality management: quality assurance, peer review and quality improvement.

b) Quality assurance monitors structural, procedural and outcome indicators as they relate to accepted standards. Health care systems should include midwives in an established quality assurance program. Midwives who are not included in an existing program are encouraged to develop their own program.

c) Quality improvement modifies the process for providing care in order to improve outcomes. Modifications are based upon the measurement of parameters such as patient satisfaction, clinical outcomes, population-specific care, appropriate use of technology and resources, and access to care.

2) ACNM Standards for Midwifery Care (2003): **STANDARD VII**

a) *MIDWIFERY CARE IS EVALUATED ACCORDING TO AN ESTABLISHED PROGRAM FOR QUALITY MANAGEMENT THAT INCLUDES A PLAN TO IDENTIFY AND RESOLVE PROBLEMS.*

The midwife:

(1) Participates in a program of quality management for the evaluation of practice within the setting in which it occurs.

(2) Provides for a systematic collection of practice data as part of a program of quality management.

(3) Seeks consultation to review problems, including peer review of care.

(4) Acts to resolve problems identified.

3. **Continued competency activities**

   a. **ACNM Standards for Midwifery Care 2003: STANDARD I**

   MIDWIFERY CARE IS PROVIDED BY QUALIFIED PRACTITIONERS

   The midwife:

   1) Is certified by the ACNM designated certifying agent.
   2) Shows evidence of continuing competency as required by the ACNM designated certifying agent.
   3) Is in compliance with the legal requirements of the jurisdiction where the midwifery practice occurs.

   b. **Continuing Competency Assessment (CCA) of the ACNM**

   1) Voluntary recognition program developed to provide CNM/CMs an opportunity to demonstrate competency in the provision of health care to women, newborns and their families.
   2) The ACNM CCA Program is not connected to certification as a CNM or CM, however, some employers, accreditation agencies, and/or state licensing bodies may require participation in the CCA Program in order to practice.
   3) Options for completing CCA 5 year cycles include
      a) Taking the National Certification Examination
      b) Accrual of CEUs/Acceptable Alternatives
         (1) 5 CEUs (50 contact hours) or more of ACNM or ACCME Category I approved CEUs in all areas of practice including antepartum, intrapartum, postpartum, neonatal, gynecology, family planning, primary care and professional practice issues.
         (2) **Continuing education is defined as an educational experience whose content goes beyond basic midwifery education**. Education activities include workshops, home study programs, video or computer assisted programs, grand rounds, etc.

c. **Certificate Maintenance Program (CMP)**

1) For CNM/CMs certified after January 1, 1996
2) Eight-year cycle
3) Administered by the AMCB
4) **There are 2 options for recertification**:

a) **Option 1: AMCB Certificate Maintenance Module Method**

(1) Successfully complete 3 AMCB Certificate Maintenance Modules during the eight-year certification cycle. The eight-year cycle begins with the year of certification. One module must be completed in EACH of the three areas of practice: Antepartum including Primary Care during Pregnancy; Intrapartum/Postpartum/Newborn; and Gynecological and Primary Care of the Well-Woman. **AND**

(2) Obtain 20 contact hours (2.0 CEUs) of ACNM or ACCME Category 1 approved continuing education units. The Certificate Maintenance Modules completed cannot count toward the required 20 contact hours (2.0 CEUs).

b) Option 2: Reexamination Method

(1) Take the current AMCB Certification Examination no sooner than the seventh (7th) year of the current eight-year certification cycle.

(a) Once the exam is taken, the CNM/CM may not change to Option 1.

(b) The exam must be passed by the end of the eighth (8th) year of the certification cycle.

(c) Criteria for passing and retaking the exam will be the same as those in effect for first time candidates at the time the exam is taken. **AND**

(2) Obtain 20 contact hours and (2 CEUs) of ACNM or ACCME Category 1 approved continuing education activities.

d. Refer to 2005 ACNM Code of Ethics, statement #7: Midwives, in all areas of professional practice will maintain the necessary knowledge, skills, and behaviors needed for ***competence***.

e. Adding new skills to scope of practice: ACNM Standards for Midwifery Practice 2003 Standard VIII: *MIDWIFERY PRACTICE MAY BE EXPANDED BEYOND THE ACNM CORE COMPETENCIES TO INCORPORATE NEW PROCEDURES THAT IMPROVE CARE FOR WOMEN AND THEIR FAMILIES.* The midwife:

1) Identifies the need for a new procedure taking into consideration consumer demand, standards for safe practice, and availability of other qualified personnel.
2) Ensures that there are no institutional, state, or federal statutes, regulations, or bylaws that would constrain the midwife from incorporation of the procedure into practice.

3) Demonstrates knowledge and competency, including:
    a) Knowledge of risks, benefits, and client selection criteria.
    b) Process for acquisition of required skills.
    c) Identification and management of complications.
    d) Process to evaluate outcomes and maintain competency.
4) Identifies a mechanism for obtaining medical consultation, collaboration, and referral related to this procedure.
5) Reports the incorporation of this procedure to the ACNM

Standards for the Practice of Midwifery 2003

Midwifery practice as conducted by certified nurse-midwives (CNMs) and certified midwives (CMs) is the independent management of women's health care, focusing particularly on pregnancy, childbirth, the post partum period, care of the newborn, and the family planning and gynecologic needs of women. The CNM and CM practice within a health care system that provides for consultation, collaborative management, or referral, as indicated by the health status of the client. CNMs and CMs practice in accord with the Standards for the Practice of Midwifery, as defined by the American College of Nurse-Midwives (ACNM).

STANDARD I

MIDWIFERY CARE IS PROVIDED BY QUALIFIED PRACTITIONERS

The midwife:

1. Is certified by the ACNM designated certifying agent.
2. Shows evidence of continuing competency as required by the ACNM designated certifying agent.
3. Is in compliance with the legal requirements of the jurisdiction where the midwifery practice occurs.

STANDARD II

MIDWIFERY CARE OCCURS IN A SAFE ENVIRONMENT WITHIN THE CONTEXT OF THE FAMILY, COMMUNITY, AND A SYSTEM OF HEALTH CARE.

The midwife:

1. Demonstrates knowledge of and utilizes federal and state regulations that apply to the practice environment and infection control.
2. Demonstrates a safe mechanism for obtaining medical consultation, collaboration, and referral.
3. Uses community services as needed.
4. Demonstrates knowledge of the medical, psychosocial, economic, cultural, and family factors that affect care.
5. Demonstrates appropriate techniques for emergency management including arrangements for emergency transportation.
6. Promotes involvement of support persons in the practice setting.

STANDARD III

MIDWIFERY CARE SUPPORTS INDIVIDUAL RIGHTS AND SELF-DETERMINATION WITHIN BOUNDARIES OF SAFETY

The midwife:

1. Practices in accord with the Philosophy and the Code of Ethics of the American College of Nurse-Midwives.
2. Provides clients with a description of the scope of midwifery services and information regarding the client's rights and responsibilities.

3. Provides clients with information regarding, and/or referral to, other providers and services when requested or when care required is not within the midwife's scope of practice.
4. Provides clients with information regarding health care decisions and the state of the science regarding these choices to allow for informed decision-making.

STANDARD IV

MIDWIFERY CARE IS COMPRISED OF KNOWLEDGE, SKILLS, AND JUDGMENTS THAT FOSTER THE DELIVERY OF SAFE, SATISFYING, AND CULTURALLY COMPETENT CARE.

The midwife:

1. Collects and assesses client care data, develops and implements an individualized plan of management, and evaluates outcome of care.
2. Demonstrates the clinical skills and judgments described in the ACNM Core Competencies for Basic Midwifery Practice.
3. Practices in accord with the ACNM Standards for the Practice of Midwifery.
4. Practices in accord with service/practice guidelines that meet the requirements of the particular institution or practice setting.

STANDARD V

MIDWIFERY CARE IS BASED UPON KNOWLEDGE, SKILLS, AND JUDGMENTS WHICH ARE REFLECTED IN WRITTEN PRACTICE GUIDELINES

The midwife:

1. Describes the parameters of service for independent and collaborative midwifery management and transfer of care when needed.
2. Establishes practice guidelines for each specialty area which may include, but is not limited to, primary health care of women, care of the childbearing family, and newborn care.
3. Includes the following information in each specialty area:
   a) Client selection criteria
   b) Parameters and methods for assessing health status
   c) Parameters for risk assessment
   d) Parameters for consultation, collaboration, and referral
   e) Appropriate interventions including treatment, medication, and/or devices.

STANDARD VI

MIDWIFERY CARE IS DOCUMENTED IN A FORMAT THAT IS ACCESSIBLE AND COMPLETE.

The midwife:

1. Uses records that facilitate communication of information to clients, consultants, and institutions.
2. Provides prompt and complete documentation of evaluation, course of management, and outcome of care.

3. Promotes a documentation system that provides for confidentiality and transmissibility of health records.
4. Maintains confidentiality in verbal and written communications.

STANDARD VII

MIDWIFERY CARE IS EVALUATED ACCORDING TO AN ESTABLISHED PROGRAM FOR QUALITY MANAGEMENT THAT INCLUDES A PLAN TO IDENTIFY AND RESOLVE PROBLEMS.

The midwife:

1. Participates in a program of quality management for the evaluation of practice within the setting in which it occurs.
2. Provides for a systematic collection of practice data as part of a program of quality management.
3. Seeks consultation to review problems, including peer review of care.
4. Acts to resolve problems identified.

STANDARD VIII

MIDWIFERY PRACTICE MAY BE EXPANDED BEYOND THE ACNM CORE COMPETENCIES TO INCORPORATE NEW PROCEDURES THAT IMPROVE CARE FOR WOMEN AND THEIR FAMILIES.

The midwife:

1. Identifies the need for a new procedure taking into consideration consumer demand, standards for safe practice, and availability of other qualified personnel.
2. Ensures that there are no institutional, state, or federal statutes, regulations, or bylaws that would constrain the midwife from incorporation of the procedure into practice.
3. Demonstrates knowledge and competency, including:
   a) Knowledge of risks, benefits, and client selection criteria.
   b) Process for acquisition of required skills.
   c) Identification and management of complications.
   d) Process to evaluate outcomes and maintain competency.
4. Identifies a mechanism for obtaining medical consultation, collaboration, and referral related to this procedure.
5. Reports the incorporation of this procedure to the ACNM.

Source: Division of Standards and Practice

Approved: ACNM Board of Directors, March 8, 2003

(Supersedes the ACNM's Functions, Standards and Qualifications, 1983 and Standards for the Practice of Nurse-Midwifery 1987, 1993. Standard VIII has been adapted from the ACNM's Guidelines for the Incorporation of New Procedures into Nurse-Midwifery Practice)

Philosophy of the American College of Nurse-Midwives

We, the midwives of the American College of Nurse-Midwives, affirm the power and strength of women and the importance of their health in the well-being of families, communities and nations. We believe in the basic human rights of all persons, recognizing that women often incur an undue burden of risk when these rights are violated.

We believe every person has a right to:

· Equitable, ethical, accessible quality health care that promotes healing and health

· Health care that respects human dignity, individuality and diversity among groups

· Complete and accurate information to make informed health care decisions

· Self-determination and active participation in health care decisions

· Involvement of a woman's designated family members, to the extent desired, in all health care experiences

We believe the best model of health care for a woman and her family:

· Promotes a continuous and compassionate partnership

· Acknowledges a person's life experiences and knowledge

· Includes individualized methods of care and healing guided by the best evidence available

· Involves therapeutic use of human presence and skillful communication

We honor the normalcy of women's lifecycle events. We believe in:

· Watchful waiting and non-intervention in normal processes

· Appropriate use of interventions and technology for current or potential health problems

· Consultation, collaboration and referral with other members of the health care team as needed to provide optimal health care

We affirm that midwifery care incorporates these qualities and that women's health care needs are well-served through midwifery care.

Finally, we value formal education, lifelong individual learning, and the development and application of research to guide ethical and competent midwifery practice. These beliefs and values provide the foundation for commitment to individual and collective leadership at the community, state, national and international level to improve the health of women and their families worldwide.

Revised last: September, 2004

(Replaces version updated October, 1989)

NOTES

References

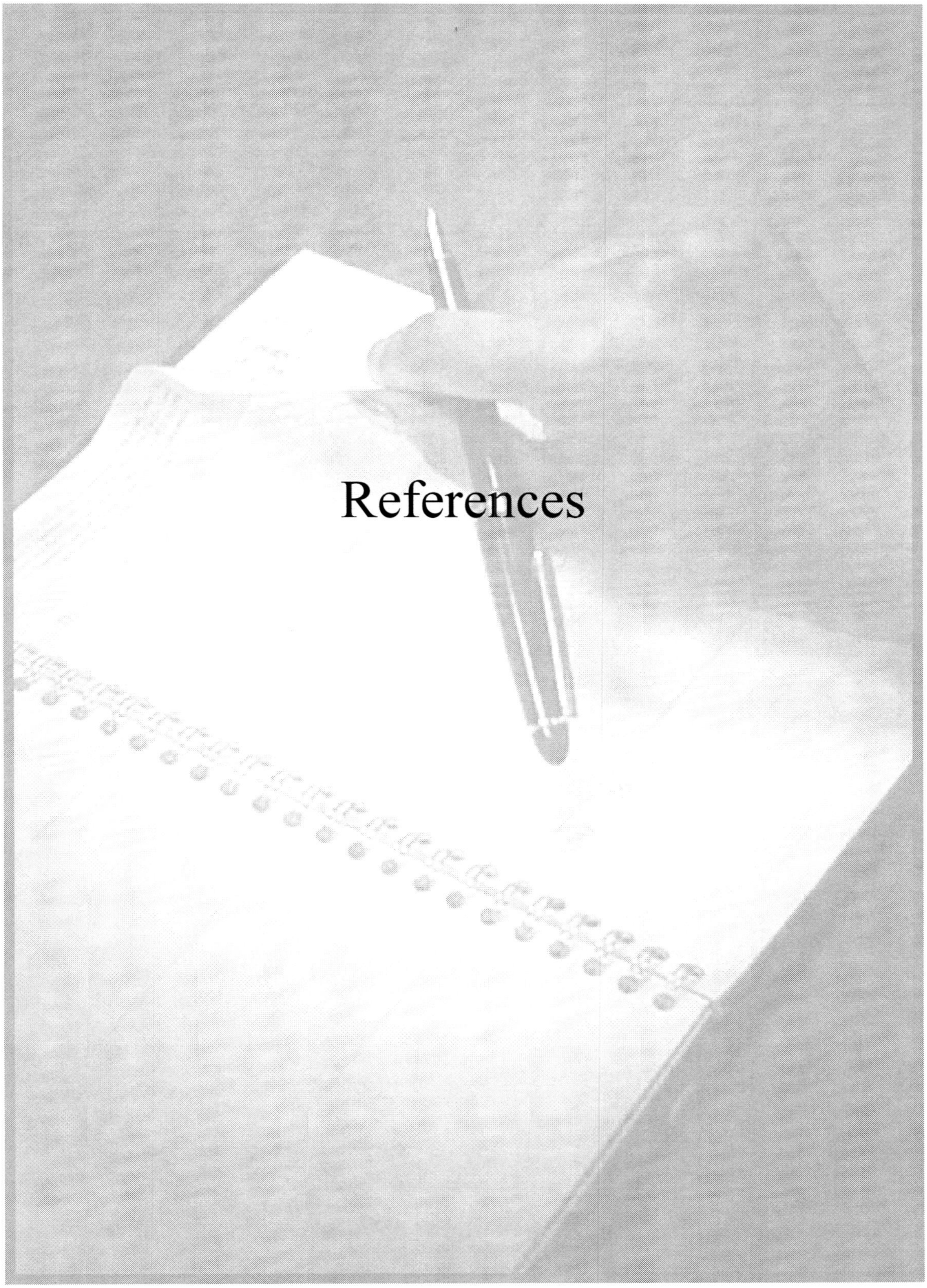

American Academy of Pediatrics and American Heart Association. 2000. *Textbook of Neonatal Resuscitation, 4th Edition.*

Blackburn ST. 2003. *Maternal, Fetal, and Neonatal Physiology: A Clinical Perspective, Second Edition*. Saunders.

Coad J & Dunstall M. 2001. *Anatomy and Physiology for Midwives*. Mosby.

Cunningham FG, Leveno KJ, Bloom SL, Hauth JC, Gilstrap L III, Wenstrom KD. 2005. *Williams Obstetrics, Twenty-Second Edition*. McGraw-Hill Companies.

DeCherney AH, Nathan L. 2003. *Current Obstetric and Gynecologic Diagnosis & Treatment, Ninth Edition*. McGraw-Hill Companies.

Gabbe SG, Niebyl JR, Simpsom JL. 2002. *Obstetrics: Normal and Problem Pregnancies. Fourth Edition*. Churchill Livingstone.

Hacker NF, Moore, JG, Gambone, JC. 2004. *Essentials of Obstetrics and Gynecology, Fourth Edition.* Elsevier-Saunders.

Hatcher RA, Trussell J, Stewart F, Nelson AL, Cates Jr W, Guest F, Kowal D. 2004. *Contraceptive Technology, 18th Revised Edition*. Ardent Media.

Hatcher RA, Zieman M, Cwiak C, Darney PD, Creinin MD, Stosur HR. 2004. *A Pocket Guide to Managing Contraception: 2004-2005 Edition*. The Bridging the Gap Foundation.

McCance KL & Huether SE. 2006. *Pathophysiology: The Biologic Basis for Disease in Adults and Children.* Elsevier Mosby.

Mosby's Medical, Nursing, and allied Health Dictionary, Sixth Edition. 2002. Mosby.

Nichols FH & Humenick SS. (2000). *Childbirth Education: Practice, Research, And Theory, Second Edition.* WB Saunders

Oxorn H. 1986. *Oxorn-Foote Human Labor and Birth, Fifth Edition*. Appleton Lange.

Seidel HM, Ball JW, Dains JE, Benedict GW. 2003. *Mosby's Guide to Physical Examination, Fifth Edition*. Mosby.

Sinclair C. 2004. *A Midwife's Handbook*. Elsevier.

Skidmore-Roth, L (2001). *Mosby's_Handbook of Herbs and Natural Supplements*. Mosby

Speroff L & Darney PD. 2001. *A Clinical Guide for Contraception, Third Edition*. Lippincott Williams & Wilkins.

Spratto FR & Woods AL. (2003) *2003 Edition PDR Nurses Drug Handbook.* Clifton Park NY: Delmar Learning.

Varney H, Kriebs JM, Gegor CL. 2004. *Varney's Midwifery, Fourth Edition*. Jones and Bartlett.

Walsh L. 2001. *Midwifery: Community-Based Care During the Childbearing Year*. W.B. Saunders Company.

Wheeler L. 2002. *Nurse-Midwifery handbook: A Practical Guide to Prenatal and Postpartum Care, Second Edition*. Lippincott Williams & Wilkins.

Youngkin EL & Davis MS. 2004. *Women's Health: A Primary Care Clinical Guide*. Pearson Prentice Hall.

